Management of Non-Muscle Invasive Bladder Cancer

Sanchia S. Goonewardene · Raj Persad ·
Hanif Motiwala · David Albala

Management of Non-Muscle Invasive Bladder Cancer

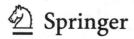 Springer

Sanchia S. Goonewardene
East of England Deanery
Norfolk and Norwich University Hospital
Norwich, UK

Hanif Motiwala
Southend University Hospital
Westcliff-on-Sea, UK

Raj Persad
North Bristol NHS Trust
Bristol, UK

David Albala
Boston University
Boston, MA, USA

ISBN 978-3-030-28648-4   ISBN 978-3-030-28646-0   (eBook)
https://doi.org/10.1007/978-3-030-28646-0

This Springer imprint is published by the registered company Springer Nature Switzerland AG
The registered company address is: Gewerbestrasse 11, 6330 Cham, Switzerland

Preface

Welcome to Management of Non-Muscle Invasive Bladder Cancer (NMIBC). The concept of this book first came to me as a young trainee, whilst assisting with cystectomies. I had often read papers, but very rarely understood principles behind management of NMIBC. Clearly, there were hundreds and hundreds of papers out there, but which were the right ones to read?

Bladder cancer is often considered the 'Cinderella' of all the cancers—underfunded for research. Within this book, my team and I have pulled together some of the controversies in non-muscle invasive bladder cancer. The aim of this book is to use the knowledge to further develop your practice and improve patient care.

Bladder cancer has a significant impact on both patients and the healthcare world. Very often, the presentation of bladder cancer is unfathomable—presenting in a variety of different ways. This is what makes it so unpredictable.

Years later, again when opening for a cystectomy, I realised this book needed to be written. The most important lesson to take away from this is to always seek like-minded people to train with (much like my team and I). Do this, and you will succeed.

Norwich, UK   Sanchia S. Goonewardene

Acknowledgements

For my family and friends, for always supporting me in what I do.

For my team at Springer Nature, for always giving myself and my team a chance to get published.

For Prof. Hanif Motiwala and my crew at Southend—I hope I have done you proud with this book.

For Prof. Raj Persad—for all the support from my time at Bristol—still going strong.

For my mentor, coach, Editor in Chief, Prof. David Albala—I couldn't have achieved all of this without you.

For Mark Rochester, Vivek Kumar, Robert Mills, Edwin Hoe and Prof. Sethia—the amazing Team 1 at Norfolk and Norwich University Hospital. For Georgina Wilson and East of England Deanery—for always supporting me in my academic endeavours.

Contents

About the Authors

Miss. Sanchia S. Goonewardene, MBChB (Hons.Clin.Sc), BMedSc (Hons), PG-CGC, Dip.SSc, MRCS (Ed and Eng) MPhil, Spr, East of England Deanery qualified from Birmingham Medical School with Honours in Clinical Science and a BMedSc Degree in Medical Genetics and Molecular Medicine. She has a specific interest in academia during her spare time, with over 530 publications to her name with 2 papers as a number 1 most cited in fields (Biomedical Library), and has significantly contributed to the Urological Academic World—she has since added a section to the European Association of Urology Congress on Prostate Cancer Survivorship and Supportive Care and is an associate member of an EAU guidelines panel on Chronic Pelvic Pain. She has been the UK lead in an EAU-led study on Salvage Prostatectomy. She has also contributed to the BURST IDENTIFY study as a collaborator.

Her background with research entails an MPhil, the work from which went on to be drawn up as a document for PCUK then, NICE endorsed. She gained funding from the Wellcome Trust for her Research Elective. She is also an Alumni of the Urology Foundation, who sponsored a trip to USANZ trainee week. She also has 3 books published—Core Surgical Procedures for Urology Trainees (7794 downloads), Prostate Cancer Survivorship (5528 downloads) and her third book, Basic Urological Management (8158 downloads).

She has supervised her first thesis with Kings College London and Guys Hospital, (BMedSci Degree gained first class, students' thesis score 95%). Recently, she has gained her first Associate Editor position with the Journal of Robotic Surgery. She is an Editorial board member of the World Journal of Urology and was invited to be Guest Editor for a Special Issue on Salvage Therapy in Prostate Cancer. She is also a review board member for BMJ case reports. Additionally, she is on The International Continence Society Panel on Pelvic Floor Dysfunction, ICS abstract reviewer and has been an EPoster Chair at ICS. She has also chaired semi-live surgery at ERUS and presented her work as part of the Young Academic Urology Section at ERUS. In her spare time, she enjoys working for Rotary International.

Prof. Raj Persad, MB, BS, Ch.M., FRCS (Eng.), FRCS (Urol.), FEBU appointed in 1996, is a Consultant Urological Surgeon and Andrologist in Bristol.

In his clinical role, he is one of the most experienced pelvic cancer surgeons in the UK and was one of te first in the UK to practice female neobladder reconstruction following cystectomy for invasive bladder cancer. He has subspecialised over many years in precise surgical techniques, which improve both oncologic and functional outcomes. This includes techniques ranging from (1) the use of the Da Vinci Robot for performing Robot-Assisted Laparoscopic Radical Prostatectomy, (2) High-Intensity Focused Ultrasound for minimally invasive non-surgical treatment of prostate cancer and (3) Rectal Spacer and Fiducial Marker precision placement for optimizing the outcomes of Image-Guided Radiotherapy for prostate cancer.

In the field of Diagnostics, he has been one of the National Leads in developing the prostate pre-biopsy MRI pathway for patients with elevated PSA. This has optimized the accuracy of cancer diagnosis minimized clinical risk and sepsis associated with transrectal biopsy. He has developed to a fine art both cognitive transperineal biopsies of the prostate as well as Fusion Biopsy of the prostate.

Professor Persad has been a National pioneer in minimally invasive techniques for the treatment of Symptomatic Benign Prostatic as an alternative to Transurethral Prostatectomy (TURP). These techniques include Urolift (prostatic urethral lift) procedure, which he does under general or local anaesthetic depending on patient preference as well as REZUM, steam treatment of the prostate. He also treats BPH with Green Light Laser. All these techniques are offered by Prof. Persad for BPH as well as traditional TURP if tablet therapy has failed or cannot be tolerated by the patient.

Professor Persad is also a National Authority in the treatment of Erectile Dysfunction. He practices optimum medical therapies for all male patients and has a large cohort of patients, who are diabetic or who have had prostatectomy and in need of erectile function restoration. If conservative therapy fails with erectogenic pharmacotherapy or use of medical devices, he can offer the insertion of state-of-the-art penile prosthetic devices. Professor Persad also treats deformity due to Peyronies across a range of severity, offering therapeutic injection in its early phases and various types of surgical correction if this fails according to patient needs.

Professor Persad has a 25-year experience in the restoration of fertility through microsurgical reversal of vasectomy and has some of the best results nationally. He also for more complex cases offers epididymo-vasovasostomy. In combination with the Bristol Centre for Reproductive Medicine, he will soon be offering male infertility procedures such as micro-TESE (testicular extraction of sperm) in order to optimize assisted conception techniques.

Academically, Prof. Persad is involved in an extensive range of research with the Universities of Bristol, Pittsburgh, London and Oxford. These include the detection of early bladder and prostate cancer and novel imaging and treatment strategies for these diseases. He formerly led a team of researchers engaged in improving strategies for treatment of advanced prostate cancer in areas of hormonal treatment and immunotherapy (BPCRN). He has been Principal Investigator, Chief Investigator, and Collaborator in many National and International studies sponsored by the MRC, EORTC, CRUK, and NCRN. He has been a recipient of £4.5 m research grants from UK bodies as well as the NIH USA, and has published over 300 scientific articles and 7 books in the field of Urology.

Together with Scientists and Clinicians in Bristol, he is part of the productive BRC (Biomed Research Centre), which has a number of far-reaching clinical and scientific goals in the field of cancer and is Surgical Principle Investigator for the PreVent and Pre-Empt trials of lifestyle intervention in prostate cancer. He has an innovative research programme with Prof. Chris Melhuish in Medical Robotics to enhance surgery and radiotherapy modalities with Robotic assistance.

In addition to his University and NHS Clinical commitments, he spends time visiting hospital units in the developing world (e.g. Tanzania), where he helps to train junior doctors and other healthcare professionals.

Mr. Hanif Motiwala, MB, BS, ChM, FRCS (Eng.), FRCS (Urol), FEBU is well known to the community worldwide. He was Professor of Urology in India and has also served as an FRCS Urol Examiner. He has been training programme director for the London Deanery, Imperial Rotation, and was well liked by all of his trainees. He has also been a Lecturer for Institute of Urology and Oxford Trainees.

He has over 25 years' experience as a Consultant in urology and extensive exposure to senior leadership roles within healthcare provision and professional institutions including Chairman of the surgical division at Wexham Park Hospital. He also has a strong track record of achieving clinical targets within tightly controlled budgets, developing innovative strategies to improve patient care and optimise the use of resources, for which he received a Bronze Award.

He is a dedicated and committed surgeon, utilising teaching, surgical and medical skills for the greater good through international voluntary work, building capability and skills in reconstructive surgery in India and Africa. He was conferred a position as Visiting Professor—University of Khartoum, Sudan, 2009 in recognition of voluntary work in Sudan, conducting final Urology Examinations to train qualified surgeons, providing training to surgeons in reconstruction and carrying out complex surgery.

Dr. David Albala, MD, graduated with a geology degree from Lafayette College in Easton, Pennsylvania. He completed his medical school training at Michigan State University and went on to complete his surgical residency at the Dartmouth-Hitchcock Medical Center. Following this, Dr. Albala was an endourology fellow at Washington University Medical Center under the direction of Ralph V. Clayman. He practiced at Loyola University Medical Center in Chicago and rose from the ranks of Instructor to full Professor in Urology and Radiology in 8 years. After 10 years, he became a tenured Professor at Duke University Medical Center in North Carolina. At Duke, he was Co-Director of the Endourology fellowship and Director for the Center of Minimally Invasive and Robotic Urological Surgery. He has over 180 publications in peer-reviewed journals and has authored five books in endourology and general urology. He is the Editor-in-Chief of the Journal of Robotic Surgery. He serves on the editorial board for Medical Reviews in Urology, Current

Opinions in Urology and Urology Index and Reviews. He serves as a reviewer for eight surgical journals.

Presently, he is Chief of Urology at Crouse Hospital in Syracuse, New York and a physician at Associated Medical Professionals (a group of 29 urologists). He is considered a national and international authority in laparoscopic and robotic urological surgery and has been an active teacher in this area for over 20 years. His research and clinical interests have focused on robotic urological surgery. In addition, other clinical interests include minimally invasive treatment of benign prostatic hypertrophy (BPH) and the use of fibrin sealants in surgery. He has been a Visiting Professor at numerous institutions across the United States as well as overseas in countries such as India, China, Iceland, Germany, France, Japan, Brazil, Australia, and Singapore. In addition, he has done operative demonstrations in over 32 countries and 23 states. He has trained 16 fellows in endourology and advanced robotic surgery.

In addition, Dr. Albala is a past White House Fellow who acted as a special assistant to Federico Pena, Secretary of Transportation, on classified and unclassified public health related issues.

Part I
Background and Pathology on Bladder Cancer

Chapter 1
Background on Bladder Cancer

Bladder Cancer (BC) is the 7th most common cancer worldwide in men and the 17th most common cancer worldwide in women (Burger 2013). Approximately 75% of newly diagnosed bladder cancers are non-invasive (NMIBC). Each year, approximately 110,500 men and 70,000 women are diagnosed with new cases and 38,200 patients in the European Union and 17,000 US patients die from BC (Burger 2013).

Incidence rates are consistently lower in women than men. Diverging incidence trends were also observed by sex in many countries, with stabilising or declining rates in men but some increasing trends seen for women. Bladder cancer ranks 13th in terms of deaths ranks, with overall mortality rates decreasing particularly in the most developed countries (Antoni et al. 2017). Despite its prevalence, morbidity, mortality and associated cost of management, BC remains grossly under-recognized as a public health concern and underfunded scientifically (Kaplan 2014). Although 5-year survival rates for patients with prostate or kidney cancer have improved tremendously in the past 30 years, progress in BC is not comparable to this.

References

Antoni S, Ferlay J, Soerjomataram I, Znaor A, Jemal A, Bray F. Bladder cancer incidence and mortality: a global overview and recent trends. Eur Urol. 2017;71(1):96–108. https://doi. org/10.1016/j.eururo.2016.06.010, Epub 2016 Jun 28.
Burger M, Catto JW, Dalbagni G, Grossman HB, Herr H, Karakiewicz P, Kassouf W, Kiemeney LA, La Vecchia C, Shariat S, Lotan Y. Epidemiology and risk factors of urothelial bladder cancer. Eur Urol. 2013;63(2):234–41.
Kaplan AL, Litwin MS, Chamie K. The future of bladder cancer care in the USA. Nat Rev Urol. 2014;11(1):59–62.

© Springer Nature Switzerland AG 2020
S. S. Goonewardene et al., *Management of Non-Muscle Invasive Bladder Cancer*,
https://doi.org/10.1007/978-3-030-28646-0_1

Chapter 2
Introduction to Bladder Cancer Type and Therapy

The most common histological type of BC is urothelial cell carcinoma (Amin et al. 2013). Bladder cancer can be muscle invasive or non-muscle invasive, treatment is divided according to this (Witjes et al. 2014). If non-muscle invasive, treatment can be endoscopic, intravesical immunotherapy or intravesical chemotherapy or surgery. However, if muscle invasive, more radical therapy e.g. radical cystectomy with neoadjuvant chemotherapy and lymph node dissection or radical radiotherapy, is required.

Bladder cancer is a heterogeneous disease with a variable natural history. 70% present with NMI tumours (stages Ta, T1, or carcinoma in situ) (Sun and Trinh 2015). 30% present with muscle-invasive disease (T2–4) associated with a high risk of death from distant metastases (Sun and Trinh 2015). Yet 50 and 70% of NMI tumors do recur, and approximately 10–20% of them progress to muscle-invasive disease (Sun and Trinh 2015).

Active curative treatment for patients diagnosed with BC, include radical radiotherapy (radiation directed at the bladder) or radical surgery (surgical removal of the bladder and surrounding lymph nodes) and BCG (Witjes et al. 2014). Surgery can be conducted as open, laparoscopic or robotic. There is no gold standard yet. If a patient is fit enough for surgery and the bladder cancer is localised, cystoprostatectomy can be conducted. Smoking and work-related carcinogens remain the most important risk factors for bladder cancer (Witjes et al. 2014). Open radical cystectomy with lymph node dissection (LND) remains the treatment of choice for treatment failures in NMIBC and T2–T4a N0 M0 BCa.

Diagnosis, grading and pathological staging is made using cystoscopy, tumor biopsy, and urine cytology (Pashos et al. 2002). Transurethral resection (TUR) of bladder tumor is the basis of pathological staging (Pashos et al. 2002). If histology demonstrates muscle invasive disease, radical therapy-radiotherapy or cystectomy is the gold standard, although trimodality therapy (TUR, radiation, systemic chemotherapy) can be considered as a bladder-preserving strategy (Pashos et al. 2002). Intravesical immunotherapy is effective for preventing disease recurrence, although

S. S. Goonewardene et al., *Management of Non-Muscle Invasive Bladder Cancer*, https://doi.org/10.1007/978-3-030-28646-0_2

its role in slowing disease progression is uncertain. Chemotherapy and radiation plus cystectomy can be used to treat or prevent pelvic recurrence of invasive disease or to prolong life in patients with metastatic disease (Pashos et al. 2002).

For well-informed, well-selected patients, multimodality treatment could be offered as an alternative, especially if cystectomy is not an option (Witjes et al. 2014). For fit patients, cisplatinum-based neoadjuvant chemotherapy should always be discussed, since it improves overall survival. However, this implies patients must have a level of fitness to undergo radical cystectomy. For patients with metastatic disease, cisplatin-containing combination chemotherapy is recommended. For unfit patients, carboplatin combination chemotherapy or single agents can be used.

References

Amin MB, McKenney JK, Paner GP, Hansel DE, Grignon DJ, Montironi R, Lin O, Jorda M, Jenkins LC, Soloway M, Epstein JI, Reuter VE. ICUD-EAU international consultation on bladder cancer 2012: pathology. Eur Urol. 2013;63(1):16–35.
Pashos CL, Botteman MF, Laskin BL, Redaelli A. Bladder cancer: epidemiology, diagnosis, and management. Cancer Pract. 2002;10(6):311–22.
Sun M, Trinh QD. Diagnosis and staging of bladder cancer. Hematol Oncol Clin North Am. 2015;29(2):205–18, vii.
Witjes JA, Compérat E, Cowan NC, De Santis M, Gakis G, Lebret T, Ribal MJ, Van der Heijden AG, Sherif A. EAU guidelines on muscle-invasive and metastatic bladder cancer: summary of the 2013 guidelines. Eur Urol. 2014;65(4):778–92.

Part II
Histological Variants in Bladder Cancer

Chapter 3
Histological Variants in Bladder Cancer— Sqaumous Cell Carcinoma and Squamous Differentiation

Bladder squamous cell carcinoma, squamous metaplasia, and transitional cell carcinoma with squamous differentiation are rare findings (Rausch et al. 2014). A common risk factor is chronic bladder irritation and inflammation (Rausch et al. 2014). The prognostic and clinical relevance and natural history of squamous cell lesions has been under investigation, revealing individual premalignant characteristics (Rausch et al. 2014).

Urothelial carcinoma (UC) with squamous differentiation (UC w/SD) is the most common variant (Raman and Jafri 2015). Accurate identification is key although barriers exist; tumor heterogeneity, sampling limitation and pathologic interpretation of specimens (Raman and Jafri 2015). Although many cases of UC w/SD present with muscle-invasive bladder cancer, those cancers that are confirmed to be truly non-muscle invasive can be managed with endoscopic resection, adjuvant intravesical therapies (i.e., Bacillus Calmette-Guérin), and close surveillance (Raman and Jafri 2015). Radical cystectomy series suggest that UC w/SD tends to present at a more advanced stage than pure UC does although survival outcomes are similar when controlling for standard clinicopathologic factors (Raman and Jafri 2015).

Abdollah et al. (2012) tested the effect of histological subtype (NBSCC vs. UC) on cancer-specific mortality (CSM), after adjusting for other-cause mortality (OCM) (Abdollah et al. 2012). Abdollah identified 12,311 patients who were treated with radical cystectomy (RC) between 1988 and 2006, within 17 Surveillance, Epidemiology and End Results (SEER) registries (Abdollah et al. 2012). Histological subtype was NBSCC in 614 (5%) patients versus UC in 11,697 (95%) patients (Abdollah et al. 2012). At RC, the rate of non-organ confined (NOC) disease was higher in NBSCC than UC (71.7% vs. 52.2%; $p<0.001$). (Abdollah et al. 2012). After adjustment for OCM, the 5-year cumulative CSM rates were 25.0% versus 19.8% ($p=0.2$) for patients with NBSCC versus UC organ confined (OC) BCa, respectively (Abdollah et al. 2012). The same rates were 46.3% versus 49.3% in patients with NOC BCa ($p=0.1$). At RC, the rate of

© Springer Nature Switzerland AG 2020
S. S. Goonewardene et al., *Management of Non-Muscle Invasive Bladder Cancer*,
https://doi.org/10.1007/978-3-030-28646-0_3

NOC bladder cancer is higher in NBSCC patients than in their UC counterparts (Abdollah et al. 2012). Despite a more advanced stage at surgery, NBSCC histological subtype is not associated with a less favourable CSM than UC histological subtype, after accounting for OCM and the extent of the disease (OC vs. NOC) (Abdollah et al. 2012).

The true clinical significance of variant histology is challenging, especially with nonmuscle invasive disease (Porten et al. 2014). This tends to identify a high-risk population with a worse prognosis and better suited for early aggressive intervention (i.e., radical cystectomy), then treatment recommendations should reflect this notion (Porten et al. 2014). High-risk NMIBC or variant histology should be offered early cystectomy, especially if pure squamous, adenocarcinoma, sarcomatoid, plasmacytoid, or micropapillary disease (Porten et al. 2014). For squamous differentiation, intravesical therapy is an option based on standard risk stratification in NMIBC (Porten et al. 2014). With variant histology, there is a risk of understating and also have close surveillance to not compromise the opportunity of cure (Porten et al. 2014). The management of NMIBC and variant histology is difficult due to understaging and clinical controversies in management of high-risk NMIBC disease for standard urothelial cell carcinoma (early cystectomy vs. intravesical therapy) (Porten et al. 2014).

References

Abdollah F, Sun M, Jeldres C, Schmitges J, Thuret R, Djahangirian O, Tian Z, Shariat SF, Perrotte P, Montorsi F, Karakiewicz PI. Survival after radical cystectomy of non-bilharzial squamous cell carcinoma vs urothelial carcinoma: a competing-risks analysis. BJU Int. 2012;109(4):564–9.

Porten SP, Willis D, Kamat AM. Variant histology: role in management and prognosis of nonmuscle invasive bladder cancer. Curr Opin Urol. 2014;24(5):517–23.

Raman JD, Jafri SM. Surgical management of bladder urothelial carcinoma with squamous differentiation. Urol Oncol. 2015;33(10):429–33.

Rausch S, Lotan Y, Youssef RF. Squamous cell carcinogenesis and squamous cell carcinoma of the urinary bladder: a contemporary review with focus on nonbilharzial squamous cell carcinoma. Urol Oncol. 2014;32(1):32.e11–6.

Chapter 4
Histological Variants in Bladder Cancer— Adenocarcinoma

Primary adenocarcinomas of the bladder and urachus are extremely rare, accounting for 0.5–2.0% of all bladder malignancies (Williams and Chavda 2015). During fetal development, the urachus develops into the median umbilical ligament that stretches from the umbilicus to the bladder. Adenocarcinoma accounts for 90% of all cases of urachal carcinoma (Williams and Chavda 2015).

4.1 Histopathology of Bladder Adenocarcinoma

Non-Urothelial cell carcinoma and variants of urothelial cancer (UC) account for up to 25% of all bladder cancers (Klaile et al. 2016). Most of the non-UCs are of epithelial origin (approximately 90%) including adenocarcinoma. Primary bladder adenocarcinoma (PBA) is an epithelial malignancy with pure glandular differentiation, without evidence of typical urothelial (transitional cell) carcinoma (Pokuri et al. 2016).

PBA is rare, accounting for 0.5–2%, more common in men than in women and diagnosed in the sixth decade of life (Pokuri et al. 2016). Additional variant histology might prognosticate an impaired prognosis (Klaile et al. 2016). Accordingly, aggressive behavior and often advanced stages at primary presentation are frequently observed in non-UC arguing for radical and sometimes different treatment strategies as compared to pure UC (Klaile et al. 2016).

Clinical symptoms maybe haematuria and an irritative bladder (Pokuri et al. 2016). PBA is common in schistosomiasis-endemic regions and in congenital bladder exstrophy (ectopia vesicae). It is common in the trigone and posterior bladder wall (Pokuri et al. 2016). Urachal adenocarcinoma however, arises within urachal remnants (residual tissues from the embryonic allantoic stalk connecting the umbilicus and bladder), close to the dome and anterior wall of the bladder (Pokuri et al. 2016). Morphologically, PBA is classified into enteric and

S. S. Goonewardene et al., *Management of Non-Muscle Invasive Bladder Cancer*, https://doi.org/10.1007/978-3-030-28646-0_4

nonenteric types, which includes mucinous, signet-ring cell variant, clear-cell type, hepatoid, and mixed forms. Currently, there is no standard of care in the management of PBA (Pokuri et al. 2016).

Adenocarcinoma is a rare, often aggressive variant of bladder cancer (Burnett et al. 1991). 28 patients with vesical adenocarcinoma were reviewed to determine best management (Burnett et al. 1991). Excluded were mixed transitional cell carcinoma and adenocarcinoma (Burnett et al. 1991). Three major classes of tumor were identified: primary vesical adenocarcinoma, urachal adenocarcinoma, and extravesical adenocarcinoma (Burnett et al. 1991). Signet ring cell tumors appeared to behave more aggressively than other cell types (Burnett et al. 1991). Radical surgery was the most effective treatment (Burnett et al. 1991).

This clearly highlights the importance of surgical management in adenocarcinoma of the bladder.

Mesonephric adenocarcinoma of the bladder may be the malignant counterpart of nephrogenic adenoma (Schultz et al. 1984). The invasive potential of nephrogenic neoplasms changed the management of this disease (Schultz et al. 1984). Nephrogenic adenoma and mesonephric adenocarcinoma appear cytologically similar on a NMI bladder biopsy. The latter is excluded by deeper bladder biopsies (Schultz et al. 1984). Muscular invasion may indicate a more aggressive behavior and may require radical cystectomy for cure (Schultz et al. 1984).

4.2 Survival Outcomes in Adenocarcinoma of the Urinary Bladder

Dutta et al. investigated the prognostic significance of tumor location on survival outcomes in bladder adenocarcinoma (BAC) (Dutta et al. 2016). A total of 1,361 cases of BAC with known tumor location were identified (Dutta et al. 2016). Most tumors were low grade (grade I and II; 51%). 5-year overall survival (OS) and disease-specific survival (DSS) rates were 37.3% and 49.0%, respectively (Dutta et al. 2016). The 5-year OS rates were 42.3%, 35.9%, and 28.4% for UD, LW, and BL lesions, respectively ($p < 0.0001$), whereas the 5-year DSS rates were 50.2%, 51.7%, and 42.1% for UD, LW, and BL lesions, respectively ($p = 0.0097$) (Dutta et al. 2016). Multivariate Cox regression analysis controlling for tumor stage and grade demonstrated that both tumors of the LW (hazards ratio [HR] = 1.52 for OS and 1.30 for DSS) and BL (HR = 1.71 for OS and 1.57 for DSS) conferred a worse prognosis relative to those of the UD ($p < 0.05$) (Dutta et al. 2016). Tumor location of BAC is an independent prognostic factor for disease outcome (Dutta et al. 2016). Our results suggest that the urachal and dome locations are associated with relatively favorable survival and oncological outcomes, whereas basal location confers poorer outcomes (Dutta et al. 2016).

4.3   Surgical Management of Adenocarcinoma of the Bladder

Busto Martín present reviewed management of signet-ring cell bladder adeno-carcinoma (Busto Martín et al. 2010). There were 9 cases of primary signet ring cell adenocarcinomas (4 pure and 5 mixed) (Busto Martín et al. 2010). Definitive treatment was radical cystectomy with Bricker's urinary diversion in four patients, cystectomy with Mainz's II diversion in one patient and palliative management with TURB in three cases and percutaneous nephrostomy in the remaining case (Busto Martín et al. 2010). Adjuvant chemotherapy was used in three cases (Busto Martín et al. 2010). Only two patients were alive at the time of the study. Mean survival was 327 days for pure tumors and 586 for the mixed ones (Busto Martín et al. 2010). This demonstrates pure signet-ring cell primary adenocarcinoma of the bladder has a worse prognosis than transitional cell cancer. Radical cystectomy is the treatment of choice, with adjuvant chemotherapy if possible (Busto Martín et al. 2010). Five-year survival is less than 11% (Busto Martín et al. 2010).

Three cases of adenocarcinoma involving the bladder and consisting mainly of signet-ring-shaped cells were reviewed by DeFilipo et al. (1987). This unusual neoplasm has a worse prognosis than transitional cell carcinoma of the bladder, possibly because of factors that lead to delays in management (DeFilipo et al. 1987). Radiation therapy is ineffective, and the results of treatment with segmental resection of the involved area of the bladder are equivalent to those of total cystectomy (DeFilipo et al. 1987).

4.4   Urachal Adenocarcinoma—Surgical Management

Urachal adenocarcinoma is a rare and aggressive form of bladder cancer that arises from the urachus (Aoun et al. 2015). An en bloc resection of the urachus and umbilicus is recommended with either a total or partial cystectomy (Aoun et al. 2015). However, there is no standard laparoscopic or robotic surgical technique for the operative management of these tumors. Robotic-assisted laparoscopic technique for the treatment of a primary malignant urachal tumor can be conducted (Aoun et al. 2015).

Correa reported two cases of urachal adenocarcinoma managed with robotic-assisted partial cystectomy (Correa et al. 2010). The robotic approach is safe and an alternative to traditional open or laparoscopic-assisted partial cystectomy for this uncommon aggressive malignancy (Correa et al. 2010).

There is no consensus regarding management of adenocarcinoma. Whilst wide local excision with partial or radical cystectomy may be preferable, bladder-sparing management is increasing (Williams and Chavda 2015). Williams et al.

reported a case of robot-assisted laparoscopic partial cystectomy with en bloc resection of the urachus and bilateral pelvic lymphadenectomy for urachal carcinoma (Williams and Chavda 2015). The robot-assisted laparoscopic technique allowed decreased morbidity, postoperative pain, and recovery time, whilst allowing oncological principles to be followed (Williams and Chavda 2015).

The treatment of choice for urachal carcinoma has traditionally been an open approach, either by radical cystectomy or the more recently adopted bladder-sparing approach of extended partial cystectomy and umbilectomy. Milboua, reported for the first time a laparoscopic technique for an extended partial cystectomy with en bloc umbilectomy for the management of urachal carcinoma in a 41-year-old man (Milhoua et al. 2006). This demonstrated reasonable outcomes, with an often aggressive tumour.

4.5 Chemotherapy in Metastatic Adenocarcinoma of the Bladder

Teo et al. have used chemotherapy in metastatic adenocarcinoma of the bladder (Teo et al. 2011). Owing to the histologic similarity between this patient's tumor and colorectal cancer, palliative FOLFOX6 (folinic acid, 5-fluorouracil and oxaliplatin) chemotherapy plus bevacizumab was administered (Teo et al. 2011). After 3 months of treatment the patient showed a good response, which was sustained for more than 10 months after diagnosis (Teo et al. 2011).

References

Aoun F, Peltier A, van Velthoven R. Bladder sparing robot-assisted laparoscopic en bloc resection of urachus and umbilicus for urachal adenocarcinoma. J Robot Surg. 2015;9(2):167–70.

Burnett AL, Epstein JI, Marshall FF. Adenocarcinoma of urinary bladder: classification and management. Urology. 1991;37(4):315–21.

Busto Martín LA, Janeiro Pais M, González Dacal J, Chantada Abal V, Busto Castañón L. Signet-ring cell adenocarcinoma of the bladder: case series between 1990–2009. Arch Esp Urol. 2010;63(2):150–3.

Correa JJ, Hakky TS, Spiess PE, Chuang T, Sexton WJ. Robotic-assisted partial cystectomy with en bloc excision of the urachus and the umbilicus for urachal adenocarcinoma. J Robot Surg. 2010;3(4):235–8.

DeFillipo N, Blute R, Klein LA. Signet-ring cell carcinoma of bladder. Evaluation of three cases with review of literature. Urology. 1987;29(5):479–83.

Dutta R, Abdelhalim A, Martin JW, Vernez SL, Faltas B, Lotan Y, Youssef RF. Effect of tumor location on survival in urinary bladder adenocarcinoma: a population-based analysis. Urol Oncol. 2016;34(12):531.e1–6.

Klaile Y, Schlack K, Bocgcmann M, Steinestel J, Schrader AJ, Krabbe LM. Variant histology in bladder cancer: how it should change the management in non-muscle invasive and muscle invasive disease? Transl Androl Urol. 2016;5(5):692–701.

Milhoua PM, Knoll A, Bleustein CB, Ghavamian R. Laparoscopic partial cystectomy for treatment of adenocarcinoma of the urachus. Urology. 2006;67(2):423.e15–7.

Pokuri VK, Sule N, Perfetto C, Duff M, Kopp C, Guru K, Shah D, George S. A novel treatment approach prolonging survival in an uncommon metastatic primary bladder adenocarcinoma. J Community Support Oncol. 2016;14(2):72–5.

Schultz RE, Bloch MJ, Tomaszewski JE, Brooks JS, Hanno PM. Mesonephric adenocarcinoma of the bladder. J Urol. 1984;132(2):263–5.

Teo M, Swan NC, McDermott RS. Sustained response of adenocarcinoma of the urinary bladder to FOLFOX plus bevacizumab. Nat Rev Urol. 2011;8(5):282–5.

Williams CR, Chavda K. En bloc robot-assisted laparoscopic partial cystectomy, urachal resection, and pelvic lymphadenectomy for urachal adenocarcinoma. Rev Urol. 2015;17(1):46–9.

Chapter 5
Histological Variants in Bladder Cancer— Sarcomatoid Differentiation

5.1 Histopathology of Sarcomatoid Bladder Tumours

Urothelial cancer has a significant ability to differentiate (Pompas-Veganzones et al. 2014). Neuroendocrine tumors arise as a result. Neuroendocrine tumors of the bladder have hormone secretion and often a poor outcome (Pompas-Veganzones et al. 2014). These tend to be either pure neuroendocrine neoplasms or a neuroendocrine counterpart mixed with classical urothelial bladder cell carcinomas, adenocarcinoma, sarcomatoid carcinoma or mixtures of these components (Pompas-Veganzones et al. 2014) Their clinical aggressiveness remain a challenge for pathological staging and treatment (Pompas-Veganzones et al. 2014). Sarcomas and sarcomatoid carcinomas exhibited cellular atypia, mitotic activity with atypical mitosis, in the presence of necrosis (Spiess et al. 2007).

5.2 Management in Paediatric Cases

Wang et al. reviewed a case of sarcomatoid differentiation in a paediatric patient. The case presented with painless hematuria and urinary frequency (Wang et al. 2016). The tumor displayed sarcomatoid differentiation and an aggressive behaviour. Post surgical management included adjuvant chemotherapy (Wang et al. 2016). However, given the aggressive nature of sarcomatoid disease, the disease progressed (Wang et al. 2016).

The greater proportion of bladder cancers in paediatric patients are low-grade and present at an early stage, whereas sarcomatoid differentiation in the setting of a high-grade urothelial carcinoma is indicative of a poor prognosis (Wang et al. 2016). It is recommended that the management of urothelial neoplasia in young patients should be predominantly decided on the basis of the grade and stage of the tumor rather than the age of the patient.

© Springer Nature Switzerland AG 2020
S. S. Goonewardene et al., *Management of Non-Muscle Invasive Bladder Cancer*,
https://doi.org/10.1007/978-3-030-28646-0_5

5.3   Clinical Presentation, Biphasic, Monophasic Components of Sarcomatoid Bladder Cancer

Patients tend to present with gross hematuria and irritative symptoms (Matsuoka et al. 2008). The tumour is aggressive and spreads quickly, where presentation is with advanced disease. This disease had local recurrences and partial and total cystectomies were performed, respectively. This disease can be monophasic or biphasic (Matsuoka et al. 2008). The recurrent tumors were monophasic sarcomatoid carcinoma purely composed of spindle cell component (Matsuoka et al. 2008). Sarcomatoid carcinoma demands radical resection at the initial surgical treatment because of aggressive potential of spindle cell component (Matsuoka et al. 2008). In this case, biphasic sarcomatoid carcinoma of the bladder has recurred as monophasic tumor, demonstrating tumours can flip from biphasic to monophasic (Matsuoka et al. 2008).

Carcinosarcoma and sarcomatoid carcinoma of the bladder after organ transplantation is higher in comparison to the healthy population, but overall occurrence is still rare (McCrea et al. 2012). Due to the decreased immunitary response effects of antirejection drugs, these cancers have aggressive course and respond poorly to treatment (McCrea et al. 2012). Bladder drained pancreatic transplants are associated with a number of urologic challenges that can delay the diagnosis and the treatment of malignancies of the genito-urinary system (McCrea et al. 2012).

5.4   Surgical Management of Sarcomatoid Differentiation of Bladder Cancer

Sarcomatoid carcinoma should be resected radically at initial resection because of aggressive potential of spindle cell component (Matsuoka et al. 2008). Local recurrences and distant metastases frequently occurred with primary sarcoma and sarcomatoid carcinoma despite aggressive surgical management, which was often combined with neoadjuvant chemotherapy (50% and 65% disease-specific mortality, respectively) (Spiess et al. 2007).

5.5   Survival Outcomes in Sarcomatoid Differentiation of Bladder Cancer

Sarcomatoid carcinoma and carcinosarcoma of the bladder are rare aggressive tumors that contain epithelial and mesenchymal elements. These have a worse prognosis than conventional urothelial carcinoma (Wright et al. 2007). Cases were identified from the Surveillance, Epidemiology and End Results Program (Wright et al. 2007). Overall unadjusted survival rates for 46,515 cases of urothelial carcinoma, 135 with sarcomatoid carcinoma and 166 with carcinosarcoma were 77%, 54% and 48% at 1 year, and 47%, 37% and 17% at 5 years, respectively (Wright et al. 2007). Sarcomatoid carcinoma and carcinosarcoma present with a more aggressive T stage and with more frequent regional and distant metastases compared to urothelial carcinoma (Wright et al. 2007). Overall mortality was worse with carcinosarcoma than with sarcomatoid carcinoma (HR 1.70, 95% CI 1.23–2.34) (Wright et al. 2007). Compared to patients with urothelial carcinoma those with sarcomatoid carcinoma and carcinosarcoma present at a more advanced stage and with greater mortality risk after adjusting for stage at presentation (Wright et al. 2007). The survival rate of sarcomatoid carcinoma is better than that of carcinosarcoma, offering some justification for the continued differentiation of these tumor types for clinical prognostication.

Sarcomatoid urothelial carcinoma is a dedifferentiated biphasic tumor that exhibits morphological and/or immunohistochemical evidence of epithelial and mesenchymal differentiation (Fatima et al. 2015).

Fatima, examined thirty-seven cases of sarcomatoid urothelial carcinoma (Fatima et al. 2015). Twenty-six of 37 (70%) were male and 11/37 (30%) patients were female. Twenty-five cases were from cystectomy/cystoprostatectomy specimens, 8 cases from transurethral resection of bladder tumor specimens and 4 cases were from biopsy specimens (Fatima et al. 2015). Four of 37 (10%) cases had focal heterologous components; 1 case with both chondroid and osteoid, 2 cases with chondroid and 1 case rhabdoid elements (Fatima et al. 2015). Twenty-one of 37 (56%) died within a year of presentation (Fatima et al. 2015). Sarcomatoid urothelial carcinoma is an aggressive variant of urothelial carcinoma which commonly presents at an advanced stage, and over 50% of patients in this series died of disease within 1 year of presentation (Fatima et al. 2015).

References

Fatima N, Canter DJ, Carthon BC, Kucuk O, Master VA, Nieh PT, Ogan K, Osunkoya AO. Sarcomatoid urothelial carcinoma of the bladder: a contemporary clinicopathologic analysis of 37 cases. Can J Urol. 2015;22(3):7783–7.

Matsuoka Y, Hirokawa M, Chiba K, Hashiba T, Tomoda T, Sugiura S. Biphasic and monophasic sarcomatoid carcinoma of the urinary bladder. Can J Urol. 2008;15(3):4106–8.

McCrea PH, Chang M, Bailley G, Molinari M. Sarcomatoid carcinoma of the bladder after simultaneous kidney-pancreas transplant: a case report and review of the literature. BMJ Case Rep. 2012;28:2012.

Pompas-Veganzones N, Gonzalez-Peramato P, Sanchez-Carbayo M. The neuroendocrine component in bladder tumors. Curr Med Chem. 2014;21(9):1117–28.

Spiess PE, Tuziak T, Tibbs RF, Bassett R, Tamboli P, Brown GA, Grossman HB, Ayala AG, Czerniak B. Pseudosarcomatous and sarcomatous proliferations of the bladder. Hum Pathol. 2007;38(5):753–61.

Wang Z, Xiong W, Pan C, Zhu L, Wang X, Huang Z, Zhao X, Zhong Z. Aggressive muscle-invasive bladder cancer with sarcomatoid differentiation in a 10-year-old girl: a case report. Exp Ther Med. 2016;11(3):985–7.

Wright JL, Black PC, Brown GA, Porter MP, Kamat AM, Dinney CP, Lin DW. Differences in survival among patients with sarcomatoid carcinoma, carcinosarcoma and urothelial carcinoma of the bladder. J Urol. 2007;178(6):2302–6; discussion 2307.

Chapter 6
Histological Variants in Bladder Cancer— Carcinosarcoma

6.1 Histopathology of Carcinosarcoma of the Bladder

The carcinomatous element consisted of urothelial and squamous cell carcinomas (Nishikawa et al. 2011). The sarcomatous element was composed of osteosarcoma, chondrosarcoma and spindle cell sarcoma (Nishikawa et al. 2011). Immunohistochemical examination demonstrated the carcinomatous component was positive for cytokeratin and the sarcomatous component was positive for S-100 protein (Nishikawa et al. 2011). Carcinosarcoma of the urinary bladder is a rare neoplasm that is composed of malignant epithelial and mesenchymal components (Atılgan and Gençten 2013). NMI carcinosarcoma of the bladder is aggressive and has always invaded the lamina propria, since in addition to the carcinomatous degeneration of the mucosa, sarcomatous degeneration of the underlying submucosal stroma is also present (Kuntz et al. 1993). The tumour's pathoanatomical study can be mixed with an epithelial pattern of transitional and squamous cells and a sarcomatous pattern composed of rabdomiosarcoma, osteochondrosarcoma and pleomorphous indifferentiated sarcoma with giant multinuclear cells (Pena Outeiriño et al. 1995).

Carcinosarcomas are histologically malignant biphasic neoplasms with an epithelial and a spindle cell component (Torenbeek et al. 1999). Both a polyclonal and a monoclonal origin have been postulated for these tumours, but the latter has been favoured (Torenbeek et al. 1999). For carcinosarcoma, the stem cell from which the epithelial and mesenchymal components are derived is expected to be more immature than the epithelial stem cell from which different components of sarcomatoid carcinoma originate, since in the latter, immunohistochemical or ultrastructural epithelial characteristics are still detectable (Torenbeek et al. 1999).

© Springer Nature Switzerland AG 2020
S. S. Goonewardene et al., *Management of Non-Muscle Invasive Bladder Cancer*,
https://doi.org/10.1007/978-3-030-28646-0_6

6.2   Clinical Presentation of Carcinosarcoma
of the Bladder

Carcinosarcoma is a rare tumor which represent less than 0.5% of all cancers of the bladder (Bennani et al. 1994). It is three times more frequent in men than in women (Bennani et al. 1994). Hematuria is the most frequent alarming symptom and pathogenesis is still a matter of debate. Diagnosis is based on the pathological examination including immunohistochemical study and, if necessary, with electron microscopy examination (Bennani et al. 1994). The tumor contains two highly malignant cellular components: one is epithelial and the other is mesenchymal. Management can often be controversial. Early diagnosis and radical cystectomy are key (Bennani et al. 1994).

Carcinosarcoma of the urinary bladder ca present with symptoms of pain irritative urinary symptoms and macroscopic hematuria (Nishikawa et al. 2011; Atılgan and Gençten 2013). Gross hematuria nearly always was the presenting symptom (Sen et al. 1985). In a case such as this, cystoscopy revealed a non-papillary tumor covered with necrotic tissue on the right side of the posterior wall of the bladder (Nishikawa et al. 2011).

6.3   Surgical Management of Carcinoma of the Bladder

Atilgan investigated the impact of surgical management on carcinosarcoma. Transurethral resection of the tumour (TURBT) revealed a carcinosarcoma (Atılgan and Gençten 2013). Despite the radical resection, the patient underwent radical cystectomy, and there was no tumor recurrence for 15 months after treatment (Atılgan and Gençten 2013). Transurethral resection was performed, histologically, the tumor was found to be composed of carcinomatous and sarcomatous elements (Nishikawa et al. 2011). Total cystectomy with ileal conduit is most commonly the definitive form of management (Nishikawa et al. 2011). Pathological examination showed no residual tumor (Nishikawa et al. 2011). Patients with carcinosarcoma, should be referred to specialists or centers with extensive experience with this rare and serious disease (Atılgan and Gençten 2013). Patients treated by partial cystectomy fared poorly, while 7 treated by radical cystectomy and supravesical urinary diversion had an excellent prognosis: 6 (86%t) have been free of disease for more than 1 year, including 4 who have survived more than 45 months without evidence of recurrence or metastasis (Sen et al. 1985).

Transurethral resection (TUR) of urothelial carcinoma (UC) of the bladder and adjuvant intravesical chemotherapy with pirarubicin 10 years ago recurred with a gross hematuria (Hirano et al. 2018). Pelvic MRI showed the tumor without extending the base of the bladder wall. The tumor could be completely removed with TUR (Hirano et al. 2018). The malignant epithelial elements consisted of high-grade UC and the majority of mesenchymal components were fibrosarcomatous differentiation based on immunohistochemical studies (Hirano et al. 2018). The tumor could be pathologically also suspected to be an early stage on TUR specimens (Hirano et al. 2018). Although he has received no additional intervention due to the occurrence of myocardial infarction at three weeks after the TUR, he has been alive with no evidence of recurrence of the disease 27 months after the TUR (Hirano et al. 2018).

Kuntz reviewed the case of a female patient is presented who had a large carcinosarcoma of the urinary bladder that became clinically manifest only 2 months before treatment (Kuntz et al. 1993). The initial treatment by transurethral resection was followed by radical cystectomy; 7 months postoperatively the patient died of local tumour recurrence with widespread metastases (Kuntz et al. 1993). Carcinosarcoma of the urinary bladder is a rare tumour with a poor prognosis. The majority of such tumours are not diagnosed until tumour growth is already far advanced (Kuntz et al. 1993). Owing to the small number of cases there is no clinically proven form of management. Any local surgical treatment, such as TUR or partial cystectomy, involves the risk of incomplete tumor removal, because the sarcomatous elements typically invade the submucosa while the overlying mucosa remains intact (Kuntz et al. 1993). Therefore, radical cystectomy appears to be the treatment of choice for both NMI and invasive carcinosarcoma of the urinary bladder (Kuntz et al. 1993).

The Surveillance, Epidemiology, and End Results (SEER) Program database was used to identify cases by tumor site and histology codes (Wang et al. 2010). A total of 221 histology confirmed cases were identified between 1973 and 2004, this accounted for approximately 0.11% of all primary bladder tumors during the study period (Wang et al. 2010). Multiple primary tumors were indentified in about 40% of study subjects (Wang et al. 2010). The majority of patients (95.9%) received surgery, 35.8% had radical or partial cystectomy, 15.8% received radiation therapy combination with surgery (Wang et al. 2010). The median overall survival was 14 months (95% CI 7–21 months). 1-, 5-, and 10-year cancer specific survival rate were 53.9, 28.4 and 25.8% (Wang et al. 2010). Urinary bladder carcinosarcoma commonly presented as high grade, advanced stage and aggressive behavior with a poor prognosis (Wang et al. 2010).

Carcinosarcoma of the prostate is an extremely rare tumor (Dallinger and Würnschimmel 2010). In the case of rapid tumor progression, especially after radiation therapy to the pelvis or after hormone deprivation therapy because of prostate cancer, this tumor entity should be considered, and immediate histological confirmation is required (Dallinger and Würnschimmel 2010). The only curative therapy is immediate radical surgical excision (Dallinger and Würnschimmel 2010).

The histopathologic diagnosis of the TURBT specimens was sarcoma (Shirai et al. 1999). Radical cystectomy was performed under the diagnosis clinical stage III, T3bN0M0 (Shirai et al. 1999). The post-operative histopathologic diagnosis of the tumor was sarcomatoid carcinoma, composed of nests of transitional cell carcinoma (G3) and predominant areas of spindle cell sarcomatoid transformation (Shirai et al. 1999).

6.4 Survival Outcomes and Prognosis in Carcinosarcoma of the Bladder

Guo, analysed the prognosis of Chinese patients diagnosed with sarcomatoid carcinoma (SC) of the bladder (Guo et al. 2013). Carcinosarcoma of the bladder was most common in older males and most patients had high-grade or late-stage disease at diagnosis (Guo et al. 2013). The 6-month, 1-year, 2-year, and 5-years survival rates were 78.9%, 42.7%, 28.0%, and 21.0%, respectively. Pathologic tumor stage was unrelated to prognosis (Guo et al. 2013). Early diagnosis and surgical intervention are preferred strategies for improvement of prognosis (Guo et al. 2013). The association between clinical stage and survival time requires further analysis (Guo et al. 2013).

The effect of bladder cancer histological subtypes other than transitional cell carcinoma (nonTCC) on clinical outcomes remains uncertain (Rogers et al. 2006). Rogers conducted a multi-institutional retrospective study of patients with bladder cancer treated with radical cystectomy to assess the impact of nonTCC histology on bladder cancer specific outcomes (Rogers et al. 2006). Patients with nonTCC and nonSCC bladder cancer were at significantly increased risk for progression and death compared to patients with TCC or SCC ($p < 0.001$) (Rogers et al. 2006). This association remained statistically significant in patients with organ confined disease (stage pT2 or lower) and patients with nonorgan confined disease (stage pT3 or higher) ($p < 0.001$) (Rogers et al. 2006). NonTCC and nonSCC histological subtype is an independent predictor of bladder cancer progression and mortality in patients undergoing radical cystectomy for bladder cancer (Rogers et al. 2006). Patients with bladder TCC and SCC share similar stage specific clinical outcomes (Rogers et al. 2006).

References

Atılgan D, Gençten Y. Carcinosarcoma of the bladder: a case report and review of the literature. Case Rep Urol. 2013;2013:716704.

Bennani S, Louahlia S, Aboutaieb R, el Mrini M, Benjelloun S. Carcinosarcoma of the bladder. Apropos of two cases. J Urol (Paris). 1994;100(4):210–6.

Dallinger B, Würnschimmel E. Appearance of carcinosarcoma after radiotherapy for local recurrence after radical prostatectomy. Case report and review of the literature. Urologe A. 2010;49(6):750–4.

Guo AT, Huang H, Wei LX. Clinicopathological characteristics and prognosis of Chinese patients with sarcomatoid carcinoma of the bladder. Histol Histopathol. 2013;28(9):1167–74.

Hirano D, Yoshida T, Funakoshi D, Sakurai F, Ohno S, Kusumi Y. A case of early stage bladder carcinosarcoma in late recurrence of urothelial carcinoma after transurethral resection. Case Rep Urol. 2018;15(2018):1405108.

Kuntz RM, Geyer V, Savvas V, Grosse G. Carcinosarcoma of the urinary bladder. Urologe A. 1993;32(1):59–63.

Nishikawa R, Fujimura M, Endo Y, Sekita N, Suzuki H, Sugano I, Mikami K. A case of carcinosarcoma of the urinary bladder. Hinyokika Kiyo. 2011;57(4):199–202.

Pena Outeiriño JM, León Dueñas E, Romero Gil JR, Leal López A. Bladder carcinosarcoma. A clinical case. Actas Urol Esp. 1995;19(3):234–7.

Rogers CG, Palapattu GS, Shariat SF, Karakiewicz PI, Bastian PJ, Lotan Y, Gupta A, Vazina A, Gilad A, Sagalowsky AI, Lerner SP, Schoenberg MP. Clinical outcomes following radical cystectomy for primary nontransitional cell carcinoma of the bladder compared to transitional cell carcinoma of the bladder. J Urol. 2006;175(6):2048–53; discussion 2053.

Sen SE, Malek RS, Farrow GM, Lieber MM. Sarcoma and carcinosarcoma of the bladder in adults. J Urol. 1985;133(1):29–30.

Shirai S, Kawakami S, Yoshida M, Ueda S, Nakamura T, Honda Y. Sarcomatoid carcinoma of the urinary bladder in a hemodialysis patient: a case report. Nihon Hinyokika Gakkai Zasshi. 1999;90(10):847–50.

Torenbeek R, Hermsen MA, Meijer GA, Baak JP, Meijer CJ. Analysis by comparative genomic hybridization of epithelial and spindle cell components in sarcomatoid carcinoma and carcinosarcoma: histogenetic aspects. J Pathol. 1999;189(3):338–43.

Wang J, Wang FW, Lagrange CA, Hemstreet Iii GP, Kessinger A. Clinical features of sarcomatoid carcinoma (carcinosarcoma) of the urinary bladder: analysis of 221 cases. Sarcoma. 2010;2010. pii: 454792.

Chapter 7
Histological Variants in Bladder Cancer— Small Cell Carcinoma

7.1 Variant Histology in Bladder Cancer—Small Cell Incidence and Histopathology

Small-cell carcinoma of the urinary bladder is a rare and aggressive type of bladder cancer that has a poor prognosis (Thota et al. 2013). The incidence has been gradually increasing because of the aging population (Thota et al. 2013). Owing to its rarity there are no available treatment guidelines (Thota et al. 2013).

Small cell carcinoma of the urinary bladder (SCC-BL) is an extremely rare malignancy, accounting for <1% of all bladder tumors. Its prognosis is very poor because of its highly aggressive behavior and high metastatic potential (Gkirlemis et al. 2013).

It is associated with rapid progression, early metastases formation and high mortality rates (Heidegger et al. 2016). Prior series have shown a significant male predominance, occurs mainly during the 7th and 8th decade of life and macroscopic haematuria is the most common presenting symptom (Gkirlemis et al. 2013).

Small cell carcinoma of the urinary bladder (SCCUB) is a rare and aggressive cancer of the bladder. SCCUB is part of neuroendocrine family of tumors that affect several organ systems including respiratory, gastrointestinal and male and female genitourinary tract (Pant-Purohit et al. 2010). SCCUB affect males predominantly with common risk factors include smoking, bladder calculi, bladder manipulation, and chronic cystitis (Pant-Purohit et al. 2010). Prognosis of SCCUB remains poor due to high metastatic potential and lack of symptoms in earlier stages of the disease (Pant-Purohit et al. 2010). Pathogenesis of the disease is linked to loss of genetic material, hypermethylation of tumor suppressors and at times amplification of the chromosomal regions carrying oncogenes (Pant-Purohit et al. 2010).

© Springer Nature Switzerland AG 2020   27
S. S. Goonewardene et al., *Management of Non-Muscle Invasive Bladder Cancer*,
https://doi.org/10.1007/978-3-030-28646-0_7

Small cell, LCNEC and mixed-NEC are a morphological spectrum of high-grade neuroendocrine carcinoma with overlapping histological features, identical immunophenotype, Ki-67 proliferative rate and patient outcomes. Finally, the nuclear size criteria is misleading as HGNEC, particularly cases of LCNEC and mixed-NEC, may have enlarged nuclei compared to small cell carcinomas and are more prone to be misdiagnosed as UC, thereby preventing appropriate management.

7.2   Histological Variants in Bladder Cancer—Small Cell Treatment

Small cell carcinoma is an aggressive malignancy often associated with poor prognosis due to the presence of advanced disease (Shatagopam et al. 2015). Small cell malignancies, although in initially described in the lung, can occur in extrapulmonary sites such as bladder, with similar clinicopathologic outcomes (Shatagopam et al. 2015). There has been a paradigm shift in the management of lung SCC from initial surgical excision to use of chemotherapy followed by local therapies (Shatagopam et al. 2015). Patients with small cell neuroendocrine tumors of the bladder should be offered chemotherapy before surgery (Alanee et al. 2018).

The premise for doing this is to improve patient survival. Use of platinum-based combination chemotherapy then surgical resection and/or radiation offers the best outcome (Shatagopam et al. 2015). A multimodal approach that includes chemotherapy, local radiation therapy, and definitive surgery in resectable cases appears to be an optimal management approach (Thota et al. 2013). Majority of cases are treated with local resection of the tumor with neoadjuvant or adjuvant platinum-based chemotherapy (Pant-Purohit et al. 2010). Radiation therapy is used as alternative to radical cystectomy or as palliative measure (Pant-Purohit et al. 2010).

High grade neuroendocrine carcinomas (HGNEC) treated by cystectomy often carry an original diagnosis of typical urothelial carcinoma (UC) and may be of a mixed nature (Gupta et al. 2015). The correct diagnosis of HGNEC is critical in influencing the decision for early chemotherapy, potentially followed by cystectomy (Gupta et al. 2015). According to the most important studies, cystectomy alone seems not to be efficient enough for the management of the disease (Gkirlemis et al. 2013). On the other hand, radiation therapy when combined with chemotherapy is highly effective with increased survival rates (Gkirlemis et al. 2013).

Choong performed a retrospective study at Mayo Clinic (Rochester, MN) to characterize the clinical and pathologic features of patients with SCC of the urinary bladder diagnosed between 1975 and 2003 with emphasis on management (Choong et al. 2005). Forty-four patients were identified who had primary bladder SCC, 61.4% of whom had pure SCC (Choong et al. 2005). The 5-year survival rates for patients with Stage II, III, and IV disease were 63.6%, 15.4%, and 10.5%, respectively (Choong et al. 2005). Six of eight patients with Stage II bladder SCC achieved a cure with radical cystectomy. Five patients with Stage IV disease had obvious metastases and received chemotherapy (Choong et al. 2005). Fourteen patients underwent radical cystectomy and were diagnosed later with locally advanced disease (T4b) or lymph node metastasis (N1–N3; Stage IV disease) (Choong et al. 2005). Only 2 of 19 patients with Stage IV disease who received adjuvant chemotherapy were alive at 5 years (Choong et al. 2005).

Heidegger et al. presented long-term disease-free survival of a 60 year-old man who was diagnosed with SCBC two and a half years ago. He underwent four cycles of cisplatin/etoposide chemotherapy as well as a prophylactic whole-brain radiotherapy followed by a radical cystoprostatectomy and ileal neobladder with extended pelvic lymphadenectomy (Heidegger et al. 2016). Since 33 months the patient is now recurrence-free (Heidegger et al. 2016). Early multimodal therapy results in long-term disease-free survival, therefore it is highly recommended to give neoadjuvant chemotherapy as a part of multimodal management of a primary metastases-free, localized and surgically resectable SCBC.

Majority of cases are treated with local resection of the tumor with neoadjuvant or adjuvant platinum-based chemotherapy regimen (Pant-Purohit et al. 2010). Radiation therapy is used as alternative to radical cystectomy or as palliative measure (Pant-Purohit et al. 2010).

Small cell carcinoma of the urinary bladder (SCCB) is difficult to characterize and study because of its rarity (Koay et al. 2011). Koay analysed the SEER-Medicare database (1991–2005) was used to estimate chemotherapy use (Koay et al. 2011). There were 642 patients in the SEER limited dataset. Patients who had stage IV disease without distant metastasis (i.e., positive lymph node status) had overall and cancer-specific survival rates similar to those of patients who had stage I through III disease, but they had significantly better survival compared with patients who had distant metastasis ($p<0.0001$) (Koay et al. 2011). Transurethral resection of the bladder tumor became the most common surgical treatment ($p<0.0001$), representing 55% of patients from 2001 to 2005 (Koay et al. 2011). The receipt of radiation and chemotherapy did not change significantly during the study period (Koay et al. 2011). These comprehensive data delineated the patient population for this rare disease, described several independent prognostic variables, and demonstrated clear treatment trends for this disease (Koay et al. 2011). The results suggest that a simpler staging system (i.e., limited stage vs. extensive stage) may be appropriate for patients with SCCB (Koay et al. 2011).

Neuroendocrine tumors of the bladder comprise a small subset of all bladder tumors (Siefker-Radtke et al. 2004). For patients treated with initial cystectomy median cancer specific survival (CSS) was 23 months, with 36% disease-free at 5 years (Siefker-Radtke et al. 2004). For patients receiving preoperative chemotherapy median CSS has not been reached ($p=0.026$), although CSS at 5-years was 78% with no cancer related deaths observed beyond 2 years (Siefker-Radtke et al. 2004). Notably 7 of 25 patients treated with initial cystectomy received chemotherapy after surgery but their survival was no better than those treated with cystectomy alone (Siefker-Radtke et al. 2004). As others have observed, the pathological stage was higher than clinically appreciated for 56% of patients treated with initial cystectomy (Siefker-Radtke et al. 2004). Moreover, there were no cancer related deaths among patients with disease down staged to pT2 or less (Siefker-Radtke et al. 2004).

7.3   Bladder Sparing in Small Cell Carcinoma

Consolidation thoracic irradiation and prophylactic cranial irradiation (PCI) both increase 3-year absolute survival by 5.4% in SCLC patients with limited disease and a complete response to chemotherapy. Lester et al. report their experience using this strategy (Lester et al. 2006). Seven patients were identified. In total, six out of seven had platinum-based chemotherapy. Four patients received consolidation radiotherapy (CRT) to the bladder after a complete response to chemotherapy, and non have locally relapsed to date (Lester et al. 2006). The three patients with limited disease remain alive and disease free 14, 30 and 36 months after diagnosis (Lester et al. 2006). Combined modality therapy using platinum-based combination chemotherapy and consolidation radiotherapy may provide effective local control and allow a bladder-preserving approach to the management of SCC of the bladder (Lester et al. 2006). The role of PCI is controversial, and should be discussed with patients on an individual basis (Lester et al. 2006).

Bex evaluate the feasibility and efficacy of a therapeutic algorithm for the management of small cell carcinoma of the bladder derived from the treatment of small cell lung cancer (Bex et al. 2005). During a 10-year period, 25 patients (23 men and 2 women; median age 64 years, with 8 [32%] older than 75 years) with small cell carcinoma of the bladder were defined as having limited disease (LD) or extensive disease (ED) in analogy to the classification of small cell lung cancer (Bex et al. 2005). Patients with LD were eligible for chemotherapy and sequential radiotherapy (Bex et al. 2005). Patients unfit for chemotherapy were offered complete transurethral resection and radiotherapy or cystectomy for large symptomatic tumors. Patients with ED were offered palliative chemotherapy (Bex et al. 2005). Of the 25 patients, 17 (68%) had LD and 8 (32%) ED (Bex et al. 2005). Without regard to stage, the median survival of those receiving chemotherapy was 15 months versus 4 months for those who did not. The median survival for those with LD was 12 months versus 5 months for those with ED (Bex et al. 2005). Nine patients (52.9%) with LD could not undergo chemoradiotherapy because of comorbidity and reduced performance ($n = 7$), progression ($n = 1$), or drug-related death ($n = 1$) (Bex et al. 2005). Five of those patients underwent TUR and radiotherapy and two cystectomy (Bex et al. 2005). This treatment algorithm offers bladder sparing for most patients, with few long-term remissions in patients with small, confined tumors. None of the patients died of locoregional tumor progression, supporting that cystectomy is not the treatment of choice for those with LD (Bex et al. 2005). With a significant proportion of elderly patients with comorbidities, chemoradiotherapy was not feasible in more than one half of the patients with LD (Bex et al. 2005).

Small cell carcinoma of the bladder is an uncommon but clinically aggressive disease (Eswara et al. 2015). There is no standard surgical or medical management for the disease (Eswara et al. 2015). The median follow-up for survivors was 34 months. Patients presented most often with muscle-invasive disease (T2–4: 89%), and 21% had lymph node/distant metastases (Eswara et al. 2015). Tobacco use and chemical exposure were noted in 64 and 4% of patients, respectively. Patients with T1–2N0M0 had a median survival of 22 months compared to 8 months for those with more advanced disease ($p = 0.03$). Patients with T3–4 or nodal/metastatic disease who were given chemotherapy had an improved survival compared to those with T3–4 or nodal/metastatic disease who did not undergo chemotherapy (13 vs. 4 months, $p = 0.005$) (Eswara et al. 2015). The median time to recurrence of the entire cohort was 8 months, overall and cancer-specific survival was 14 months, and 5-year survival was 11% (Eswara et al. 2015). Small cell carcinoma of the bladder is an aggressive disease with poor outcomes. Patients with T1–2N0M0 disease survived longer than those with advanced disease (Eswara et al. 2015). Patients with T3–4 or nodal/metastatic disease had improved survival with chemotherapy.

7.4   Histological Variants in Bladder Cancer—Small Cell Survival Outcomes

Mukesh reported the clinical experience and management of patients with small cell carcinoma (SCC) of the bladder, treated in the Anglia Cancer network from 1992 to 2007, and to review published studies, as SCC is a rare condition, accounting for <1% of all bladder tumours, and there is no established treatment strategy for managing these patients (Mukesh 2007). Twenty patients were identified with primary bladder SCC (male: female ratio 3:1; mean age 68 years; mean follow-up 15.8 months). Nine patients (45%) had extensive-stage disease at diagnosis (Mukesh 2007). Four patients received best supportive care, three had a radical cystectomy, one radical radiotherapy and six sequential chemo-radiotherapy (Mukesh 2007). In all, 13 patients were treated with chemotherapy, with six receiving cyclophosphamide, doxorubicin and vincristine, three receiving carboplatin and etoposide, and the remainder receiving alternative platinum-based regimens (Mukesh 2007). For 12 patients with assessable disease, six had a complete response, three a partial response and three had progressive disease after chemotherapy (Mukesh 2007). No patient received prophylactic cranial irradiation (PCI). At the time of analysis, 14 (70%) patients had died, with one (5%) developing brain metastasis. The median survival was 33 months for patients receiving chemotherapy, versus 3 months with no chemotherapy (Mukesh 2007). SCC of the bladder tends to occur in an older population, more commonly in men (Mukesh

2007). It is an aggressive tumour with a propensity for early metastasis. The response rate to chemotherapy is high but the overall prognosis is poor (Mukesh 2007).

Poor prognosis and rarity render disease management complicated (Gkirlemis et al. 2013). A definitive treatment is not yet established but combined therapy with systemic platinum-based chemotherapy and adjuvant local radiotherapy seems to be the most effective therapeutic approach for limited-stage SCC-BL (Gkirlemis et al. 2013). Further research is required in order to clarify whether prophylactic cranial irradiation (PCI) should be performed on a regular basis (Gkirlemis et al. 2013).

Small-cell carcinomas (sccs) of the genitourinary (gu) tract are rare systemic diseases, and there is no standard treatment strategy for patients with this malignancy. Pervez et al. reported outcomes on GU small cell carcinoma (Pervez et al. 2013). The 58 patients identified had scc in the following primary sites: urinary bladder ($n = 35$), prostate ($n = 17$), and upper urinary tract ($n = 6$). In 38 patients (66%), the scc was of pure histology; in the remainder, histology was mixed (Pervez et al. 2013). Overall, 28 patients had limited-stage disease; 24 had extensive-stage disease; and staging was unknown in 6 patients. Median survival for the entire cohort was 7.5 months, with extensive-stage disease being identified as a poor prognostic factor (survival was 22.0 months for limited-stage patients and 4.1 months for extensive-stage patients, $p < 0.001$) (Pervez et al. 2013). Based on site, prostate patients fared worst, with a median survival of only 5.1 months. Compared with best supportive care, treatment was associated with better outcomes (median survival: 12.3 months vs. 2.3 months, $p < 0.0001$) (Pervez et al. 2013).

Small-cell cancer of the gu tract is an aggressive cancer, with a poor prognosis overall. Although there is no standard of care, patients should be treated using a multimodality approach analogous to that used in the treatment of small-cell lung cancer.

7.5 Histological Variants in Small Cell Carcinoma of the Urinary Bladder—Radiotherapy

Small cell carcinoma of the urinary bladder (SCCB) is rare (Mattes et al. 2015). Mattes reported their experience with definitive external beam radiation therapy (EBRT) as part of multimodality management of SCCB. Nineteen patients with locoregional SCCB were treated (Mattes et al. 2015). Five patients had radiographic nodal disease (Mattes et al. 2015). Eighteen patients received neoadjuvant (17/19; 89%) or concurrent (11/19: 58%) platinum-based chemotherapy (Mattes et al. 2015). Three patients had in-bladder recurrence (2-year local recurrence, 25%), 2 being noninvasive and successfully managed with transurethral resection and the third being invasive but managed with chemotherapy alone due to simultaneous distant metastases (Mattes et al. 2015). Six patients had recurrence distantly (2-year distant recurrence, 40%), predominantly bone metastases ($n = 3$). No patients developed brain metastases (Mattes et al. 2015). Actuarial 2-year disease-free and overall survival was 51% and 78%, respectively. The 2-year distant metastasis-free survival for node-negative and node-positive patients was 76% and 26%, respectively ($p = 0.04$) (Mattes et al. 2015). The 2-year incidence of distant metastases for patients receiving ≥4 cycles of doublet chemotherapy was 27%, compared with 75% with less chemotherapy ($p = 0.01$) (Mattes et al. 2015). The incidence of grade ≥2 acute and late genitourinary or gastrointestinal toxicity was 69 and 7%, respectively (Mattes et al. 2015). Definitive chemoradiation for locoregional SCCB is well tolerated, with encouraging local control and overall survival at 2 years (Mattes et al. 2015).

7.6 Cranial Irradiation in Small Cell Bladder Cancer

Extrapulmonary small-cell carcinoma (EPSCC) is a rare disease (Naidoo et al. 2013). Management is based on small-cell lung carcinoma (Naidoo et al. 2013). Prophylactic cranial irradiation (PCI) is not routinely administered in EPSCC (Naidoo et al. 2013). Two hundred eighty patients were identified; 141 (50.4%) were men and 139 (49.6%) were women (Naidoo et al. 2013). One hundred eighty six patients (66.4%) had extensive-stage disease, 65 (23.2%) had limited-stage disease, and in 29 patients (10.3%) the stage was unknown (Naidoo et al. 2013). Eighteen patients (6.4%) developed brain metastases, with a median overall survival of 10.1 months (Naidoo et al. 2013). Eleven (61%) received cranial irradiation, and 12 (67%) received palliative chemotherapy (Naidoo et al. 2013). Median overall survival was 15.2 months (10.2–20.6) for limited-stage disease, 2.3 months (1.7–3.1) for extensive-stage EPSCC, and 3.7 months (1.3–8.3) for disease of unknown stage (Naidoo et al. 2013). Brain metastases were uncommon in EPSCC compared with small-cell lung carcinoma.

The incidence of symptomatic brain metastases in small-cell carcinoma of the urinary bladder (SCBC) is unknown (Bex et al. 2010). Among 39 patients with LD, median disease-specific survival was 35 months (Bex et al. 2010). Four developed symptomatic brain metastases after a median follow-up of 15 months (range 3–24) and were treated with whole-brain radiotherapy (Bex et al. 2010). No patient with ED developed symptomatic brain metastases during a median follow-up of 6 months (Bex et al. 2010). The reported incidence of brain metastases in SCBC in the literature ranges between 0 and 40% (Bex et al. 2010). On the basis of all reported series, the pooled estimate of the cumulative incidence of brain metastases is 10.5% (95% confidence interval 7.5–14.1%) (Bex et al. 2010). The incidence of symptomatic brain metastases from SCBC is significantly lower than that from small-cell lung cancer.

References

Alanee S, Alvarado-Cabrero I, Murugan P, Kumar R, Nepple KG, Paner GP, Patel MI, Raspollini MR, Lopez-Beltran A, Konety BR. Update of the international consultation on urological diseases on bladder cancer 2018: non-urothelial cancers of the urinary bladder. World J Urol. 2018.

Bex A, Nieuwenhuijzen JA, Kerst M, Pos F, van Boven H, Meinhardt W, Horenblas S. Small cell carcinoma of bladder: a single-center prospective study of 25 cases treated in analogy to small cell lung cancer. Urology. 2005;65(2):295–9.

Bex A, Sonke GS, Pos FJ, Brandsma D, Kerst JM, Horenblas S. Symptomatic brain metastases from small-cell carcinoma of the urinary bladder: The Netherlands Cancer Institute experience and literature review. Ann Oncol. 2010;21(11):2240–5.

Choong NW, Quevedo JF, Kaur JS. Small cell carcinoma of the urinary bladder. The Mayo Clinic experience. Cancer. 2005;103(6):1172–8.

Eswara JR, Heney NM, Wu CL, McDougal WS. Long-term outcomes of organ preservation in patients with small cell carcinoma of the bladder. Urol Int. 2015;94(4):401–5.

Gkirlemis K, Miliadou A, Koukourakis G, Sotiropoulou-Lontou A. Small cell carcinoma of the bladder: a search of the current literature. J Buon. 2013;18(1):220–6.

Gupta S, Thompson RH, Boorjian SA, Thapa P, Hernandez LP, Jimenez RE, Costello BA, Frank I, Cheville JC. High grade neuroendocrine carcinoma of the urinary bladder treated by radical cystectomy: a series of small cell, mixed neuroendocrine and large cell neuroendocrine carcinoma. Pathology. 2015;47(6):533–42.

Heidegger I, Tulchiner G, Schäfer G, Horninger W, Pichler R. Long term disease free survival with multimodal therapy in small cell bladder cancer. Eur J Med Res. 2016;21(1):40.

Koay EJ, Teh BS, Paulino AC, Butler EB. A surveillance, epidemiology, and end results analysis of small cell carcinoma of the bladder: epidemiology, prognostic variables, and treatment trends. Cancer. 2011;117(23):5325–33.

Lester JF, Hudson E, Barber JB. Bladder preservation in small cell carcinoma of the urinary bladder: an institutional experience and review of the literature. Clin Oncol (R Coll Radiol). 2006;18(8):608–11.

Mattes MD, Kan CC, Dalbagni G, Zelefsky MJ, Kollmeier MA. External beam radiation therapy for small cell carcinoma of the urinary bladder. Pract Radiat Oncol. 2015;5(1):e17–22.

Naidoo J, Teo MY, Deady S, Comber H, Calvert P. Should patients with extrapulmonary small-cell carcinoma receive prophylactic cranial irradiation? J Thorac Oncol. 2013;8(9):1215–21.

Pant-Purohit M, Lopez-Beltran A, Montironi R, MacLennan GT, Cheng L. Small cell carcinoma of the urinary bladder. Histol Histopathol. 2010;25(2):217–21.

Pervez N, El-Gehani F, Joseph K, Dechaphunkul A, Kamal M, Pertschy D, Venner P, Ghosh S, North S. Genitourinary small-cell carcinoma: a single-institution experience. Curr Oncol. 2013;20(5):258–64.

Shatagopam K, Kaimakliotis HZ, Cheng L, Koch MO. Genitourinary small cell malignancies: prostate and bladder. Future Oncol. 2015;11(3):479–88.

Siefker-Radtke AO, Dinney CP, Abrahams NA, Moran C, Shen Y, Pisters LL, Grossman HB, Swanson DA, Millikan RE. Evidence supporting preoperative chemotherapy for small cell carcinoma of the bladder: a retrospective review of the M. D. Anderson cancer experience. J Urol. 2004;172(2):481–4.

Thota S, Kistangari G, Daw H, Spiro T. A clinical review of small-cell carcinoma of the urinary bladder. Clin Genitourin Cancer. 2013;11(2):73–7.

Chapter 8
Histological Variants—Plasmacytoid Bladder Cancer

8.1 Diagnostics in Plasmacytoid Bladder Cancer

Plasmacytoid urothelial carcinoma (PUC) is a rare tumor of the urinary bladder (Mai et al. 2006). Mai reported seven cases of PUC (Mai et al. 2006). Cases of urothelial carcinoma (UC) were reviewed for a period of seven years to identify PUC (Mai et al. 2006). Representative sections from each case of PUC were submitted for immunohistochemical studies (Mai et al. 2006). There were a total of seven cases of PUC out of 260 cases of invasive urothelial carcinoma (Mai et al. 2006). The common type of urothelial carcinoma (CUC) was present in focal areas in five cases (Mai et al. 2006). Cases with extensive PUC showed coarse and indurated mucosal folds and thickened bladder walls, with no grossly identifiable tumor (Mai et al. 2006). Urine cytology showed a scant number of atypical single cells, frequently without tumor diathesis, leading to a shortfall in the positive cytological diagnosis (Mai et al. 2006). Histologically, PUC appeared as dyscohesive, plasmacytoid cells with eccentric nuclei, extending widely into the bladder walls and extensively into adjacent pelvic organs (Mai et al. 2006). PUC is a distinct clinical and pathological subtype of urothelial carcinoma. The clinical presentation is frequently late due to the frequent absence of hematuria and indurated mucosal surface at cystoscopy. The disease followed an ominous course with recurrence in all the patients, and with patient death.

Makise review two cases of urinary bladder urothelial carcinoma (UC) and rold of CA19-9 in diagnostics. In both, histological examination of a transurethral resection specimen of the bladder tumor revealed UC with plasmacytoid and micropapillary differentiations (Makise et al. 2015). Elevated serum carbohydrate antigen 19-9 (CA19-9) returned to near normal levels after radical cystectomy, but they increased shortly before death with metastatic disease. In Case 2, no residual carcinoma was found in the radical cystectomy specimen or lymph nodes. Postoperative serum CA19-9 was maintained at normal levels, and the patient

© Springer Nature Switzerland AG 2020
S. S. Goonewardene et al., *Management of Non-Muscle Invasive Bladder Cancer*,
https://doi.org/10.1007/978-3-030-28646-0_8

remains alive without recurrence or metastasis (Makise et al. 2015). Although plasmacytoid is a known aggressive variants of UC, plasmacytoid UC may be more aggressive (Makise et al. 2015). Serum CA19-9 could serve as a useful biomarker to monitor progression of plasmacytoid UC.

8.2   Histological Variants—Clinical Presentation of Plasmacytoid Bladder Cancer

Qin reported a 74-year-old male who presented with hematuria (Qin et al. 2014). Zhang studied the clinicopathologic features and prognosis of plasmacytoid urothelial carcinoma (PUC) of the urinary bladder (Zhang et al. 2013). Most patients (15/16) presented with hematuria (Zhang et al. 2013).

The index case was a patient with complaint of lower abdominal pain but without any urological symptoms (Wang et al. 2012). The authors report a case of a 57-year-old male patient with a 3-month history of hematuria and pelvic pain (da Fonseca et al. 2014).

Post surgery and chemotherapy, patients have also presented with extensive spread to the scrotal wall (Wang et al. 2016).

PUC is a rare tumor associated with poor prognosis due to its advanced clinical stage upon its diagnosis. The delayed diagnosis is mainly due to the late occurrence of hematuria and absence of papulary mucosal surface at cystoscopy (Wang et al. 2012) can be achieved based on its typical histological features, clinical history and immunohistochemical results.

8.3   Histological Variants—Histopathology of Plasmacytoid Bladder Cancer

Plasmacytoid urothelial carcinoma (PUC) of the urinary bladder is an uncommon and aggressive variant of urothelial carcinoma associated with late presentation and poor prognosis (Qin et al. 2014). The pattern of tumor spread along fascial planes, the tendency for initial understaging, and the rapid recurrence after initially response to chemotherapy (Wang et al. 2016). Immunohistochemical examination showing expression of epithelial markers, CD138, and losing the membranous expression of E-cadherin confirms evidence of PUC (Qin et al. 2014). Histologically, PUC appeared to be dyscohesive, plasmacytoid cells with eccentric nuclei and abundant eosinophilic cytoplasm with characteristics of plasmacytoid morphology (Wang et al. 2016).

Bladder plasmacytoid carcinoma is an invasive urothelial carcinoma subtype that is emphasized for its morphological overlap with plasma cells and metastatic carcinoma (Ricardo-Gonzalez et al. 2012). Frequent intraperitoneal spread that is not typical of conventional urothelial carcinoma (Ricardo-Gonzalez et al. 2012).

A plasmacytoid variant of urothelial carcinoma has been recently recognized in the World Health Organization classification system (Raspollini et al. 2011). This is characterized by a discohesive growth of plasmacytoid cells with eccentric nuclei, extending in the bladder wall and often in the perivesical adipose tissue (Raspollini et al. 2011). The electron microscopic examination showed the presence of divergent squamous and glandular differentiation (Raspollini et al. 2011). At variance with conventional urothelial carcinoma, the analysis of exons 4–9 of TP53 gene revealed no alteration in all the 4 tumors tested, and this can be of value in choosing additional chemotherapy after surgery (Raspollini et al. 2011). Plasmacytoid carcinoma of the bladder is a tumor entity, which can be characterized by specific immunohistochemical markers, including positivity for GATA-3, and presents phenotypic and genotypic peculiarities (Raspollini et al. 2011).

The tumor cells were small to medium in size and contained eccentric nuclei and moderate to abundant eosinophilic cytoplasm, assuming a plasmacytoid appearance (Zhang et al. 2013). The architectural pattern varied from loosely cohesive sheets to cords, papillae, small nests or gland-like structures. Most tumors invaded into the lamina propria or muscularis propria (Zhang et al. 2013). Twelve of the 16 cases had concurrent conventional urothelial carcinoma component. Immunohistochemical study showed that the tumor cells in all cases were strongly positive for AE1/AE3, epithelial membrane antigen, CK7 and CK18. CK20 and uroplakin III were also expressed in 9 cases (Zhang et al. 2013). CEA, p53, CD138, p63 and E-cadherin were positive in 12, 13, 15, 11 and 10 cases, respectively. Ki-67 index ranged from 5 to 70% (mean = 30%) (Zhang et al. 2013).

Microscopically, all tumors contained plasmacytoid cells, which composed 30–100% of the entire tumor (Ro et al. 2008). The plasmacytoid tumor cells were characterized by eccentrically located nuclei and abundant eosinophilic cytoplasm (Ro et al. 2008). Immunohistochemical staining demonstrated that both plasmacytoid and conventional TCC components were positive for cytokeratins 7 and 20 (Ro et al. 2008). The mean Ki-67 labeling index was 30% (range, 10–50%), and p53 expression in the majority of cases was low (5–10%), except for in 2 cases (70 and 80%) (Ro et al. 2008).

8.4   Histological Variants—Surgical Management of Plasmacytoid Bladder Cancer

A transurethral biopsy revealed urothelial carcinoma with plasmacytoid appearance (Qin et al. 2014). The pathological diagnosis was PUC (High-grade, pT4N2M0) with diffuse muscle, small tracts, and vascular invasion, in which almost of the areas studied on the tissue section showed Plasmacytoid differentiation.

Kawarhara reported a case of high-grade invasive urothelial carcinoma with plasmacytoid differentiation of the urinary bladder (Kawahara et al. 2011). A 75-year-old woman was referred to our hospital because of macroscopic hematuria. Cystoscopy detected a solid pedunculated bladder tumor, and a transurethral resection of the bladder tumor (TUR-Bt) and the image findings showed pT1N0M0 bladder cancer (Kawahara et al. 2011). Following the TUR-Bt, external beam radiotherapy and chemotherapy with gemcitabine and nedaplatin were carried out. The bladder tumor has not recurred for 2 years after the TUR-Bt (Kawahara et al. 2011).

Wang et al. had a patient that underwent cystectomy (Wang et al. 2012). Other than radical cystectomy, postoperative adjuvant treatment could be a good approach to prolong the survival time of PUC patients.

Radical cystectomy with lymphadenectomy was performed and pathological examination showed a pT3pN0 PVUC of the bladder (da Fonseca).

8.5   Metastatic Spread of Plasmacytoid Bladder Cancer

Ricardo-Gonzalez identified cases of plasmacytoid urothelial carcinoma diagnosed on radical cystectomy (Ricardo-Gonzalez et al. 2012). A total of 10 male and 5 female patients 42–81 years old were identified. One tumor was pT2, 11 pT3 and 3 pT4. Six of 15 patients (40%) presented with lymph node metastasis and 5 (33%) had intraperitoneal metastasis at cystectomy (Ricardo-Gonzalez et al. 2012). These initial sites of metastatic spread included the prerectal space, ovary and vagina, ovary and fallopian tube, bowel serosa, and omentum and bowel serosa in 1 case each (Ricardo-Gonzalez et al. 2012). Three patients had subsequent metastasis involving the prerectal space, pleural fluid and small bowel serosa, and bowel serosa in 1 each. Eight patients had followup information available, including 3 who died of disease, 3 with disease and 2 with no evidence of disease (Ricardo-Gonzalez et al. 2012). Of the patients 33% with the plasmacytoid variant of urothelial carcinoma presented with intraperitoneal disease spread and 20% had subsequent metastasis involving serosal surfaces. The possibility of noncontiguous intraperitoneal spread involving serosal surfaces should be recognized to ensure proper intraoperative staging and clinical followup for patients with plasmacytoid carcinoma.

8.6   Surgical and Adjuvant Management in Plasmacytoid Bladder Cancer

Keck reviewed 205 tumor samples of patients with locally advanced bladder cancer mainly treated within the randomized AUO-AB05/95 trial with radical cystectomy and adjuvant cisplatin-based chemotherapy for histologic subtypes (Keck et al. 2013). 178 UC, 18 plasmacytoid (PUC) and 9 micropapillary (MPC) carcinomas of the bladder were identified (Keck et al. 2013). Patients suffering from PUC have the worst clinical outcome regarding overall survival compared to conventional UC and MPC of the bladder that in turn seem have to best clinical outcome (27.4 months, 62.6 months, and 64.2 months, respectively; $p = 0.013$ by Kaplan Meier analysis) (Keck et al. 2013). Histopathological diagnosis of rare variants of urothelial carcinoma can identify patients with poor prognosis (Keck et al. 2013).

8.7   Prognosis in Plasmacytoid Bladder Cancer

Plasmacytoid variant (PCV) urothelial cancer (UC) of the bladder is rare, with poor clinical outcomes (Kaimakliotis et al. 2014). A retrospective analysis of the Indiana University Bladder Cancer Database between January 2008 and June 2013 was performed comparing 30 patients with PCV UC at cystectomy to 278 patients with nonvariant (NV) UC at cystectomy who underwent surgery for muscle-invasive disease (Kaimakliotis et al. 2014). Patients with PCV UC who were diagnosed with a higher stage at cystectomy (73% pT3–4 vs. 40%, $p = 0.001$) were more likely to have lymph node involvement (70% vs. 25%, $p < 0.001$), and positive surgical margins were found in 40% of patients with PCV UC versus 10% of patients with NV UC ($p < 0.001$) (Kaimakliotis et al. 2014). Median overall survival and disease-specific survival were 19 and 22 months for PCV, respectively. Median overall survival and disease specific survival had not been reached for NV at 68 months ($p < 0.001$) (Kaimakliotis et al. 2014). Presence of PCV UC on transurethral resection of bladder tumor was associated with non-organ-confined disease (odds ratio = 4.02; 95% CI: 1.06–15.22; $p = 0.040$), and PCV at cystectomy was associated with increased adjusted risk of mortality (hazard ratio = 2.1; 95% CI: 1.2–3.8; $p = 0.016$) (Kaimakliotis et al. 2014). PCV is an aggressive UC variant, predicting non-organ-confined disease and poor survival. Differentiating between non-muscle- and muscle-invasive disease in patients with PCV UC seems less important than the aggressive nature of this disease. Instead, any evidence of PCV on transurethral resection of bladder tumor may warrant aggressive therapy.

8.8   Metastatic Pattern of Spread—Plasmacytoid Bladder Cancer

Kaimakliotis examined differences in disease progression and nature of tumor invasion that may lead to more accurate expectations of tumor behavior and improved management options for plasmacytoid variant (PCV) histology Urothelial cell carcinoma patients (Kaimakliotis et al. 2014). Using the Indiana University Bladder Cancer Database, a retrospective analysis radical cystectomies was conducted.

Of 510 patients who met inclusion criteria, 30 had +UM on final pathology. The incidence of +UM in NV patients was 17 of 457 (3.7%), in MPV 5 of 28 (17.9%), and in PCV 8 of 25 (32.0%) ($p < 0.001$) (Kaimakliotis et al. 2014). Carcinoma in situ on the luminal margin was noted for all cases, except in 5 of the 8 PCV patients with +UM, in whom retrograde longitudinal invasion along the subserosal and adventitia was noted (Kaimakliotis et al. 2014). +PSM and +LN were significantly higher for both PCV (28.0%, 72.0%) and MPV (10.7%, 64.3%) than NV (2.6%, 18.6%, $p < 0.001$, each) (Kaimakliotis et al. 2014).

PCV exhibits a unique pattern of spread along the ureter. This proposes a new mode of invasion along the fascial sheath (Kaimakliotis et al. 2014). The incidence of +PSM and +LN liken PCV to the known aggressive MPV, and in conjunction with the increased incidence of +UM, may lead to a paradigm shift, with surgeons and pathologists being more vigilant with surgical margins (Kaimakliotis et al. 2014).

8.9 Systematic Chemotherapy in Plasmacytoid Bladder Cancer

Hayashi report two cases of the plasmacytoid variant of urothelial carcinoma of urinary bladder in which systemic chemotherapy was effective (Hayashi et al. 2011). In the first case resection of the brain tumor and transurethral resection of the bladder tumor were performed. Three cycles of adjuvant MVAC (methotrexate, vinblastine, adriamycin, and cisplatin) chemotherapy were given (Hayashi et al. 2011). He has no evidence of recurrence 96 months after resection of brain metastasis. In the second case, MRI revealed a bladder tumor with abdominal wall invasion, and a transurethral biopsy was performed. The pathological diagnosis was plasmacytoid variant of urothelial carcinoma of urinary bladder (cT4bN0M0). After three cycles of neoadjuvant GC (gemcitabine and cisplatin) chemotherapy, MRI demonstrated a complete response. Radical cystectomy was performed, and the pathological diagnosis was pT0pN0.

References

da Fonseca LG, Souza CE, Mattedi RL, Girardi DM, Sarkis ÁS, Hoff PMG. Plasmacytoid urothelial carcinoma: a case of histological variant of urinary bladder cancer with aggressive behavior. Autops Case Rep. 2014;4(4):57–61.

Hayashi T, Tanigawa G, Fujita K, Imamura R, Nakazawa S, Yamamoto Y, Hosomi M, Shimazu K, Fushimi H, Yamaguchi S. Two cases of plasmacytoid variant of urothelial carcinoma of urinary bladder: systemic chemotherapy might be of benefit. Int J Clin Oncol. 2011;16(6):759–62.

Kaimakliotis HZ, Monn MF, Cary KC, Pedrosa JA, Rice K, Masterson TA, Gardner TA, Hahn NM, Foster RS, Bihrle R, Cheng L, Koch MO. Plasmacytoid variant urothelial bladder cancer: is it time to update the treatment paradigm? Urol Oncol. 2014;32(6):833–8.

Kawahara T, Oshiro H, Sekiguchi Z, Ito H, Makiyama K, Uemura H, Kubota Y. High-grade invasive urothelial carcinoma with focal plasmacytoid differentiation successfully treated by transurethral resection followed by chemoradiotherapy. Int J Urol. 2011;18(12):851–3.

Keck B, Wach S, Stoehr R, Kunath F, Bertz S, Lehmann J, Stöckle M, Taubert H, Wullich B, Hartmann A. Plasmacytoid variant of bladder cancer defines patients with poor prognosis if treated with cystectomy and adjuvant cisplatin-based chemotherapy. BMC Cancer. 2013;8(13):71. https://doi.org/10.1186/1471-2407-13-71.

Mai KT, Park PC, Yazdi HM, Saltel E, Erdogan S, Stinson WA, Cagiannos I, Morash C. Plasmacytoid urothelial carcinoma of the urinary bladder report of seven new cases. Eur Urol. 2006;50(5):1111–4.

Makise N, Morikawa T, Takeshima Y, Fujimura T, Homma Y, Fukayama M. Urinary bladder urothelial carcinoma with concurrent plasmacytoid and micropapillary differentiations: a report of two cases with an emphasis on serum carbohydrate antigen 19-9. Pathol Int. 2015;65(9):495–500.

Qin M, Wang G, Sun Y, He Q. Plasmacytoid urothelial carcinoma of the bladder. Indian J Pathol Microbiol. 2014;57(2):320–2.

Raspollini MR, Sardi I, Giunti L, Di Lollo S, Baroni G, Stomaci N, Menghetti I, Franchi A. Plasmacytoid urothelial carcinoma of the urinary bladder: clinicopathologic, immunohistochemical, ultrastructural, and molecular analysis of a case series. Hum Pathol. 2011;42(8):1149–58.

Ricardo-Gonzalez RR, Nguyen M, Gokden N, Sangoi AR, Presti JC Jr, McKenney JK. Plasmacytoid carcinoma of the bladder: a urothelial carcinoma variant with a predilection for intraperitoneal spread. J Urol. 2012;187(3):852–5.

Ro JY, Shen SS, Lee HI, Hong EK, Lee YH, Cho NH, Jung SJ, Choi YJ, Ayala AG. Plasmacytoid transitional cell carcinoma of urinary bladder: a clinicopathologic study of 9 cases. Am J Surg Pathol. 2008;32(5):752–7.

Wang YG, Perera M, Gleeson J. Plasmacytoid urothelial carcinoma of the bladder with extensive scrotal wall invasion. Urol Ann. 2016;8(3):381–3

Wang Z, Lu T, Du L, Hu Z, Zhuang Q, Li Y, Wang CY, Zhu H, Ye Z. Plasmacytoid urothelial carcinoma of the urinary bladder: a clinical pathological study and literature review. Int J Clin Exp Pathol. 2012;5(6):601–8.

Zhang W, Jiang YX, Liu Y, Yu WJ, Zhao H, Li YJ. Plasmacytoid urothelial carcinoma of the urinary bladder: a clinicopathologic study of 16 cases. Zhonghua Bing Li Xue Za Zhi. 2013;42(7):433–7.

Part III
Epidemiology and Risk Factors in Bladder Cancer

Chapter 9
Introduction to Epidemiology of Bladder Cancer

9.1 Smoking

A significant risk factors for urothelial tumor is tobacco smoking (Cigarette smoking) is the prevalent risk factor for the development of BC (Simonis et al. 2014). In those who already have BC, smoking increases the risk of both disease recurrence and progression. Smoking cessation may limit these effects (Simonis et al. 2014) and therefore it is the duty of each urologist to raise awareness regarding the dangers of smoking with respect to BC. Many epidemiological studies and reviews have been performed to identify the causes of bladder cancer (Letašiová et al. 2012). Smoking, mainly cigarette smoking, is a well known risk factor for various diseases, including bladder cancer (Letašiová et al. 2012).

There are also data suggesting an effect from of other types of smoking besides cigarettes (cigar, pipe, Egyptian waterpipe, smokeless tobacco and environmental tobacco smoking), and other sources of arsenic exposure such as air, food, occupational hazards, and tobacco (Letašiová et al. 2012). Other studies show that hairdressers and barbers with occupational exposure to hair dyes experience enhanced risk of bladder cancer (Letašiová et al. 2012).

Worldwide incidence of BC may reflect differences in tobacco usage, changes in coding practices, prevalence of schistosomiasis (Africa), and occupational exposure (Chavan et al. 2014). Reduction of incidence of bladder tumors is based on elimination of these risk factors and bladder cancer screening in high-risk patients.

Ferris demonstrated the variable combination of constitutional and environmental risk factors, the majority of which are unknown (Ferris et al. 2013). The most significant constitutional risk factors are related to age, gender, race, ethnicity geographic location and genetic polymorphisms (Ferris et al. 2013). The main occupational risk factors are those related to aromatic amines and polycyclic aromatic hydrocarbons.

© Springer Nature Switzerland AG 2020
S. S. Goonewardene et al., *Management of Non-Muscle Invasive Bladder Cancer*,
https://doi.org/10.1007/978-3-030-28646-0_9

9.2   Occupational Exposure

The most notable risk factor for development of bladder cancer is occupational exposure to aromatic amines (2-naphthylamine, 4-aminobiphenyl and benzidine) and 4,4′-methylenebis(2-chloroaniline), which can be found in the products of the chemical, dye and rubber industries as well as in hair dyes, paints, fungicides, cigarette smoke, plastics, metals and motor vehicle exhaust (Letašiová et al. 2012). Exposure to polycyclic aromatic hydrocarbons, nitrosamines, aromatic amines and arsenic also contribute (Guillaume et al. 2014). Occupational exposure to chemicals such as o-toluidine, aniline and nitrobenzene increase the risk of BC in rubber and dye factory workers (Carreón et al. 2014). Other risk factors include urinary schistosomiasis (specific to squamous cell cancer), pelvic radiation therapy, the use of cyclophosphamide (Guillaume et al. 2014). Occupational exposure, which represent 5–10% of BC risk factors and occupations with high risk exposure, such as aluminium production, the manufacture of dyes, paints and colourings, the rubber industry and the extraction and industrial use of fossil fuels (Ferris et al. 2013).

9.3   Age and Gender Related Disease

Ferris et al. identified risk factors for BC including age and gender (diagnosed at age 65 and over, with a 4:1 ratio of males to females); race, ethnicity and geographic location (predominantly in Caucasians and in Southern European countries); genetic basis (N-acetyltransferase-2 and glutathione s-transferase M1 gene mutations, which significantly increase the risk for BC) (Ferris et al. 2013).

Bladder cancer incidence is higher in old men, shows geographic variation, and is mostly an environmental disease (Malats and Real 2015). This reflects and outline of age and gender factors. Cigarette smoking, occupational exposures, water arsenic, Schistosoma haematobium infestation (a risk factor for squamous cell carcinoma), and some medications are the best-established risk factors (Malats and Real 2015). Data on environmental and genetic factors involved in the disease outcome are as yet not fully conclusive (Malats and Real 2015).

Among men, triglycerides and BP were positively associated with bladder cancer risk overall (Teleka et al. 2018) among women, BMI was inversely associated with risk. This again reflects disparities in gender between risk of bladder cancer. The associations for BMI and BP differed between men and women (Teleka et al. 2018). Among men, BMI, cholesterol and triglycerides were positively associated with risk for NMIBC and BP was positively associated with MIBC (Teleka et al. 2018). Among women, glucose was positively associated with MIBC (Teleka et al. 2018). This highlights risk factors that needed to be assessed in bladder cancer. Apart from cholesterol, HRs for metabolic factors did not significantly differ between MIBC and NMIBC, and there were no interactions between smoking and metabolic factors on BC (Teleka et al. 2018).

Martini et al. assessed the strength of the online tool RiskCheck Bladder Cancer (RCBC) for early detection of bladder cancer (BC) (Martini et al. 2013). 141 patients were diagnosed with bladder cancer (Martini et al. 2013). This test demonstrated a sensitivity of 71.6%, a specificity of 56.5%, a positive predictive value of 67.8%, a negative predictive value of 52% and an accuracy of 63.5% (Martini et al. 2013). Risk factors ranked by importance are time of smoking, gender, occupational toxin exposure, and amount of consumed cigarettes resulting in a 95% association with BC. The high predictive power of RCBC for the identification of asymptomatic patients living under risk could be demonstrated.

References

Carreón T, Hein MJ, Hanley KW, Viet SM, Ruder AM. Bladder cancer incidence among workers exposed to o-toluidine, aniline and nitrobenzene at a rubber chemical manufacturing plant. Occup Environ Med. 2014;71(3):175–82.

Chavan S, Bray F, Lortet-Tieulent J, Goodman M, Jemal A. International variations in bladder cancer incidence and mortality. Eur Urol. 2014;66(1):59–73. https://doi.org/10.1016/j.eururo.2013.10.001.

Ferris J, Garcia J, Berbel O, Ortega JA. Constitutional and occupational risk factors associated with bladder cancer. Actas Urol Esp. 2013;37(8):513–22.

Guillaume L, Guy L. Epidemiology of and risk factors for bladder cancer and for urothelial tumors. Rev Prat. 2014;64(10):1372–4, 1378–80.

Letašiová S, Medve'ová A, Šovčíková A, Dušinská M, Volkovová K, Mosoiu C, Bartonová A. Bladder cancer, a review of the environmental risk factors. Environ Health. 2012;11(Suppl 1):S11.

Malats N, Real FX. Epidemiology of bladder cancer. Hematol Oncol Clin North Am. 2015;29(2):177–89, vii.

Martini T, Mayr R, Lodde M, Seitz C, Trenti E, Comploj E, Palermo S, Pycha A, Mian C, Zywica M, Weidner W, Lüdecke G. Validation of RiskCheck Bladder Cancer©, version 5.0 for risk-adapted screening of bladder cancer. Urol Int. 2013;91(2):175–81.

Simonis K, Shariat S F, Rink M. Smoking and smoking cessation effects on oncological outcomes in nonmuscle invasive bladder cancer. Curr Opin Urol. 2014;24(5):492 9.

Teleka S, Häggström C, Nagel G, Bjørge T, Manjer J, Ulmer H, Liedberg F, Ghaderi S, Lang A, Jonsson H, Jahnson S, Orho-Melander M, Tretli S, Stattin P, Stocks T. Risk of bladder cancer by disease severity in relation to metabolic factors and smoking; a prospective pooled cohort study of 800,000 men and women. Int J Cancer. 2018.

Chapter 10
Epidemiology, Risk Factors and Occupational Hazards—A Systematic Review

A systematic review relating to bladder cancer epidemiology, risk factors and occupational hazards was conducted. This was to identify the bladder cancer epidemiology, risk factors and occupational hazards. The search strategy aimed to identify all references related to bladder cancer AND screening. Search terms used were as follows: (Bladder cancer) AND (Epidemiology) AND (Risk Factors) AND (Occupational Hazards). The following databases were screened from 1989 to June 2019:

- CINAHL
- MEDLINE (NHS Evidence)
- Cochrane
- AMed
- EMBASE
- PsychINFO
- SCOPUS
- Web of Science.

In addition, searches using Medical Subject Headings (MeSH) and keywords were conducted using Cochrane databases. Two UK-based experts in bladder cancer were consulted to identify any additional studies.

Studies were eligible for inclusion if they reported primary research focusing on bladder cancer and screening. Papers were included if published after 1984 and had to be in English. Studies that did not conform to this were excluded. Only primary research was included (Fig. 10.1). The overall aim was to identify the role and components of bladder cancer screening.

Abstracts were independently screened for eligibility by two reviewers and disagreements resolved through discussion or third party opinion. Agreement level was calculated using Cohen's Kappa to test the intercoder reliability of this screening process. Cohens' Kappa allows comparison of inter-rater reliability between papers using relative observed agreement. This also takes account of

© Springer Nature Switzerland AG 2020
S. S. Goonewardene et al., *Management of Non-Muscle Invasive Bladder Cancer*,
https://doi.org/10.1007/978-3-030-28646-0_10

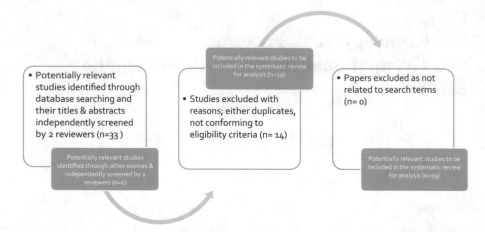

Fig. 10.1 Flow chart of studies identified through the systematic review (adapted from PRISMA)

the comparison occurring by chance. The first reviewer agreed all 19 papers to be included, the second, agreed on 19.

Data extraction was piloted by the researcher and amended in consultation with the research team (author and two academic supervisors). Data collected included authors, year and country of publication, study aims, setting, intervention aims, number of participants, study design, intervention components and delivery methods, comparison groups and outcome measures, notes and follow-up questions for the authors. Studies were quality assessed using the PRISMA criteria for randomised controlled trials, Mays et al. (Moher et al. 2009; Moher, Liberati et al. 2009, 154, 153; Mays et al. 2005) for the action research and qualitative studies and the Critical Skills Appraisal programme for cohort studies. This was also applied to randomised controlled trials and qualitative studies.

The search identified 19 papers (Fig. 10.1). All 19 mapped to the search terms and eligibility criteria. The current systematic reviews were examined to gain further knowledge about the subject. 14 papers were excluded due to not conforming to eligibility criteria or adding to the evidence for bladder cancer screening. Of the 19 papers left, relevant abstracts were identified and the full papers obtained (all of which were in English), to quality assure against search criteria. There was considerable heterogeneity of design among the included studies therefore a narrative review of the evidence was undertaken. There was significant heterogeneity within studies, including clinical topic, numbers, outcomes, as a result a narrative review was thought to be best. There were 19 cohort studies, with a moderate level of evidence. These were from a range of countries with minimal loss to follow-up. All participants were identified appropriately.

References

Moher D, Liberati A, Tetzlaff J, Altman DG. Preferred reporting items for systematic reviews and meta-analyses: the prisma statement. BMJ. 2009;339(7716):332–6.

Mays N, Pope C, Popay J. Systematically reviewing qualitative and quantitative evidence to inform management and policy-making in the health field. J Health Serv Res Policy. 2005;10(Suppl. 1):6–20.

Chapter 11
Systematic Review Results on Bladder Cancer Epidemiology, Occupational Hazards and Risk Factors

11.1 Bladder Cancer Survival

Bladder cancer survival has been examined in detail (Dement et al. 1998). The cause-specific mortality (1940–1993) of 2,985 male workers employed in oil refineries was examined (Dement et al. 1998). Separate analyses were undertaken by race, refinery, employment status (active and retired), and time since entry into employment (Dement et al. 1998). Proportionate cancer mortality ratio (PCMR) analyses also were conducted. Significantly decreased mortality was observed for cancers of the bladder (PMR = 40) (Dement et al. 1998). However, this may be explained by length of time in employment and exposure to carcinogens.

Darby, 1993, studied the long term effects of participation in the United Kingdom's atmospheric nuclear weapon tests and experimental programmes (Darby et al. 1993). Greater than 10 years after initial participation the relative risk of death in participants was raised for bladder cancer. However, the overall conclusion was participation in nuclear weapon tests had no detectable effect on expectation of life or on subsequent risk of developing cancer or other fatal diseases (Darby et al. 1993).

Exposure to occupational hazards among firefighters may lead to increased mortality from cancer (Ma et al. 2005). Mortality from bladder cancer was increased and approached statistical significance (SMR = 1.79; 95% CI: 0.98–3.00). Firefighters certified between 1972 and 1976 had excess mortality from bladder cancer (SMR = 1.95; 95% CI: 1.04–3.33) (Ma et al. 2005). This demonstrates the impact of exposure to occupational risk factors can have on mortality from cancer.

© Springer Nature Switzerland AG 2020
S. S. Goonewardene et al., *Management of Non-Muscle Invasive Bladder Cancer*,
https://doi.org/10.1007/978-3-030-28646-0_11

11.2   Carcinogenic Agents—Population Studies

Pukkala examined up to 45 years of cancer incidence data by occupational category for the Nordic populations (Pukkala et al. 2009). 15 million people aged 30–64 years in the 1960, 1970, 1980/1981 and/or 1990 censuses in Denmark, Finland, Iceland, Norway and Sweden were inlcuded. High risk occupations were examined. The occupations with the highest risk factors included workers producing tobacco and chimney sweeps. Low risk factors were demonstrated in farmers, gardeners and teachers (Pukkala et al. 2009). Waiters had the highest risk of bladder cancer in men and tobacco workers in women. This can be attributed to smoking (Pukkala et al. 2009). Hairdressers also had a high risk factor for bladder cancer—this may be due to exposure from hiar dye. Chimney sweeps are exposed to carcinogens such as polycyclic aromatic hydrocarbons from the chimney soot, and hairdressers' work environment is also rich in chemical agents (Pukkala et al. 2009).

11.3   Populations Studies with Women

The relation between occupation and bladder cancer in women was examined during the National Bladder Cancer Study (Silverman et al. 1990). This was a population-based, case-control study conducted in 10 areas of the United States (Silverman et al. 1990). Increased risk of bladder cancer occurred in metal working and fabrication occupations (relative risk (RR) = 1.5; 95% confidence interval (CI) 0.9–2.6) (Silverman et al. 1990). Punch and stamping press operatives had a significant trend in risk with increasing duration of employment and an increased risk for women employed as chemical processing workers was also shown. The authors estimate that 11% of bladder cancer diagnosed among white women in the United States is attributable to occupational exposures (Silverman et al. 1990).

The incidence of cancer of the urinary bladder is three- to five-fold lower in women than in men (Kabat et al. 2013). Kabat assessed the association of menstrual and reproductive factors and exogenous hormone use with the risk of incident transitional cell cancer of the urinary bladder in a cohort of 145,548 postmenopausal women (ages 50–79 years at baseline) enrolled in the Women's Health Initiative (Kabat et al. 2013). Relative to nulliparous women, parous women had a reduced risk of transitional cell cancer, however, there was no clear trend with increasing number of births. Risk was significantly increased in women with a history of at least two miscarriages (HR 1.52, 95% CI 1.15–2.00) (Kabat et al. 2013). In conclusion Kabat found limited evidence for associations of reproductive factors or exogenous hormone use with the risk of bladder cancer (Kabat et al. 2013).

11.4 Population Studies with Men

In nearly all populations studied, the risk of bladder cancer is two to four times as great in men as in women (Hartge et al. 1990). Hartge examined gender-specific incidence rates without known carcinogenic factors (Harge et al. 1990). The data used were obtained from the National Bladder Cancer Study. Even in the absence of exposure to cigarettes, occupational hazards, or urinary tract infection, the gender-related risk persisted; the incidence of bladder cancer was 11.0 in men and 4.1 in women, yielding a ratio of 2.7 (Hartge et al. 1990). Possible explanations for the excessive risk in men include environmental and dietary exposures not yet identified and innate sexual characteristics such as anatomic differences, urination habits, or hormonal factors (Hartge et al. 1990).

11.5 Arylamines

Cancer incidence was investigated in a cohort of 700 workers employed at a Connecticut chemical plant between mid-1965 and 1989 (Ouellet-Hellstrom and Rench 1996). The plant produced a variety of chemicals, including arylamines such as dichlorobenzidine (DCB), o-dianisidine, o-tolidine, but not benzidine. The principal finding was a statistically significant increase in the standardized incidence ratio (SIR) for bladder cancer in men (SIR = 8.3; confidence interval, 3.3–17.0) (Ouellet-Hellstrom and Rench 1996). Based on an exposure classification system developed by a panel of former and current employees, the observed association between bladder cancer cases and exposure to arylamines increased with increasing exposure (SIRs = 0.0, 5.5, 16.4, for none, low, or moderate levels of exposure, respectively) (Ouellet-Hellstrom and Rench 1996). Smoking probably contributed to the bladder cancer risk, as all case subjects were known to be current or former cigarette smokers (Ouellet-Hellstrom and Rench 1996).

Tomioka evaluate non-urological cancer risks associated with benzidine (BZ) and beta-naphthylamine (BNA), a historical cohort study was undertaken (Tomioka et al. 2015). A total of 224 male workers exposed to BZ/BNA were followed from 1953 to 2011 (Tomioka et al. 2015). Follow-up was successful for 216 (96.4%). Follow-up duration averaged 44.0 (SD 10.7) years. DOE did not affect BC incidence (Tomioka et al. 2015). This study confirms the high risk of BC, suggesting that BZ/BNA have the potential to cause BC.

11.6   Anilene Dyes

Occupational exposure to health hazards was studied in 258 industrial work-ers who had bladder cancer against 454 matched controls (Nizamova 1991). All participants were members of Tambov Province centers of chemical industry (Nizamova 1991). Statistical significance (relative risk-4.7) was established for exposure to aromatic amines (Nizamova 1991). For those contacting with aniline dyes the relative risk (RR) made up 2.4 (Nizamova 1991). The risk to develop bladder cancer in powder shops (RR-3.2) was attributed to the hazards of dyes and diphenylamine (Nizamova 1991). In leather-shoe and textile industry the exposure to dyes was not safe (RR-6.1), neither was it to chemicals, oil products, pesticides, overheating (RR-3.2, 1.6, 3.2 and 2.9, respectively) (Nizamova 1991). It is stated that in line with a significant risk to develop bladder cancer at exposure to aro-matic amines there exist a number of occupational factors contributing to this risk.

11.7   Arsenic

Arsenic is a ubiquitous, naturally occurring metalloid that has significant risk of bladder cancer (Oberoi et al. 2014). Individuals are exposed to naturally occurring levels of arsenic in grains, vegetables, meats and fish, as well as through food pro-cessed with water containing arsenic (Oberoi et al. 2014). Oberoi 2014, examined the global burdens of disease for bladder cancers attributable to inorganic arsenic in food (Oberoi et al. 2014). Oberoi used World Health Organization estimates of food consumption in thirteen country clusters, in conjunction with reported meas-urements of total and inorganic arsenic in different foods. The conclusion was that each year 9129–119,176 additional cases of bladder cancer worldwide are attribut-able to inorganic arsenic in food.

11.8   Textile Industry

A case-control study on bladder cancer was carried out in Spain (González et al. 1989). The study included 497 cases (438 males and 59 females), 583 hospital controls and 530 population controls. These patients were matched by sex, age and residence (González et al. 1989). Among men, an increased risk of bladder can-cer was discovered for textile workers (OR = 1.97, 95% CL 1.2–3.3), mechanics, maintenance workers (OR = 1.86, 95% CL 1.2–2.8), workers in the printing indus-try (OR = 2.06, 95% CL 1.0–4.3) and for managers (OR = 2.03, 95% CL 1.2–3.5) (González et al. 1989). The risk was highest among those first employed <25 and prior to1960. Among mechanics the risk was highest working >25 and after 1960 (González et al. 1989). The OR for smokers who had also been employed in one of the high risk occupations was 7.82 (95% CL 4.4–14.0) which is compatible with a multiplicative effect of joint exposure to tobacco and occupational hazards (González et al. 1989).

In 1981–2 a retrospective study was conducted in a polyamide-polyester factory in Lyon, France. This study evaluated the effect of exposure to phthalates, nickel catalysers, and other chemicals in the work environment (Hours et al. 1989). An excess of cases of bladder cancer (based on seven cases) was noted among nylon workers (Hours et al. 1989). The cohort is still young, however, and a continued follow up is required.

11.9 Metalworking Fluids Exposure

Occupations with mineral oil exposure have been associated with bladder cancer in population-based case-control studies (Friesen et al. 2009). Friesen, 2009 examined bladder cancer incidence in relation to quantitative exposures to metalworking fluids (MWFs), based on 21,999 male automotive workers, Penalized splines were also fit to estimate the functional form of the exposure-response relation. Increased bladder cancer risk was associated with straight MWFs but not with any other exposure (Friesen et al. 2009). Calendar time windows relevant to polycyclic aromatic hydrocarbon exposure were examined but could not be distinguished from the lagged (10-, 20-year) metrics. The quantitative relation with straight MWFs strengthens the evidence for mineral oils as a bladder carcinogen (Friesen et al. 2009).

11.10 Smoking and Bladder Cancer

Bladder cancer is associated with occupational hazards and smoking (Sadetzki et al. 2000). Sadetzki, 2000, assessed risk factors for bladder cancer (Sadetzki et al. 2000). The study included 140 male patients and 280 matched controls (Sadetzki et al. 2000). This paper confirmed industrial employment as an occupational hazard (OR = 2.21; 95% CI = 1. 21–4.02) and exposure to 3 or more metals (OR = 3.65; 95% CI = 1.21–11. 08) as risk factors. Smoking had infrequent association with higher rates in theose smoking <18 years (OR = 2.64; 95% CI = 1.4–4.99) and smoking >30 cigarettes per day (OR = 1.82; 95% CI = 0.95–3.49) (Sadetzki et al. 2000). This paper suggests prevention of bladder cancer has a long way to go (Sadetzki et al. 2000).

Occupation and bladder cancer in women was examined with the National Bladder Cancer Study, a population-based, case-control study (Silverman et al. 1990). Increased risk was apparent for women ever employed in metal working and fabrication occupations (relative risk (RR) = 1.5; 95% confidence interval (CI) 0.9–2.6) (Silverman et al. 1990). Stamping press operatives had a significant increase in risk with increasing duration of employment. There was also an increased risk for women employed as chemical processing workers. 11% of bladder cancer diagnosed among women is attributable to occupational exposures (Silverman et al. 1990).

11.11   Impact of Occupational Risk Factors on Prognosis of Recurrent Bladder Cancer

The influence of occupational risk factors on bladder cancer is well known, studies on the influence on bladder cancer prognosis are rare. Primary relapses were examined in three case-control series (Selinski et al. 2016). Recurrent bladder tumour was noted in 416 cases (52%). Workers in the leather industry ($n=4$), printing industry ($n=4$), transportation ($n=43$), and chemical industry ($n=40$) and locksmiths/mechanics ($n=44$) demonstrated shorter relapse-free times.

Mortality at two engine plants was analysed to review bladder cancer mortality among workers exposed to machining fluids (Park and Mirer 1996). Causes of death and work histories were available for 1870 decendents. Elevated mortality ratios for bladder cancer was not statistically significant in plantwide populations. Nitrosamines were probably present in camshaft and crankshaft grinding, which can also increase bladder cancer risk. Bladder cancer increased was also associated with duration among workers grinding in straight oil MF (OR $= 3.0$, 95% CI $= 1.15$, 7.8) and in machining/heat-treat operations (OR $= 2.9$, 95% CI $= 1.14$, 7.2).

11.12   Results from the Literature and Other Reviews on Bladder Cancer Epidemiology, Risk Factors, Occupational Exposure

Many epidemiological studies and reviews have been performed to identify the causes of bladder cancer (Letašiová et al. 2012). Letašiová reviewed the links between various environmental risk factors and cancer of the bladder. Risks identified include smoking, arsenic in drinking water at concentrations higher than 300 µg/l, exposure to aromatic amines (2-naphthylamine, 4-aminobiphenyl and benzidine) and 4,4′-methylenebis(2-chloroaniline). These are commonly found in chemical, dye and rubber industries as well as in hair dyes, paints, fungicides, cigarette smoke, plastics, metals and motor vehicle exhausts (Letašiová et al. 2012). Other types of smoking besides cigarettes e.g. cigar, pipe, Egyptian water-pipe, smokeless tobacco and environmental tobacco smoking, can also have an effect. Other sources of arsenic exposure such as air, food, occupational hazards, and tobacco were also demonstrated as a risk (Letašiová et al. 2012). This study highligjhted it may be several years or decades between exposure and subsequent presntation of bladder cancer (Letašiová et al. 2012).

Each year, 430,000 people are diagnosed with bladder cancer (Al-Zalabani et al. 2016). This is a significant proporation of the population. Due to the aggressiveness of disease, prevention is paramount. Al-zalabani, 2016 reviewed all meta-analyses on modifiable risk factors of primary bladder cancer (Al-Zalabani et al. 2016). Statistically significant associations were found for current (RR 3.14) or former (RR 1.83) cigarette smoking, pipe (RR 1.9) or cigar (RR 2.3) smoking, antioxidant supplementation (RR 1.52), obesity (RR 1.10), higher physical activity levels (RR 0.86), higher body levels of selenium (RR 0.61) and vitamin D (RR 0.75), and higher intakes of: processed meat (RR 1.22), vitamin A (RR 0.82), vitamin E (RR 0.82), folate (RR 0.84), fruit (RR 0.77), vegetables (RR 0.83), citrus fruit (RR 0.85), and cruciferous vegetables (RR 0.84). Occupations with highest risk of exposure were tobacco workers (RR 1.72), dye workers (RR 1.58), and chimney sweeps (RR 1.53). Modification of lifestyle and occupational exposures can reduce this risk significantly. While smoking remains one of the key risk factors, also several diet-related and occupational factors are very relevant (Al-Zalabani et al. 2016).

Workplace exposures account for 5–25% of all bladder cancer cases (Olfert et al. 2006). A critical review of the literature between 1938 and 2004 was performed, with a focus on occupational exposures (Olfert et al. 2006). Occupational exposure to bladder carcinogens, particularly to beta-naphthylamine occur in a number of industries, including aromatic amine manufacture, rubber and cable manufacture, and dyestuff manufacture and use (Olfert et al. 2006) can have an impact on bladder cancer risk (Olfert et al. 2006).

11.13   Statement of Main Findings and Specific Areas of Unmet Needs Arising from Systematic Review

There are a number of risk factors and occupational hazards, which can result in increased risk of bladder cancer (Fig. 11.1). Most notable, smoking, aromatic amines, anilene dyes, acrylamines, arsenic, metalworking fluids, and chemicals in the textile industry. What has also been shown, is that these can impact on prognosis and recurrence of bladder cancer and must be addressed as a result.

The systematic review highlighted the requirement for a current screening pathway with a role for molecular testing. This requires further input into research to develop this area further (Fig. 11.2).

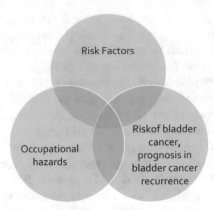

Fig. 11.1 Themes identified, based on the systematic review

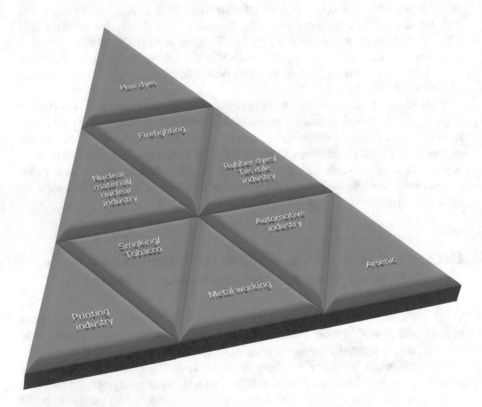

Fig. 11.2 Bladder Cancer Epidemiology—risk factors and occupational hazards in bladder cancer

References

Al-Zalabani AH, Stewart KF, Wesselius A, Schols AM, Zeegers MP. Modifiable risk factors for the prevention of bladder cancer: a systematic review of meta-analyses. Eur J Epidemiol. 2016;31(9):811–51.

Darby SC, Kendall GM, Fell TP, Doll R, Goodill AA, Conquest AJ, Jackson DA, Haylock RG. Further follow up of mortality and incidence of cancer in men from the United Kingdom who participated in the United Kingdom's atmospheric nuclear weapon tests and experimental programmes. BMJ. 1993;307(6918):1530–5.

Dement JM, Hensley L, Kieding S, Lipscomb H. Proportionate mortality among union members employed at three Texas refineries. Am J Ind Med. 1998;33(4):327–40.

Friesen MC, Costello S, Eisen EA. Quantitative exposure to metalworking fluids and bladder cancer incidence in a cohort of autoworkers. Am J Epidemiol. 2009;169(12):1471–8.

González CA, López-Abente G, Errezola M, Escolar A, Riboli E, Izarzugaza I, Nebot M. Occupation and bladder cancer in Spain: a multi-centre case-control study. Int J Epidemiol. 1989;18(3):569–77.

Hartge P, Harvey EB, Linehan WM, Silverman DT, Sullivan JW, Hoover RN, Fraumeni JF Jr. Unexplained excess risk of bladder cancer in men. J Natl Cancer Inst. 1990;82(20):1636–40.

Hours M, Cardis E, Marciniak A, Quelin P, Fabry J. Mortality of a cohort in a polyamide-polyester factory in Lyon: a further follow up. Br J Ind Med. 1989;46(9):665–70.

Kabat GC, Kim MY, Luo J, Hou L, Cetnar J, Wactawski-Wende J, Rohan TE. Menstrual and reproductive factors and exogenous hormone use and risk of transitional cell bladder cancer in postmenopausal women. Eur J Cancer Prev. 2013;22(5):409–16.

Letašiová S, Medve'ová A, Šovčíková A, Dušinská M, Volkovová K, Mosoiu C, Bartonová A. Bladder cancer, a review of the environmental risk factors. Environ Health. 2012;11(Suppl. 1):S11. https://doi.org/10.1186/1476-069X-11-S1-S11.

Ma F, Fleming LE, Lee DJ, Trapido E, Gerace TA, Lai H, Lai S. Mortality in Florida professional firefighters, 1972 to 1999. Am J Ind Med. 2005;47(6):509–17.

Nizamova RS. Occupational hazards and bladder cancer. Urol Nefrol (Mosk). 1991;(5):35–8.

Oberoi S, Barchowsky A, Wu F. The global burden of disease for skin, lung, and bladder cancer caused by arsenic in food. Cancer Epidemiol Biomarkers Prev. 2014;23(7):1187–94.

Olfert SM, Felknor SA, Delclos GL. An updated review of the literature: risk factors for bladder cancer with focus on occupational exposures. South Med J. 2006;99(11):1256–63.

Ouellet-Hellstrom R, Rench JD. Bladder cancer incidence in arylamine workers. J Occup Environ Med. 1996;38(12):1239–47.

Park RM, Mirer FE. A survey of mortality at two automotive engine manufacturing plants. Am J Ind Med. 1996;30(6):664–73.

Pukkala E, Martinsen JI, Lynge E, Gunnarsdottir HK, Sparén P, Tryggvadottir L, Weiderpass E, Kjaerheim K. Occupation and cancer—follow-up of 15 million people in five Nordic countries. Acta Oncol. 2009;48(5):646–790.

Sadetzki S, Bensal D, Blumstein T, Novikov I, Modan B. Selected risk factors for transitional cell bladder cancer. Med Oncol. 2000;17(3):179–82.

Selinski S, Bürger H, Blaszkewicz M, Otto T, Volkert F, Moormann O, Niedner H, Hengstler JG, Golka K. Occupational risk factors for relapse-free survival in bladder cancer patients. J Toxicol Environ Health A. 2016;79(22–23):1136–43.

Silverman DT, Levin LI, Hoover RN. Occupational risks of bladder cancer among white women in the United States. Am J Epidemiol. 1990;132(3):453–61.

Tomioka K, Obayashi K, Saeki K, Okamoto N, Kurumatani N. Increased risk of lung cancer associated with occupational exposure to benzidine and/or beta-naphthylamine. Int Arch Occup Environ Health. 2015;88(4):455–65.

Part IV
Assessment and Diagnostics in NMIBC

Chapter 12
Bladder Cancer—Diagnostic Pathways

Bladder cancer (BCa) is the fourth most common cancer in men (Larré et al. 2013). Survival from the disease has not improved over the last quarter century. Bladder cancer is 1 of the 10 most frequently diagnosed types of cancer. Screening could identify high-grade bladder cancer at earlier stages, when it may be more easily and effectively treated Population-based screening theoretically provides the best opportunity to improve the outcomes of aggressive BCa (Larré et al. 2013). Screening for for the disease is not standard (Pashos et al. 2002), however, any patient with haematuria is screened in the UK. Potential tests include urine cytology, haematuria on dipstick, flexible cystoscopy and upper tract imaging, USS KUB or CT Urogram (Pashos et al. 2002). Cystoscopy, commonly accepted as a gold standard for the detection of bladder cancer, is invasive and relatively expensive, while urine cytology is of limited value specifically in low-grade disease (Schmitz-Dräger et al. 2015).

Bladder cancer continues to be one of the most common and expensive malignancies (Yeung et al. 2014). This is due to the aggressive nature of disease, and progression that can happen. Ten years ago, urinary markers held the potential to lower treatment costs of bladder cancer, with earlier diagnosis. Adjunct cytology remains a part of diagnostic standard of care, but recent research suggests that it is not cost effective due to its low diagnostic yield. Analysis of intravesical chemotherapy after transurethral resection of bladder tumor (TURBT), neo-adjuvant therapy for cystectomy, and robot-assisted laparoscopic cystectomy suggests that these technologies are cost effective and should be implemented more widely for appropriate patients.

Because of its relatively low incidence, screening might have a better outcome if it is restricted to a high-risk population (Vickers et al. 2013). The 5-year probability of being diagnosed with invasive bladder cancer is 0.24% (Vickers et al. 2013). In a typical scenario, a bladder cancer risk score >6 means 25% of the population would be screened to prevent 57 invasive or high-grade bladder cancers per 100,000 population (Vickers et al. 2013). More than 25% of bladder cancer

© Springer Nature Switzerland AG 2020

S. S. Goonewardene et al., *Management of Non-Muscle Invasive Bladder Cancer*,
https://doi.org/10.1007/978-3-030-28646-0_12

(BC) cases are muscle-invasive at primary diagnosis (Zlotta et al. 2011). Screening is unproven to enable the detection of more non-muscle-invasive tumors (Zlotta et al. 2011). Bladder cancer risk was associated with aristolochic acid nephropathy (AAN) was reported after intake of slimming pills containing Chinese herbs (Zlotta et al. 2011). Zlotta et al. evaluated whether a BC screening protocol in a high-risk and unique patient population had an impact on the stage of tumor presentation.

Bladder Cancer was diagnosed in 25 patients (52%) (Zlotta et al. 2011). Among 43 patients who underwent screening cystoscopies (Zlotta et al. 2011). This demonstrated Bladder Cancer screening in high-risk groups may allow identification of tumors before muscle invasion (Zlotta et al. 2011). The optimal screening programme in smoking related disease has not yet been determined.

Cassidy et al. identify significant predictors of initial and repeated adherence with bladder cancer screening in a high-risk occupationally exposed cohort (Cassidy et al. 2011). The study analyzed longitudinal health survey data and a cross-sectional behavioral health survey from the Drake Health Registry Study over 13 years (Cassidy et al. 2011). Initial compliance and repeated adherence were examined in separate logistic regression models (Cassidy et al. 2011). "Barriers to screening" and "social influence" were associated with initial participation. Lower or no alcohol consumption, comorbidities, worry that screening would find bladder cancer, and ease of arranging schedules were associated with continued adherence (Cassidy et al. 2011). To enhance overall adherence, specific strategies should be implemented when initiating a screening program and revised accordingly over time.

To assess the positive predictive value (PPV) of microhaematuria (μH) and visible haematuria (GH) in bladder cancer screening and the influence of haematuria on tumour tests in a prospective study (Pesch et al. 2011). While the PPV of μH for bladder cancer was low, there was a strong influence of haematuria and leukocytes on the protein-based tumour test NMP22® (Pesch et al. 2011). Erythrocytes and leukocytes should be determined at least semi-quantitatively for the interpretation of positive NMP22 test results (Pesch et al. 2011). In addition, a panel of tumour tests that includes methods not affected by the presence of erythrocytes or leukocytes such as cytology and UroVysion(™) would improve bladder cancer screening (Pesch et al. 2011).

Bonberg et al. explored chromosomal changes in order to assess associations with bladder cancer for improvements of the UroVysion™ assay regarding screening (Bonberg et al. 2013). The UroVysion assay showed a reasonable performance in detecting bladder cancer in the present study population and shared positive test results with cytology (Bonberg et al. 2013). A simpler, faster and cheaper version of the UroVysion assay might rely on the very strong correlations between gains at chromosomes 3, 7 and 17, resulting in a similar performance in detecting bladder cancer (Bonberg et al. 2013).

Chou and Dana (2010), updated the 2004 U.S. Preventive Services Task Force evidence review on screening for bladder cancer (Chou and Dana 2010). No randomized trials or high-quality controlled observational studies evaluated clinical outcomes associated with screening compared with no screening or treatment of screen-detected bladder cancer (Chou and Dana 2010). No study evaluated the sensitivity or specificity of tests for hematuria, urinary cytology, or other urinary biomarkers for bladder cancer in asymptomatic persons without a history of bladder cancer (Chou and Dana 2010). The positive predictive value of screening is less than 10% in asymptomatic persons, including higher-risk populations (Chou and Dana 2010). No study evaluated harms associated with treatment of screen-detected bladder cancer compared with no treatment (Chou and Dana 2010). This clearly highlights an area for further investigation.

References

Bonberg N, Taeger D, Gawrych K, Johnen G, Banek S, Schwentner C, Sievert KD, Wellhäußer H, Kluckert M, Leng G, Nasterlack M, Stenzl A, Behrens T, Brüning T, Pesch B; UroScreen Study Group. Chromosomal instability and bladder cancer: the UroVysionn(™) test in the UroScreen study. BJU Int. 2013;112(4):E372–82.

Cassidy LD, Marsh GM, Talbott EO, Kelsey SF. Initial and continued adherence with bladder cancer screening in an occupationally exposed cohort. J Occup Environ Med. 2011;53(4):455–6.

Chou R, Dana T. Screening adults for bladder cancer: a review of the evidence for the U.S. preventive services task force. Ann Intern Med. 2010;153(7):461–8.

Larré S, Catto JW, Cookson MS, Messing EM, Shariat SF, Soloway MS, Svatek RS, Lotan Y, Zlotta AR, Grossman HB. Screening for bladder cancer: rationale, limitations, whom to target, and perspectives. Eur Urol. 2013;63(6):1049–58.

Pashos CL, Botteman MF, Laskin BL, Redaelli A. Bladder cancer: epidemiology, diagnosis, and management. Cancer Pract. 2002;10(6):311–22.

Pesch B, Nasterlack M, Eberle F, Bonberg N, Taeger D, Leng G, Feil G, Johnen G, Ickstadt K, Kluckert M, Wellhäusser H, Stenzl A, Brüning T; UroScreen Group. The role of haematuria in bladder cancer screening among men with former occupational exposure to aromatic amines. BJU Int. 2011;108(4):546–52.

Schmitz-Dräger BJ, Droller M, Lokeshwar VB, Lotan Y, Hudson MA, van Rhijn BW, Marberger MJ, Fradet Y, Hemstreet GP, Malmstrom PU, Ogawa O, Karakiewicz PI, Shariat SF. Molecular markers for bladder cancer screening, early diagnosis, and surveillance: the WHO/ICUD consensus. Urol Int. 2015;94(1):1–24. https://doi.org/10.1159/000369357 Epub 2014 Dec 10.

Vickers AJ, Bennette C, Kibel AS, Black A, Izmirlian G, Stephenson AJ, Bochner B. Who should be included in a clinical trial of screening for bladder cancer? A decision analysis of data from the prostate, lung, colorectal and ovarian cancer screening trial. Cancer. 2013;119(1):143–9.

Yeung C, Dinh T, Lee J. The health economics of bladder cancer: an updated review of the published literature. Pharmacoeconomics. 2014;32(11):1093–104.

Zlotta AR, Roumeguere T, Kuk C, Alkhateeb S, Rorive S, Lemy A, van der Kwast TH, Fleshner NE, Jewett MA, Finelli A, Schulman C, Lotan Y, Shariat SF, Nortier J. Select screening in a specific high-risk population of patients suggests a stage migration toward detection of non-muscle-invasive bladder cancer. Eur Urol. 2011;59(6):1026–31.

Chapter 13
Systematic Review Method—Bladder Cancer Screening

A systematic review relating to literature on survivorship programmes for men with bladder cancer and screening was conducted. This was to identify the role of screening in bladder cancer. The search strategy aimed to identify all references related to bladder cancer AND screening. Search terms used were as follows: (Bladder cancer) AND (screening). The following databases were screened from 1989 to June 2019:

- CINAHL
- MEDLINE (NHS Evidence)
- Cochrane
- AMed
- EMBASE
- PsychINFO
- SCOPUS
- Web of Science.

In addition, searches using Medical Subject Headings (MeSH) and keywords were conducted using Cochrane databases. Two UK-based experts in bladder cancer were consulted to identify any additional studies.

Studies were eligible for inclusion if they reported primary research focusing on bladder cancer and screening. Papers were included if published after 1984 and had to be in English. Studies that did not conform to this were excluded. Only primary research was included. The overall aim was to identify the role and components of bladder cancer screening.

Abstracts were independently screened for eligibility by two reviewers and disagreements resolved through discussion or third party opinion. Agreement level was calculated using Cohen's Kappa to test the intercoder reliability of this screening process. Cohens' Kappa allows comparison of inter-rater reliability between papers using relative observed agreement. This also takes account of

© Springer Nature Switzerland AG 2020   69
S. S. Goonewardene et al., *Management of Non-Muscle Invasive Bladder Cancer*,
https://doi.org/10.1007/978-3-030-28646-0_13

the comparison occurring by chance. The first reviewer agreed all 43 papers to be included, the second, agreed on 43.

Data extraction was piloted by the researcher and amended in consultation with the research team (author and two academic supervisors). Data collected included authors, year and country of publication, study aims, setting, intervention aims, number of participants, study design, intervention components and delivery methods, comparison groups and outcome measures, notes and follow-up questions for the authors. Studies were quality assessed using the PRISMA criteria for randomised controlled trials, Mays et al. (Moher et al. 2009; Moher, Liberati et al. 2009, 154, 153; Mays et al. 2005) for the action research and qualitative studies and the Critical Skills Appraisal programme for cohort studies. This was also applied to randomised controlled trials and qualitative studies.

The search identified 289 papers (Fig. 13.1). However, only 43 mapped to the search terms and eligibility criteria. The current systematic reviews were examined to gain further knowledge about the subject. 246 papers were excluded due to not conforming to eligibility criteria or adding to the evidence for bladder cancer screening. Of the 43 papers left, relevant abstracts were identified and the full papers obtained (all of which were in English), to quality assure against criteria. There was considerable heterogeneity of design among the included studies therefore a narrative review of the evidence was undertaken. There was significant heterogeneity within studies, including clinical topic, numbers, outcomes, as a results a narrative review was thought to be best.

There were 43 papers in total. 1 case control study, 42 were cohort studies. The cohort studies were of a moderate quality.

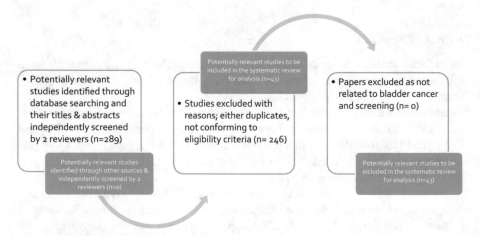

Fig. 13.1 Flow chart of studies identified through the systematic review (adapted from PRISMA)

References

Mays N, Pope C, Popay J. Systematically reviewing qualitative and quantitative evidence to inform management and policy-making in the health field. J Health Serv Res Policy. 2005;10 Suppl 1:6–20.

Moher D, Liberati A, Tetzlaff J, Altman DG. Preferred reporting items for systematic reviews and meta-analyses: the prisma statement. BMJ. 2009;339(7716):332–6.

Chapter 14
Bladder Cancer Screening—Systematic Review Results

14.1 Causes of Bladder Cancer

Bladder cancer is a malignancy that affects mainly the elderly and males (Rybotycka and Długosz 2015). Up to 90% of these cancers originate from urothelial epithelial cells (Rybotycka and Długosz 2015). Other types are: Squamous Cell Carcionoma (SCC), which involves about 5% of cases and Adenocarcinoma (less than 2%). The factors that may lead to the development of bladder cancer include: genetic disorders, molecular changes, environmental exposures, industrial carcinogens, chemical contaminants and chronic cystitis (Rybotycka and Długosz 2015).

14.2 Photodynamic Diagnosis in Bladder Cancer Screening

Bladder cancer often results in a large burden of care, particularly if detected late. Tumor stage and grade direct treatment pathways in bladder cancer (Eifler et al. 2014). However, the considerable heterogeneity of tumor biology in bladder cancer is incompletely characterized by stage and grade alone, and recent efforts to improve predictive models in bladder cancer may significantly improve accuracy and calibration (Eifler et al. 2014). Current nomograms and risk tables may be best used to individualize bladder cancer management.

Endoscopic treatment of bladder cancer can be based on photodynamic diagnostics (PDD). This is a specialized endoscopic technique where a narrow-band illumination causes tumors to fluoresce in a pink colour. Greater detection of tumours as compared to white light endoscopy is the result.

© Springer Nature Switzerland AG 2020   73
S. S. Goonewardene et al., *Management of Non-Muscle Invasive Bladder Cancer*,
https://doi.org/10.1007/978-3-030-28646-0_14

A downside of PDD is the low illumination power. This needs a shorter distance between endoscope and bladder, narrowing the field of view. Behrens et al. (2009) therefore describe an approach to combine several successive frames into a local PDD panorama, which provides a larger and sufficiently bright field for treatment (Behrens et al. 2009).

14.3   Human Papilloma Virus and Bladder Cancer

Among several risk factors for bladder cancer, Human Papilloma Virus (HPV) may have a role in the causation of bladder carcinoma. Abdollahzadeh evaluated the involvement of HPV infection in transitional cell carcinoma biopsies (Abdollahzadeh et al. 2017). 97 biopsy specimens including 67 patients with transitional cell carcinoma (TCC) of bladder and 30 cases of control group were studied using immunohistochemistry to identify HPV. 22.4% of patients with TCC of bladder and 3.3% of control group were positive for HPV ($p = 0.019$) (Abdollahzadeh et al. 2017). The prevalence of HPV was 4.3 fold higher in men than women. Considering the higher incidence of HPV positivity in patients with TCC of bladder compared to control group, it seems to be a meaningful association between HPV infection and TCC of bladder. However, literature can be conflicting.

Given the contradictory nature of the literature, Llewellyn et al. (2018) investigated the involvement of HPV 16 and 18 in a large cohort of primary bladder cancers (Llewellyn et al. 2018). All 689 cases were negative for HPV18. Squamous differentiation was positive for HPV16. However, within the UK, the presence of HPV is extremely rare in bladder cancer (<1% of cases). Polyomavirus DNA is more common, in 7% of cases. From this study, HPV is unlikely to be a causative agent (Llewellyn et al. 2018).

14.4   Smoking Cessation and Bladder Cancer

Smoking is a major risk factor for bladder cancer. The relationship between smoking cessation after initial treatment and bladder cancer recurrence has not been commonly investigated (Osch et al. 2018). Over 4 years, 403 NMIBC recurrences occurred in 210 patients. Only 25 current smokers at diagnosis quit smoking (14%) and smoking cessation after diagnosis did not decrease risk of recurrence compared to continuing smokers ($p = 0.352$) (Osch et al. 2018). Although quitting smoking after diagnosis might reduce the risk of recurrence based on retrospective evidence, this is not confirmed in this prospective study because the number of NMIBC patients quitting smoking before their first recurrence was too low. However, smoking cessation still has an important role in reducing rate of bladder cancer and bladder cancer recurrence.

14.5   Dietary Intake and Bladder Cancer

Greater consumption of fruit and vegetables decreases the risk of bladder cancer, however not clearly clarified (Jochems et al. 2018). 728 patients with non-muscle invasive bladder cancer (NMIBC), completed self-administrated questionnaires on diet prior to diagnosis and 1 year after diagnosis (Jochems et al. 2018). 728 NMIBC patients developed a recurrence of bladder cancer. There was no relationship between diet and bladder cancer recurrence (Jochems et al. 2018). Results from this study did not indicate a protective role for total fruit and vegetables in the development of a recurrence of NMIBC.

14.6   Risk of Bladder Cancer with Spinal Cord Injury

Life expectancy for people with spinal cord injury/disease (SCI/D) is increasing, due to modern advances, but so is the risk of bladder cancer. Bothig et al. conducted a single-centre retrospective evaluation of consecutive patient data with spinal cord injury and proven urinary bladder cancer (Böthig et al. 2018). The 27 had transitional cell carcinoma, while 5 had squamous cell carcinoma. Of the 32 patients, 25 (78%) had muscle invasive disease at $\geq$T2 when diagnosed (Böthig et al. 2018). This group had a significantly younger age at diagnosis, and the frequency of invasive, poorly differentiated tumour. This indicates SCI/D influences both bladder cancer risk and prognosis significantly. Early detection is key, but often remains a challenge.

14.7   Bladder Cancer and Androgenesis

Androgens may have a role in bladder carcinogenesis (Mäkelä et al. 2018). Mäkelä, reviewed 5-alpha-reductase inhibitors (5-ARIs) and bladder cancer (BCa)-specific mortality (Mäkelä et al. 2018). 10,720 newly diagnosed Finnish men (1997–2012) were identified from the national cancer registry. 5-ARI use prior to diagnosis was associated with lower bladder cancer risk. The risk decrease became stronger along with time used. Use of alpha-blockers prior to diagnosis was not associated with poorer bladder cancer survival (Mäkelä et al. 2018). Use of 5-ARIs post diagnosis was associated with decreased risk of bladder cancer death. Again, the use of alpha-blockers was not associated with survival. The risk decrease by 5-ARI use persisted for 5 years post diagnosis (Mäkelä et al. 2018). This supports the benefits of 5-alpha-reductase inhibition in bladder cancer.

14.8   Bladder Cancer and Trace Elements

Major and trace elements may play a role in the diagnosis of bladder cancer (Wach et al. 2018). Wach et al. (2018) investigated 26 major and trace elements in the serum by inductively coupled plasma (ICP)—optical emission spectrometry (OES) and ICP-sector field-mass spectrometry (sf-MS). Concentrations of five elements were detected as significantly increased in bladder cancer cases compared with healthy controls. These elements were calcium, lithium, potassium, nickel, and strontium (Wach et al. 2018). This demonstrates elements calcium, lithium, nickel and strontium in the serum could be a new method for diagnostics in bladder cancer (Wach et al. 2018).

14.9   Air Pollution and Bladder Cancer

Ambient air pollution contains low concentrations of carcinogens. This may be another cause of bladder cancer (BC) (Pedersen et al. 2018). It is unknown whether air pollution influences bladder cancer development. Pedersen evaluated the relationship between air pollution and bladder cancer incidence (Pedersen et al. 2018). Data was obtained from 15 population-based cohorts enrolled between 1985 and 2005 in eight European countries (N = 303431) During follow-up, 943 incident BC cases were diagnosed. Although this may seem like a large number, the overall metaanalysis did not demonstrate a link.

14.10   Risk Factors in Bladder Cancer

Bladder carcinoma (BC) is the fourth most common type of cancer in males from Western countries, with primary prevention an important healthcare challenge (Ferris et al. 2013). Prevention efforts must focus on the avoidance or cessation of cigarette smoking and on public education relating to known environmental risk factors (Pashos et al. 2002). Patient and disease factors must be considered in making treatment decisions and determining prognosis. Careful follow-up after treatment is essential (Pashos et al. 2002). It is hoped that ongoing research on potential tumor markers and tumor-specific therapies ultimately will result in improved clinical outcomes for patients with this malignancy (Pashos et al. 2002). Cigarette smoking is the best established risk factor for the development of bladder cancer (Simonis et al. 2014). The growing body of evidence indicates that smoking increases the risk of disease recurrence and potentially disease progression in patients with NMIBC (Simonis et al. 2014). Current and heavy long-term smokers seem to be at the greatest risk for both end points. Smoking cessation may limit these effects thereby improving prognosis (Simonis et al. 2014). It is the duty of each urologist to raise awareness regarding the greatest preventable cause of the development of bladder cancer, morbidity, and mortality.

The incidence of bladder cancer may reflect differences in the stage and extent of the tobacco epidemic, changes in coding practices, prevalence of schistosomiasis (Africa), and occupational exposure (Chavan et al. 2014). Studies have found o-toluidine, aniline and nitrobenzene responsible for bladder cancer, in rubber and dye factory workers (Carreón et al. 2014). The two main risk factors for urothelial tumors are tobacco smoking and occupational exposure to chemicals carcinogens such as polycyclic aromatic hydrocarbons, nitrosamines, aromatic amines and arsenic (Guillaume and Guy 2014). Other risk factors include urinary schistosomiasis, pelvic radiation therapy, the use of cyclophosphamide and probably diet and lifestyle factors (Guillaume and Guy 2014). Prevention of bladder tumors is based on the control of these risk factors and individual screening in high-risk patients. Recognition as an occupational disease is an important part of the social management of patient, which is today inadequately performed.

Ferris et al. identified risk factors including (a) age and gender (diagnosed at age 65 and over, with a 4:1 ratio of males to females); (b) race, ethnicity and geographic location (predominantly in Caucasians and in Southern European countries); (c) genetic (N-acetyltransferase-2 and glutathione s-transferase M1 gene mutations, which significantly increase the risk for BC); (d) occupational, which represent 5–10% of BC RF; and (f) occupations with high BC risk, such as aluminium production, the manufacture of dyes, paints and colourings, the rubber industry and the extraction and industrial use of fossil fuels. This study demonstrated BC is the end result of the variable combination of constitutional and environmental RF, the majority of which are unknown. The most significant constitutional RF are related to age, gender, race, ethnicity geographic location and genetic polymorphisms (Ferris et al. 2013). The main occupational RF are those related to aromatic amines and polycyclic aromatic hydrocarbons.

Bladder cancer incidence is higher in old men, shows geographic variation, and is mostly an environmental disease (Malats and Real 2015). Cigarette smoking, occupational exposures, water arsenic, Schistosoma haematobium infestation, and some medications are the best established risk factors (Malats and Real 2015). Data on environmental and genetic factors involved in the disease outcome are inconclusive (Malats and Real 2015).

Many epidemiological studies and reviews have been performed to identify the causes of bladder cancer (Letašiová et al. 2012). Smoking, mainly cigarette smoking, is a well-known risk factor for various diseases, including bladder cancer (Letašiová et al. 2012). Another factor strongly associated with bladder cancer is exposure to arsenic in drinking water at concentrations higher than 300 µg/l (Letašiová et al. 2012). The most notable risk factor for development of bladder cancer is occupational exposure to aromatic amines (2-naphthylamine, 4-aminobiphenyl and benzidine) and 4,4'-methylenebis(2-chloroaniline), which can be found in the products of the chemical, dye and rubber industries as well as in hair dyes, paints, fungicides, cigarette smoke, plastics, metals and motor vehicle exhaust

(Letašiová et al. 2012). There are also data suggesting an effect from of other types of smoking besides cigarettes (cigar, pipe, Egyptian waterpipe, smokeless tobacco and environmental tobacco smoking), and other sources of arsenic exposure such as air, food, occupational hazards, and tobacco (Letašiová et al. 2012). Other studies show that hairdressers and barbers with occupational exposure to hair dyes experience enhanced risk of bladder cancer (Letašiová et al. 2012).

Among men, triglycerides and BP were positively associated with BC risk overall (Teleka et al. 2018) among women, BMI was inversely associated with risk. The associations for BMI and BP differed between men and women (Teleka et al. 2018). Among men, BMI, cholesterol and triglycerides were positively associated with risk for NMIBC and BP was positively associated with MIBC (Teleka et al. 2018). Among women, glucose was positively associated with MIBC (Teleka et al. 2018). Apart from cholesterol, HRs for metabolic factors did not significantly differ between MIBC and NMIBC, and there were no interactions between smoking and metabolic factors on BC (Teleka et al. 2018).

Martini et al. assessed the strength of the online tool RiskCheck Bladder Cancer (RCBC) for early detection of bladder cancer (BC) (Martini et al. 2013). RCBC was evaluated retrospectively based on the data of 241 patients, of which 141 were suffering from BC (Martini et al. 2013). ROC analysis of the risk classification showed a sensitivity of 71.6%, a specificity of 56.5%, a positive predictive value of 67.8%, a negative predictive value of 52% and an accuracy of 63.5% (Martini et al. 2013). BC risk factors ranked by importance are time of smoking ($p < 0.0001$), gender (within the nonsmoking group: $p < 0.009$), occupational toxin exposure (within the group <35 years of smoking: $p < 0.048$) and amount of consumed cigarettes resulting in a 95% association with BC (within the group >35 years of smoking: $p < 0.0001$). The high predictive power of RCBC for the identification of asymptomatic patients living under risk could be demonstrated.

14.11   White Light Cystoscopy

White light cystoscopy (WLC) is considered to be a standard examination for localisation and surveillance of transitional cell cancer of urinary bladder (Szygula et al. 2004). However, post resection, sensitivity is too low for early detection of cancer recurrence (Szygula et al. 2004). Part of this, may be aided by photodynamic diagnosis. Fluorescent diagnosis highlights distinctive fluorescence of normal and pathological tissue (Szygula et al. 2004).

Currently two techniques are in clinical use: autofluorescent diagnosis (laser-induced fluorescence) (LIF) and photodynamic diagnosis (PDD) (Szygula et al. 2004). Sensitivity and specificity of PDD equalled to 90.9% and 66.6%, respectively (Szygula et al. 2004). With autofluorescence, his is 97.8% and 70.1%, respectively (Szygula et al. 2004). The overall sensitivity and specificity of fluorescent examination equalled to 96.5% and 69.5%, respectively (Szygula et al. 2004). Autofluorescence diagnosis (LIF) of pathological lesions within urinary bladder has been proven to be more sensitive than PDD as evaluated by a non-parametrical test for structure indicators comparison (LIF vs. PDD, $p = 0.0056$) (Szygula et al. 2004).

14.12   Urinary Cytology

Voided-urine cytology was analyzed to review screening potential in an asymptomatic population (Grotenhuis et al. 2015). Screening at age 55 or age 65 were analyzed for individuals of normal risk. The results predict cytology screening identifies the high-grade, aggressive bladder cancer, resulting in gains in life expectancy of more than three years for the asymptomatic true-positive case (Grotenhuis et al. 2015).

Voided-urine cytology as a screen for the early detection of urinary bladder cancer was also analysed by Ellwein and Farrow (1988). The focus here is on investigating screening from the perspective of the individual contemplating the screening decision. Results support the decision to screen (Elwein and Farrow 1988). Except for the risk of a false-positive outcome, cytology screening compares favorably with what could theoretically be obtained if a 100% accurate screening test were available.

Reported urine cytology accuracy, particular sensitivity, is highly variable. Turco evaluated the accuracy using population data linkage (Turco et al. 2011). Sensitivity (C3–C5 considered positive) ranged between 40.2 and 42.3%, and specificity was 93.7–94.1%. If C3 results are counted as negative, sensitivity estimates reduced to 24.7–26.0%. The positive predictive value of a C3, C4 or C5 report was 11.7, 39.2, and 66.6%, respectively (Turco et al. 2011). High grade tumour was associated with significantly higher sensitivity compared to low and intermediate grades ($p = 0.02$). Urine cytology is highly specific but has intermediate sensitivity. This highlighted it does not have a role in screening for primary bladder cancer. C3 results should be considered 'positive' and further investigated, and all positive results should prompt further intervention (Turco et al. 2011).

The DETECT study determined the diagnostic accuracy of urinary and the outcome of patients with a positive urine cytology and normal haematuria investigations (Tan et al. 2016). Of the 3556 patients recruited, urine cytology was performed in 567 (15.9%). Bladder cancer was diagnosed in 39 (6.9%) patients. The sensitivity was 43.5%, specificity 95.7%, positive predictive value (PPV) 47.6% and negative predictive value (NPV) 94.9% (Tan et al. 2016) of urinary cytology. High risk cancer was confirmed in 8 (38%) patients. This demonstrates urine cytology will miss a significant number of muscle invasive bladder cancer and high-risk disease.

14.13   Outcomes from Bladder Cancer Screening

Messing determined whether screening could lead to earlier detection and reduced mortality compared with unscreened men with newly diagnosed bladder cancer (Messing et al. 2006). 1575 men were recruited and had their urine tested repetitively with a chemical reagent strip for haemoglobin. Two hundred fifty-eight screening participants (16.4%) were assessed for haematuria and 21 participants (8.1%) were diagnosed with bladder cancer (Messing et al. 2006). Proportions of low-grade (Grade 1 and 2) NMI (Stage Ta and T1) versus high-grade (Grade 3) NMI or invasive (Stage>or=T2) cancers in screened men (52.4% vs. 47.7%) and in men from the tumor registry (60.3% vs. 39.7%) were similar ($p = 0.50$) (Messing et al. 2006). The proportion of high-grade NMI or invasive BCs that were invasive were lower in screened men (10%) than in unscreened men (60%; $p = 0.002$). At 14 years of follow-up, no men with screen-detected BC had died of BC, whereas 20.4% of men with unscreened BC had died of BC ($p = 0.02$). This demonstrated screening prevented mortality from bladder cancer.

The clinical course, over a period of 3 years, of 17 bladder tumours found on screening a male population (2356 individuals) aged over 60, is reported by Whelan et al. (1993). The importance of distinguishing pathologically between a pTa and a pT1 tumour is emphasised (Whelan et al. 1993). The progression rate to date of pT1 tumours (1 of 9: 11%) is significantly less than that reported in larger studies on symptomatic patients. This indicates the importance of screening for bladder tumours in populations who are known to be at risk (Whelan et al. 1993).

14.14   Technology in Diagnosis

Correct classification of cystoscopy images depends on experience (Freitas et al. 2018). In this paper, a texture analysis based approach is proposed for bladder tumor diagnosis presuming that tumors change in tissue texture. Texture information is present in the medium to high frequency range which can be chosen by using a discrete wavelet transform (DWT) (Freitas et al. 2018). Tumor enhancement can be improved by using automatic segmentation. Performances of 91% in sensitivity and 92.9% in specificity were obtained. The proposed method can achieve good performance on identifying bladder tumor frames.

Drejer investigated whether the use of narrow-band imaging (NBI) in bladder cancer diagnostics (Drejer et al. 2017). Pathology was found in 216 WL cystoscopies, and in 15 NBI cystoscopies (6.9%). Based on NBI, pathology was suspected in 23 patients (3.1%) in whom a WL cystoscopy revealed no tumor. In total, NBI changed the clinical decision relevantly in 1.9% of the patients. In hematuria patients, the calculated sensitivities of both NBI and WL were identically high, whereas sensitivity in patients with known NMIBC was significantly higher in NBI compared to WL (NBI: 100.0% vs. WL: 83.2%, p<0.05) (Drejer et al. 2017). NBI had a lower specificity compared to WL, especially in follow-up cystoscopies (NBI: 86.5% vs. WL: 92.1, p<0.05). NBI can be a useful tool in clinical decision making as a supplement to WL because it yields a significantly higher detection rate than WL cystoscopy alone. This is particularly relevant in patients with known recurrent NMIBC.

Horstmann, evaluated the role of fluorescence-guided cystoscopy in a high-risk bladder cancer population undergoing screening based on a multi-marker panel of urine-tests (UroScreen-study) (Horstmann et al. 2014). Twenty-two subjects with a mean age of 58 years (39–72) underwent PDD cystoscopy. Of those 3 had positive NMP22 tests, 14 positive FISH tests and 9 suspicious cytologies. Two had persisting microscopic hematuria only. PDD cystoscopy revealed enhanced unifocal fluorescence in 14 (Horstmann 2014). All had subsequent transurethral biopsy or resection. In total, 1 urothelial carcinoma (pTaG1, low grade) was diagnosed. In the other participants urothelial cancer of the bladder was ruled out. No higher detection rate was found using PDD than with the standard algorithm of the UroScreen study in which 17 tumors were detected by white light cystoscopy (Horstmann 2014). The use of PDD does not lead to a higher cancer detection rate in a high-risk screening population. Larger sample sizes may be needed to ultimately asses the value of PDD for bladder cancer screening.

Early diagnosis of bladder cancer is crucial for improvement of cancer specific survival and recurrence rate. Kollarik analyzed the possible role of fluorescence urine analysis in bladder cancer diagnosis (Kollarik et al. 2018). The cohort consisted of 20 healthy controls, 40 patients with hematuria and 75 patients with hematuria and histologically proven bladder tumor. Synchronous fluorescence spectra with a 70 nm wavelength difference were recorded for (1:1–1:128) urine dilutions. Concentration matrices of synchronous spectra (CMSS) were used to classify samples into tested groups. CMSS analysis allowed us to distinguish patients with tumor from patients with hematuria with a sensitivity 55% and specificity 74.7%. This is comparable to the sensitivity and specificity of other non-invasive tests like BTA stat and nmP-22 (Bladder check®) (Kollarik et al. 2018). Lower fluorescence intensity of Imax 280 nm and ratio of 280 to 450 nm was found to be associated with the presence of tumor. We have found an association of decreased fluorescence with the stage of the disease. Our data suggest that CMSS urine analysis has a potential role in the non-invasive diagnostic tests for bladder cancer, but it cannot replace the current diagnostic algorithm yet (Kollarik et al. 2018).

14.15 Blue Light Screening

Inoue et al. discovered urine porphyrin levels from tumor-bearing mice were elevated compared with those from normal mice after administration of 5-aminolevulinic acid (ALA) (Inoue et al. 2013). Almost all of the urinary porphyrin concentrations from the patients with bladder cancer were higher than those from healthy adults (Inoue et al. 2013). Moreover, 8 h after ALA administration, urinary UPI and CPI showed high sensitivity (100 for UPI and CPI) and specificity (96.4 for UPI and 91.4 for CPI) (Inoue et al. 2013).

These results indicate that the presence of urinary porphyrins after administration of ALA may function as tumor biomarkers (Inoue et al. 2013). This method represents a possible new tumor screening method called photodynamic screening (PDS) using ALA-induced porphyrins.

Hexaminolevulinate (HAL) is a tumour photosensitizer that is used in combination with blue-light cystoscopy (BLC) as an adjunct to white-light cystoscopy (WLC) in the diagnosis and management of non-muscle-invasive bladder cancer (NMIBC) (Daneshmand et al. 2014). Current data support an additional role in the reduction of recurrence of NMIBC. HAL-BLC should be considered for initial assessment of NMIBC, surveillance for recurrent tumours, diagnosis in patients with positive urine cytology but negative WLC findings, and for tumour staging (Daneshmand et al. 2014).

Blue light cystoscopy (BLC) using hexaminolevulinate (HAL/ Cysview/Hexvix) has been previously shown to improve detection of non-muscle-invasive bladder cancer (NMIBC) (Daneshmand et al. 2014). Danesmand et al. evaluated the detection of malignant lesions in a heterogenous group of patients in the real world setting and documented the change in risk category due to upstaging or upgrading.

Addition of BLC to standard WLC increased detection rate by 12% for any papillary lesion and 43% for carcinoma in situ (Daneshmand et al. 2014). Within the WLC negative group, an additional 206 lesions in 133 (25%) patients were detected exclusively with BLC. In multifocal disease, BLC resulted in AUA risk-group migration occurred in 33 (6%) patients and a change in recommended management in 74 (14%) (Daneshmand et al. 2014). False-positive rate was 25% for WLC and 30% for BLC. One mild dermatologic hypersensitivity reaction (0.2%). BLC increases detection rates of carcinoma in situ and papillary lesions over WLC alone and can change management in 14% of cases. Repeat use of HAL for BLC is safe (I et al.).

14.16   Ultrasound in Bladder Cancer Diagnostics

Bladder tumors are common and the only way to prove it is cystoscopy which is invasive and expensive. Finding noninvasive, well-accepted, and cost-effective method for early detection of bladder cancer is necessary. Gharibvand et al. evaluated the role of ultrasonography in the diagnosis and evaluation of bladder tumors (Gharibvand et al. 2017). Sensitivity and specificity of sonography in the diagnosis of bladder tumors were measured. The most common form of bladder in ultrasound was papillary tumors (86%) and the lowest was related to cystic mass (4%) (Gharibvand et al. 2017). The sensitivity, specificity, positive predictive value, and negative predictive value of sonography for the diagnosis of bladder tumors were 93.24%, 100%, 100%, and 16.66%, respectively. The results of our study showed that ultrasonography has high sensitivity and specificity in the diagnosis of bladder cancer and since that ultrasound is a noninvasive, well-accepted, and cost-effective diagnostic technique, ultrasound can be performed in suspected patients in the first stage.

14.17   Detrusor Muscle Thickness and Bladder Cancer

An experimental study demonstrated an increased risk of bladder cancer with detrusor muscle thickening (Cicione et al. 2018). This was assessed using ultrasound and if >2.5 mm this was defined as detrusor muscle thickening. One hundred patients (49.8%) thickened detrusor muscle, were significantly older, had more NMIBC than 101 (50.2%) patients with a thinner detrusor. Recurrence and progression was also associated with detrusor muscle thickening (Cicione et al. 2018). At univariate analysis, a thickened detrusor muscle was predictive of recurrence and progression, respectively: OR 4.9 (95% CI: 2.5–9.5) $p = 0.001$ and OR 2.21 (95% CI: 1.71–4.73), $p = 0.001$. Detrusor muscle thickening may have a role in NMIBC course with a higher recurrence rate.

14.18   Molecular Assays in Screening for Bladder Cancer

Due to the lack symptoms, diagnosis and follow-up of bladder cancer has remained a challenge (Schmitz-Dräger et al. 2015). Over the last decades, numerous molecular assays for the diagnosis of urothelial cancer have been developed (Schmitz-Dräger et al. 2015). All of these assays greater sensitivity compared urine cytology, yet they are not included in clinical guidelines (Schmitz-Dräger et al. 2015). The issue is, none of the assays have been included into clinical decision-making so far. Current data suggest that some of these markers may be used in screening and surveillance of bladder cancer (Schmitz-Dräger et al. 2015).

Bangma et al. looked at urinary molecular markers (Bladder Cancer Urine Marker Project [BLU-P]) as part of a Dutch population-based study to evaluate screening (Bangma et al. 2013). 1747 (88.1%) patients participated (follow-up-2 years). 409 patients (23.4%) had haematuria and had molecular testing (Bangma et al. 2013). Current (n = 295 [17%]) and ex-smokers (n = 998 [58%]) were significantly more likely to test positive than non-smokers. Seventy-one of 75 men (94.6%) with positive molecular markers underwent cystoscopy. Four bladder and one kidney tumor were detected, one bladder and one kidney tumor were missed. This mass screening program had a very low diagnostic yield in an unselected asymptomatic European male population.

Urinary cytology is limited by low sensitivity for low-grade tumors (Xylinas et al. 2014). Urine markers have been studied to improve diagnostics aiming to replace cystoscopy (Xylinas et al. 2014). Urinary markers have higher sensitivity compared with cytology, it is insufficient to replace cystoscopy (Xylinas et al. 2014). Moreover, most markers suffer from lower specificity than cytology (Xylinas et al. 2014).

Starke et al. evaluated the long-term outcomes in high risk patients participating in a screening trial (Starke et al. 2016). Definition of high risk was based on age ≥50 years, ≥10 pack-years, smoking and/or ≥15 years environmental exposure. These patients were enrolled in a screening trial using a nuclear matrix protein 22 (NMP22) assay. At initial screening, 57 patients had a positive NMP22 test and two had bladder cancer. Another nine patients (1.0%) were diagnosed with bladder cancer during the median follow-up of 78.4 months. The bladder cancers were non-invasive (Ta) and seven were low grade and four high grade. No patients died from bladder cancer. This however, demonstrates a low yield even in high risk patients.

Schmitz-Dräger reviewed molecular assays for diagnosis and surveillance (Schmitz-Dräger et al. 2014). There is a very low risk of tumor progression, the primary goal of surveillance is detection of recurrence (Schmitz-Dräger et al. 2014).

Although urine cytology is limited to the high risk cohort in diagnostics. The use of markers with high sensitivity for low-grade disease for patient follow-up has the potential to decrease cystoscopics usage, however, cystoscopy still remains the gold standard (Schmitz-Dräger et al. 2014).

14.19   DNA Methylation and RNA Gene Expression Assays

Diagnosis and surveillance of non-muscle invasive bladder cancer (NMIBC) is mainly based on endoscopic bladder evaluation and urine cytology. Several assays for determining additional molecular markers (urine-, tissue- or blood-based) have been developed in recent years but have not been included in clinical guidelines so far (Maas et al. 2018). Moreover, the potential of recent approaches such as DNA methylation assays, multi-panel RNA gene expression assays and cell-free DNA analysis have also contributed to the progression of molecular screening (Maas et al. 2018). Most studies on various molecular urine markers have mainly focused on a potential replacement of cystoscopy. New developments in high throughput technologies and urine markers may offer further advantages as they may represent a non-invasive approach for molecular characterization of the disease. The implementation of these technologies in well-designed clinical trials is essential to further promote the use of urine diagnostics in the management of patients with NMIBC (Maas et al. 2018).

14.20   TRAP Assays

The identification of molecular markers is often challenging in early detection of bladder cancer. Sachini developed a relatively simple, inexpensive, and accurate test that measures telomerase activity in voided for bladder cancer detection (Sachini et al. 2005). Urine telomerase activity was determined using a telomeric repeat amplification protocol (TRAP) assay and compared with urine cytology. Sensitivity was 90% (95% confidence interval [CI] , 83–94%) and specificity was 88% (95% CI, 79–93%). Specificity increased to 94% (95% CI, 85–98%) if <75 years (Sachini et al. 2005). This also applies to low-grade tumors or negative cytology results. This test represents a potentially useful noninvasive diagnostic innovation for bladder cancer detection in high-risk groups such as habitual smokers or in symptomatic patients (Sachini et al. 2005).

14.21 SERS Assays

This study identified the role of serum surface-enhanced Raman spectroscopy (SERS) spectra in bladder cancer diagnostics (Li et al. 2015). The improved diagnostic sensitivity of 90.9% and specificity of 100% were acquired for classifying bladder cancer patients from normal serum SERS spectra. The results are superior to the sensitivity of 74.6% and specificity of 97.2% obtained with the serum SERS spectra dataset (Li et al. 2015). This exploratory work demonstrates that the serum SERS associated with GA-LDA technique has enormous potential to characterize and non-invasively detect bladder cancer (Li et al. 2015).

14.22 Urinary Protein Markers

Soukup determined the combination of urinary protein markers for noninvasive detection of primary and recurrent urothelial bladder carcinomas (Soukup et al. 2015). Urinary concentrations of 27 biomarkers (NSE, ATT, AFABP, Resistin, Midkine, Clusterin, Uromodulin, ZAG2, HSP27, HSP 60, NCAM1/CD56,

Angiogenin, Calreticulin, Chromogranin A, CEACAM1, CXCL1, IL13Ra2, Progranulin, VEGFA, CarbAnhydIX, Annexin-V, TIM4, Galectin1, Cystatin B, Synuclein G, ApoA1 and ApoA2) were assessed by enzyme-linked immunosorbent assay or by electrochemiluminescence immunoassay (Soukup et al. 2015). For this clinical situation, the most accurate combination proved to be the combination of cytology with markers Midkine and Synuclein G (sensitivity 91.8%, specificity 97.5%) (Soukup et al. 2015). Multi-marker test can significantly improve the bladder cancer detection both during the primary diagnostics and monitoring of patients with NMIBC. This outcome should result in other, larger studies, but also identified a a combination of markers can give a more precise outcome.

14.23 Immunoassays

Urine based assays that non-invasively detect bladder cancer (BCa) have the potential to reduce invasive procedures. Shimzu developed a multiplex immunoassay that can simultaneously monitor ten diagnostic urinary protein biomarkers in bladder cancer diagnostics (Shimizu et al. 2016). A custom electrochemiluminescent multiplex assay was constructed (Meso Scale Diagnostics, LLC, Rockville,

MD, USA) to detect the following urinary proteins; IL8, MMP9, MMP10, ANG, APOE, SDC1, A1AT, PAI1, CA9 and VEGFA. Analysis of the independent 200-sample cohort using the multiplex assay achieved an overall diagnostic sensitivity of 0.85, specificity of 0.81, positive predictive value 0.82 and negative predictive value 0.84 (Shimizu et al. 2016). It is technically feasible to simultaneously monitor complex urinary diagnostic signatures in a single assay without loss of performance. The described protein-based assay has the potential to be developed for the non-invasive detection of bladder cancer prior to cystoscopy.

14.24   Survivin mRNA

Survivin mRNA in urine was measured to detect primary bladder cancer and recurrence (Kenney et al. 2007). The survivin expression had sensitivities and specificities of 79 and 93% in all patients, for detection of newly diagnosed bladder cancer 83 and 95%, for recurrence, 82 and 90%, and for bladder cancer in haematuria 80 and 90%. This demonstrates a highly specific assay both in diagnostics, screening and bladder cancer recurrence.

14.25   Capillary Electrophoresis

Minimally invasive methods of predicting muscle-invasive urothelial bladder can expedite treatment (Schiffer et al. 2009). Schiffer used capillary electrophoresis coupled mass spectrometry (Schiffer et al. 2009). Prospective assessment revealed a sensitivity of 81% [95% confidence interval (CI) , 69–90] and specificity of 57% (95% CI, 45–69) for muscle-invasive disease. Multivariate analysis revealed the panel ($p < 0.0001$) and tumor grade ($p = 0.0001$), but not cytology, predict muscle invasion (Schiffer et al. 2009). A model including grade and panel polypeptide levels improved sensitivity [92% (95% CI, 82–97)] and specificity [68% (95% CI, 55–79)] for muscle invasion. Urinary peptides can be useful in diagnosing muscle-invasive urothelial bladder cancer. However, clinical trials are required to test them further.

14.26   MiRNAs

The prognostic indicators such as tumor grade, stage, size, and multifocality may not reflect the overall clinical outcome (Ratert et al. 2013). Ratert et al. identified deregulated miRNAs in bladder cancer samples and assessed roles as diagnostic and prognostic biomarkers. Seven miRNAs (miR-20a, miR-106b, miR-130b, miR-141, miR-200a, miR-200a*, and miR-205) were found to be up-regulated and eight miRNAs (miR-100, miR-125b, miR-130a, miR-139-5p, miR-145*, miR-199a-3p, miR-214, and miR-222) were found to be down-regulated in bladder cancer. Four miRNAs previously described (miR-141, miR-199a-3p, miR-205, and miR-214) were significantly differentially expressed between NMIBS and MIBC. miRNAs provided high overall correct classification (>75%) of bladder cancer diagnosis. Two miRNAs (miR-141 and miR-205) were associated with increased overall survival time. This paper highlights the role of MiRNAS in diagnosis and prognosis of bladder cancer.

14.27   Extracellular Vesicle Associated Biomarkers

Extracellular vesicles (EVs) are present in a variety of bodily fluids. They have a role in intracellular communications and signal transduction mechanisms (Liang et al. 2017). EVs and EV-associated biomarkers (i.e., proteins, nucleic acids and lipids) can be used in diagnostics (Liang et al. 2017). Liang developed an integrated double-filtration device that detected/quantified EVs from urine via microchip ELISA (Liang et al. 2017). The concentration of EVs was significantly elevated in bladder cancer compared to healthy controls. This EV quantification device had a sensitivity of 81.3%, specificity of 90% (Liang et al. 2017). This assay, has a great role to play in diagnostics of bladder cancer, but required trials.

14.28   MMP23 Genes

Urothelial cell carcinoma (UBC) represents a public health problem because of its high incidence/relapse rates. This is hindered by having no none invasive biomarkers for bladder cancer (Allione et al. 2018). Allione, investigated the levels of MMP23 genes (microarray and qPCR) and protein (Western Blot and ELISA) in a set of samples (blood, plasma and urine) in bladder cancer. MMP23B was down regulated in blood cells in bladder cancer compared to controls (66 cases, 70 controls; adjusted p-value$=0.02$ and 0.03, respectively) (Allione et al. 2018). Yet MMP23B protein levels in plasma (53 bladder cancer cases, 49 controls) and urine (59 bladder cancer cases, 57 controls) increased in bladder cancer cases and was statistically significant in urine. There was a lack of correlation between mRNA and protein levels. Five miRNAs resulted differentially expressed between cases and controls. This suggests a role for this metalloproteinase as a biomarker in bladder cancer.

14.29   Tumour Markers in Bladder Cancer

Orywal et al. investigated alcohol and aldehyde dehydrogenase (ALDH) as tumor markers for$=$bladder cancer (Orywal et al. 2017). Serum samples were gained from 41 patients with bladder cancer and 52 healthy controls (Orywal et al. 2017). Class III and IV of ADH and total ADH activity were measured using photometric method. For measurement of class I and II ADH and ALDH activity, fluorometric method was used (Orywal et al. 2017). Significantly higher total activity of ADH was found in sera of both, low-grade and high-grade bladder cancer patients. The diagnostic sensitivity for total ADH activity was 81.5%, specificity 98.1%, positive (PPV) and negative (NPV) predictive values were 97.4% and 92.3% respectively. Area under ROC curve for total ADH activity was 0.848 (Orywal et al. 2017). A potential role of total ADH activity as a marker for bladder cancer, is herein proposed.

14.30 MicroRNAs in Bladder Cancer

Urinary bladder carcinoma contributes to 4% of newly diagnosed oncological diseases in the Czech Republic (Pospisilova et al. 2016). Biomarkers for its early non-invasive detection are therefore highly desirable. Urine is an ideal source of such biomarkers, containing cell-free nucleic acids, especially microRNAs (miR-NAs) (Pospisilova et al. 2016). To find potential biomarkers among miRNAs in urine supernatant, Pospisilova examined 109 individuals (36 controls and 73 bladder cancer patients) in three phases. In the initial phase, microarray cards with 381 miRNAs were used for miRNA analysis of 13 controls and 46 bladder cancer patients. In the second phase, the results were verified by single-target qPCR assays for the selected miRNAs. For the third phase, new independent samples of urine supernatant (23 controls and 27 bladder cancer patients) were analyzed using single-target qPCR assays for 13 verified in the previous phase. MiR-125b, miR-30b, miR-204, miR-99a, and miR-532-3p are significantly down-regulated in patients' urine. MiR-125 levels provided the highest AUC (0.801) with 95.65% specificity and 59.26% sensitivity. MiR-99a lead to AUC (0.738) with 82.61% specificity and 74.07% sensitivity. Both of these could be used successfully as urinary biomarkers.

14.31 Epigenetics in Bladder Cancer

The role of epigenetics in determining treatment has not yet been determined. Sacristan assessed methylation of tumor-suppressor genes (TSGs). This was examined for classification of non-muscle-invasive (NMI) bladder cancer subgroups to predict outcome. A retrospective design was used with primary NMI tumor types. These included pTa low grade (LG) (n = 79), pT1LG (n = 81), and pT1 high grade (HG) (n = 91). The TSGs most frequently methylated in the overall series were STK11 (96.8%), MGMT2 (64.5%), RARB (63.0%), and GATA5 (63.0%). TSG methylation correlated to clinicopathological variables in each subgroup and in the overall NMI series. Methylation of RARB, CD44, PAX5A, GSTP1, IGSF4 (CADM1), PYCARD, CDH13, TP53, and GATA5 classified pTa versus pT1 tumors. RARB, CD44, GSTP1, IGSF4, CHFR, PYCARD, TP53, STK11, and GATA5 differentiated LG versus HG tumors. Methylation of TSGs provided a molecular classification of NMIBC as per clinicopathological subgroups. Furthermore, TSG methylation predicted recurrence.

14.32   Urinary Biomarkers—Survivin

Urinary biomarkers may improve the early detection of bladder cancer (Johnen et al. 2012). Most markers have been assessed with cross-sectional design (Johnen et al. 2012). For proper validation a longitudinal design would be preferable. Johnen et al. (2012) used the prospective study UroScreen to evaluate surviving. This has multiple functions in carcinogenesis. Survivin was analyzed in 1,540 chemical workers exposed to aromatic amines. 19 bladder tumors were detected. Survivin had a sensitivity of 21.1% for all and 36.4% for high-grade tumors. Specificity was 97.5%, the positive predictive value (PPV) 9.5%, and the negative predictive value (NPV) 99.0%. Survivin demonstrated a good specificity but a low PPV and sensitivity. Therefore survivin may still be considered as a component of a multimarker panel for diagnostics.

14.33   FISH Assays—Molecular Diagnosis of Bladder Cancer

Different chromosomal aberrations have been already identified in bladder tumors. These aberrations can be detected by fluorescence in situ hybridization (I-FISH) or comparative genomic hybridization (CGH) (Houskova et al. 2007). Houskova et al. (2007) determined the diagnostic benefits of non-invasive I-FISH method and to comprehensively characterise genetic alterations using CGH in selected patients with bladder tumors (Houskova et al. 2007). Houskova examined 128 urine samples and correlated our results with histological findings. I-FISH using UroVysion kit showed positivity in 63.6% of G1 tumors, 64.3% of G2 tumors and 91.7% in G3 tumors. Houskova et al. (2007) examined also 12 bladder tissue samples by means of CGH and various genetic alterations were ascertained independent on tumor grade. The most frequent gains and losses of DNA material were detected on chromosomes 1, 8, 9, 10, 11, 13, and 14. The contribution of I-FISH is in an early and non-invasive detection of bladder cancer recurrences during follow up of patients after the surgery. CGH provides information about further genetic alterations and some of them could be ascertained as recurrent changes with prognostic significance.

The UroVysion fluorescence in situ hybridization (FISH) test demonstrated higher sensitivity over urine cytology in detecting bladder cancer by most comparative studies (Daniely et al. 2007). Daniely examined the diagnostic usefulness of a combined cytology and FISH analysis in diagnostics for recurrent urothelial carcinoma (Daniely et al. 2007). By combining cytology with molecular diagnostics, greater sensitivity is attained. All patients who had positive cystoscopy concomitantly with urine sampling were detected by combined analysis (Daniely et al. 2007). The overall sensitivity, specificity, negative predictive value (NPV) , and positive predictive values of the combined analysis test were 100%, 65%, 100%, and 44%, respectively (Daniely et al. 2007). Given the absolute sensitivity and NPV of the combined analysis test, the management of patients with a negative combined analysis result might be revised and allow for more flexible assessment and management of bladder cancer patients relying more on urine bound tests.

Fernandez determined the diagnostic benefits of non-invasive I-FISH method as part of diagnostics for bladder tumors (Fernandez et al. 2012). I-FISH using UroVysion kit showed positivity in 63,6% of G1 tumors, 64,3% of G2 tumors and 91,7% in G3 tumors (Fernandez et al. 2012). Fernandez also examined also 12 bladder tissue samples by means of CGH and various genetic alterations were ascertained independent on tumor grade (Fernandez et al. 2012). The most frequent gains and losses of DNA material were detected on chromosomes 1, 8, 9, 10, 11, 13, and 14. The contribution of I-FISH is in an early and non-invasive detection of bladder cancer recurrences during follow up of patients after the surgery (Fernandez et al. 2012).

14.34   Molecular Assays in Screening for Bladder Cancer

Due to the lack of disease-specific symptoms, diagnosis and follow-up of bladder cancer has remained a challenge to the urologic community (Schmitz-Dräger et al. 2015). Over the last decades, numerous molecular assays for the diagnosis of urothelial cancer have been developed and investigated with regard to their clinical use (Schmitz-Dräger et al. 2015). However, although all of these assays have been shown to have superior sensitivity as compared to urine cytology, none of them has been included in clinical guidelines (Schmitz-Dräger et al. 2015). The key reason for this situation is that none of the assays has been included into clinical decision-making so far. Current data suggest that some of these markers may have the potential to play a role in screening and surveillance of bladder cancer (Schmitz-Dräger et al. 2015).

Bangma et al. looked at urinary molecular markers (Bladder Cancer Urine Marker Project [BLU-P]) .

BLU-P was a Dutch population-based study initiated in 2008 to evaluate BCa screening (Bangma et al. 2013). A total of 6500 men were invited to participate in the study, 1984 (30.5%) agreed, and 1747 (88.1%) men completed the protocol and were followed for 2 yr. Overall, 409 men (23.4%) tested positive for hematuria and underwent molecular testing (Bangma et al. 2013). Current smokers (n = 295 [17%]) and past smokers (n = 998 [58%]) were significantly more likely to test positive for hematuria than nonsmokers. Seventy-one of 75 men (94.6%) with positive molecular markers underwent the recommended cystoscopy. Four BCas and one kidney tumor were detected through this sequential protocol, whereas one BCa and one kidney tumor were missed through the screening program. This mass screening program had a very low diagnostic yield in an unselected asymptomatic European male population.

Urinary cytology is limited by its low sensitivity for low-grade tumors (Xylinas et al. 2014). Urine markers have been extensively studied to help improve the diagnosis of bladder cancer with the goal of complementing or even replacing cystoscopy (Xylinas et al. 2014). Although several urinary markers have shown higher sensitivity compared with cytology, it remains insufficient to replace cystoscopy (Xylinas et al. 2014). Moreover, most markers suffer from lower specificity than cytology (Xylinas et al. 2014).

Starke et al. evaluated the long-term outcomes in patients at high risk of bladder cancer who participated in a bladder cancer screening trial (Starke et al. 2016). Patients who were classified as high risk based on age ≥ 50 years, ≥ 10 pack-years (combination of packs of tobacco per day and years of smoking) smoking and/or ≥ 15 years environmental exposure were enrolled in a one-time screening trial using a nuclear matrix protein 22 (NMP22) assay. At initial screening, 57 patients had a positive NMP22 test and two had bladder cancer. Another nine patients (1.0%) were diagnosed with bladder cancer during the median follow-up of 78.4 months. The bladder cancers were non-invasive (Ta) and seven were low grade and four high grade, respectively, and >60 pack-years smoking history (HR 4.51; $p = 0.037$).

Schmitz-Dräger et al. reviewed molecular assays for bladder cancer diagnosis and surveillance (Schmitz-Dräger et al. 2014). The conclusions made were as these patients have a very low risk of tumor progression, the primary goal of surveillance is detection of recurrent disease (Schmitz-Dräger et al. 2014).

Although urine cytology seems to be limited to detection of few patients who would develop high-grade tumors. The use of markers with high sensitivity for low-grade disease for patient follow-up has the potential to decrease the frequency of urethrocystoscopy without compromising patient prognosis (Schmitz-Dräger et al. 2014). This paper concluded markers have the potential to support clinical decision making in follow-up of patients with low-/intermediate-risk NMIBC, however, further assessment is necessary.

14.35   Blue Light Screening

Inoue et al. discovered urine porphyrin levels from tumor-bearing mice were elevated compared with those from normal mice after administration of 5-aminolevulinic acid (ALA) (Inoue et al. 2013). Almost all of the urinary porphyrin concentrations from the patients with bladder cancer were higher than those from healthy adults (Inoue et al. 2013). Moreover, 8 h after ALA administration, urinary

UPI and CPI showed high sensitivity (100 for UPI and CPI) and specificity (96.4 for UPI and 91.4 for CPI) (Inoue et al. 2013).

These results indicate that the presence of urinary porphyrins after administration of ALA may function as tumor biomarkers (Inoue et al. 2013). This method represents a possible new tumor screening method called photodynamic screening (PDS) using ALA-induced porphyrins.

Hexaminolevulinate (HAL) is a tumour photosensitizer that is used in combination with blue-light cystoscopy (BLC) as an adjunct to white-light cystoscopy (WLC) in the diagnosis and management of non-muscle-invasive bladder cancer (NMIBC) (Daneshmand et al. 2014). Current data support an additional role in the reduction of recurrence of NMIBC. HAL-BLC should be considered for initial assessment of NMIBC, surveillance for recurrent tumours, diagnosis in patients with positive urine cytology but negative WLC findings, and for tumour staging (Daneshmand et al. 2014).

Blue light cystoscopy (BLC) using hexaminolevulinate (HAL/Cysview/Hexvix) has been previously shown to improve detection of non-muscle-invasive bladder cancer (NMIBC) (Daneshmand et al. 2014). Danesmand et al. evaluated the detection of malignant lesions in a heterogenous group of patients in the real world setting and documented the change in risk category due to upstaging or upgrading.

Addition of BLC to standard WLC increased detection rate by 12% for any papillary lesion and 43% for carcinoma in situ (Daneshmand et al. 2014). Within the WLC negative group, an additional 206 lesions in 133 (25%) patients were detected exclusively with BLC. In multifocal disease, BLC resulted in AUA risk-group migration occurred in 33 (6%) patients and a change in recommended management in 74 (14%) (Daneshmand et al. 2014). False-positive rate was 25% for WLC and 30% for BLC. One mild dermatologic hypersensitivity reaction (0.2%). BLC increases detection rates of carcinoma in situ and papillary lesions over WLC alone and can change management in 14% of cases. Repeat use of HAL for BLC is safe (Daneshmand et al. 2014).

14.36   Bladder Cancer Screening

Bladder cancer (BCa) is the fourth most common cancer in men (Larré et al. 2013). Survival from the disease has not improved over the last quarter century. Population-based screening theoretically provides the best opportunity to improve the outcomes of aggressive BCa (Larré et al. 2013). Screening for the disease is not standard in the United States or Canada (Pashos et al. 2002), however, any patient with haematuria is screened in the UK. Potential tests include urine cytology, haematuria on dipstick, flexible cystoscopy and upper tract imaging, USS KUB or CT Urogram (Pashos et al. 2002). Cystoscopy, commonly accepted as a gold standard for the detection of bladder cancer, is invasive and relatively expensive, while urine cytology is of limited value specifically in low-grade disease (Schmitz-Dräger et al. 2015).

Bladder cancer continues to be one of the most common and expensive malignancies (Yeung et al. 2014). Ten years ago, urinary markers held the potential to lower treatment costs of bladder cancer/ Adjunct cytology remains a part of diagnostic standard of care, but recent research suggests that it is not cost effective due to its low diagnostic yield. Analysis of intravesical chemotherapy after transurethral resection of bladder tumor (TURBT), neo-adjuvant therapy for cystectomy, and robot-assisted laparoscopic cystectomy suggests that these technologies are cost effective and should be implemented more widely for appropriate patients.

Because of its relatively low incidence, bladder cancer screening might have a better ratio of benefits to harms if it is restricted to a high-risk population (Vickers et al. 2013). The 5-year probability of being diagnosed with invasive bladder cancer was 0.24%. In a typical scenario, a risk score >6 would result in approximately 25% of the population being screened to prevent 57 invasive or high-grade bladder cancers per 100,000 population (Vickers et al. 2013). Screening for bladder cancer can be optimized by restricting it to a subgroup of patients considered to be at elevated risk. Different eligibility criteria for a screening trial can be compared rationally using decision-analytic techniques.

More than 25% of bladder cancer (BC) cases are still muscle-invasive at first diagnosis (Zlotta et al. 2011). Screening is unproven to enable the detection of more non-muscle-invasive tumors (Zlotta et al. 2011). BC association with aristolochic acid nephropathy (AAN) was reported after intake of slimming pills containing Chinese herbs (Zlotta et al. 2011). Zlotta et al. evaluated whether a BC screening protocol in a high-risk and unique patient population had an impact on the stage of tumor presentation.

BC was diagnosed in 25 patients (52%) (Zlotta et al. 2011). Among 43 patients who underwent screening cystoscopies (Zlotta et al. 2011). This demonstrated BC screening in high-risk groups may allow identification of tumors before muscle invasion (Zlotta et al. 2011). The optimal screening schedule and the relevance of the present findings in smoking-related BC remain to be defined.

Cassidy et al. identify significant predictors of initial and repeated adherence with bladder cancer screening in a high-risk occupationally exposed cohort (Cassidy et al. 2011). The study analyzed longitudinal (13 years) health survey data and a cross-sectional behavioral health survey from the Drake Health Registry Study (Cassidy et al. 2011). Construct validity of the behavioral health survey scales was evaluated using factor analysis. Initial compliance and repeated adherence were examined in separate logistic regression models (Cassidy et al. 2011). "Barriers to screening" and "social influence" were associated with initial participation. Lower or no alcohol consumption, comorbidities, worry that screening would find bladder cancer, and ease of arranging schedules were associated with continued adherence (Cassidy et al. 2011). Factors affecting adherence with bladder cancer screening change for initial participation and for continued adherence. To enhance overall adherence, specific strategies should be implemented when initiating a screening program and revised accordingly over time.

To assess the positive predictive value (PPV) of microhaematuria (μH) and visible haematuria (GH) in bladder cancer screening and the influence of haematuria on tumour tests in a prospective study (Pesch et al. 2011). While the PPV of μH for bladder cancer was low, there was a strong influence of haematuria and leukocytes on the protein-based tumour test NMP22® (Pesch et al. 2011). Erythrocytes and leukocytes should be determined at least semi-quantitatively for the interpretation of positive NMP22 test results (Pesch et al. 2011). In addition, a panel of tumour tests that includes methods not affected by the presence of erythrocytes or leukocytes such as cytology and UroVysion(TM) would improve bladder cancer screening (Pesch et al. 2011).

Bonberg et al. explore changes at chromosomes 3, 7, 17 and 9p21 in order to assess associations with bladder cancer for possible improvements of the UroVysion™ assay regarding screening (Bonberg et al. 2013). The UroVysion assay showed a reasonable performance in detecting bladder cancer in the present study population and shared positive test results with cytology, which is much cheaper (Bonberg et al. 2013). A simpler, faster and cheaper version of the UroVysion assay might rely on the very strong correlations between gains at chromosomes 3, 7 and 17, resulting in a similar performance in detecting bladder cancer with single-probe PIs compared with the full set of these probes (Bonberg et al. 2013). Loss of 9p21 was less predictive for developing bladder cancer in UroScreen (Bonberg et al. 2013).

Bladder cancer is 1 of the 10 most frequently diagnosed types of cancer. Screening could identify high-grade bladder cancer at earlier stages, when it may be more easily and effectively treated. Chou et al. (2010), updated the 2004 U.S. Preventive Services Task Force evidence review on screening for bladder cancer in adults in primary care settings (Chou et al. 2010). No randomized trials or high-quality controlled observational studies evaluated clinical outcomes associated with screening compared with no screening or treatment of screen-detected bladder cancer compared with no treatment (Chou et al. 2010). No study evaluated the sensitivity or specificity of tests for hematuria, urinary cytology, or other urinary biomarkers for bladder cancer in asymptomatic persons without a history of bladder cancer (Chou et al. 2010). The positive predictive value of screening is less than 10% in asymptomatic persons, including higher-risk populations (Chou et al. 2010). No study evaluated harms associated with treatment of screen-detected bladder cancer compared with no treatment (Chou et al. 2010).

References

Abdollahzadeh P, Madani SH, Khazaei S, Sajadimajd S, Izadi B, Najafi F. Association between human papillomavirus and transitional cell carcinoma of the bladder. Urol J. 2017;14(6):5047–50.

Allione A, Pardini B, Viberti C, Giribaldi G, Turini S, Di Gaetano C, Guarrera S, Cordero F, Oderda M, Allasia M, Gontero P, Sacerdote C, Vineis P, Matullo G. MMP23B expression and protein levels in blood and urine are associated with bladder cancer. Carcinogenesis. 2018.

Bangma CH, Loeb S, Busstra M, Zhu X, El Bouazzaoui S, Refos J, Van Der Keur KA, Tjin S, Franken CG, van Leenders GJ, Zwarthoff EC, Roobol MJ. Outcomes of a bladder cancer screening program using home hematuria testing and molecular markers. Eur Urol. 2013;64(1):41–7.

Behrens A, Stehle T, Gross S, Aach T. Local and global panoramic imaging for fluorescence bladder endoscopy. In: Conference Proceedings of the IEEE Engineering in Medicine and Biology Society. 2009. p. 6990–3.

Bonberg N, Taeger D, Gawrych K, Johnen G, Banek S, Schwentner C, Sievert KD, Wellhäußer H, Kluckert M, Leng G, Nasterlack M, Stenzl A, Behrens T, Brüning T, Pesch B; UroScreen Study Group. Chromosomal instability and bladder cancer: the UroVysion(TM) test in the UroScreen study. BJU Int. 2013;112(4):E372–82.

Böthig R, Fiebag K, Kowald B, Hirschfeld S, Thietje R, Kurze I, Schöps W, Böhme H, Kaufmann A, Zellner M, Kadhum T, Golka K. Spinal cord injury with neurogenic lower urinary tract dysfunction as a potential risk factor for bladder carcinoma. Aktuelle Urol. 2018.

Carreón T, Hein MJ, Hanley KW, Viet SM, Ruder AM. Bladder cancer incidence among workers exposed to o-toluidine, aniline and nitrobenzene at a rubber chemical manufacturing plant. Occup Environ Med. 2014;71(3):175–82.

Cassidy LD, Marsh GM, Talbott EO, Kelsey SFInitial and continued adherence with bladder cancer screening in an occupationally exposed cohort. J Occup Environ Med. 2011;53(4):455–6.

Chavan S, Bray F, Lortet-Tieulent J, Goodman M, Jemal A. International variations in bladder cancer incidence and mortality. Eur Urol. 2014;66(1):59–73. https://doi.org/10.1016/j.eururo.2013.10.001.

Chou R, Dana T. Screening adults for bladder cancer: a review of the evidence for the U.S. preventive services task force. Ann Intern Med. 2010;153(7):461–8.

Cicione A, Manno S, Ucciero G, Cantiello F, Damiano R, Lima E, Posti A, Balloni F, De Nunzio C. A larger detrusor wall thickness increases the risk of non muscle invasive bladder cancer recurrence and progression: result from a multicenter observational study. Minerva Urol Nefrol. 2018;70(1):110–18.

Daneshmand S, Schuckman AK, Bochner BH, Cookson MS, Downs TM, Gomella LG, Grossman HB, Kamat AM, Konety BR, Lee CT, Pohar KS, Pruthi RS, Resnick MJ, Smith ND, Witjes JA, Schoenberg MP, Steinberg GD. Hexaminolevulinate blue-light cystoscopy in non-muscle-invasive bladder cancer: review of the clinical evidence and consensus statement on appropriate use in the USA 2014.

Daniely M, Rona R, Kaplan T, Olsfanger S, Elboim L, Freiberger A, Lew S, Leibovitch I. Combined morphologic and fluorescence in situ hybridization analysis of voided urine samples for the detection and follow-up of bladder cancer in patients with benign urine cytology. Cancer. 2007;111(6):517–24.

Drejer D, Béji S, Munk Nielsen A, Høyer S, Wrist Lam G, Jensen JB. Clinical relevance of narrow-band imaging in flexible cystoscopy: the DaBlaCa-7 study. Scand J Urol. 2017;51(2):120–123.

Eifler JB, Barocas DA, Resnick MJ. Predictors of outcome in bladder cancer. J Natl Compr Canc Netw. 2014;12(11):1549–54.

Ellwein LB, Farrow GM. Urinary cytology screening: the decision facing the asymptomatic patient. Med Decis Making. 1988;8(2):110–9.

Fernandez CA, Millholland JM, Zwarthoff EC, Feldman AS, Karnes RJ, Shuber AP. A noninvasive multi-analyte diagnostic assay: combining protein and DNA markers to stratify bladder cancer patients. Res Rep Urol. 2012;4:17–2.

Ferris J, Garcia J, Berbel O, Ortega JA. Constitutional and occupational risk factors associated with bladder cancer. Actas Urol Esp. 2013;37(8):513–22.

Freitas NR, Vieira PM, Lima E, Lima CS. Automatic T1 bladder tumor detection by using wavelet analysis in cystoscopy images. Phys Med Biol. 2018;63(3):035031.

Gharibvand MM, Kazemi M, Motamedfar A, Sametzadeh M, Sahraeizadeh A. The role of ultrasound in diagnosis and evaluation of bladder tumors. J Family Med Prim Care. 2017;6(4):840–43.

Grotenhuis AJ, Ebben CW, Aben KK, Witjes JA, Vrieling A, Vermeulen SH, Kiemeney LA. The effect of smoking and timing of smoking cessation on clinical outcome in non-muscle-invasive bladder cancer. Urol Oncol. 2015;33(2):65.e9–17.

Guillaume L, Guy L. Epidemiology of and risk factors for bladder cancer and for urothelial tumors. Rev Prat. 2014;64(10):1372–4, 1378–80.

Horstmann M, Banek S, Gakis G, Todenhöfer T, Aufderklamm S, Hennenlotter J, Stenzl A, Schwentner C. UroScreen study group. Prospective evaluation of fluorescence-guided cystoscopy to detect bladder cancer in a high-risk population: results from the UroScreen-Study. Springerplus. 2014;3:24.

Houskova L, Zemanova Z, Babjuk M, Melichercikova J, Pesl M, Michalova K. Molecular cytogenetic characterization and diagnostics of bladder cancer. Neoplasma. 2007;54(6):511–6.

Inoue K, Ota U, Ishizuka M, Kawada C, Fukuhara H, Shuin T, Okura I, Tanaka T, Ogura S. Porphyrins as urinary biomarkers for bladder cancer after 5-aminolevulinic acid (ALA) administration: the potential of photodynamic screening for tumors. Photodiagnosis Photodyn Ther. 2013;10(4):484–9.

Jochems SHJ, van Osch FHM, Reulen RC, van Hensbergen M, Nekeman D, Pirrie S, Wesselius A, van Schooten FJ, James ND, Wallace DMA, Bryan RT, Cheng KK, Zeegers MP. Fruit and vegetable intake and the risk of recurrence in patients with non-muscle invasive bladder cancer: a prospective cohort study. Cancer Causes Control. 2018;29(6):573–79.

Johnen G, Gawrych K, Bontrup H, Pesch B, Taeger D, Banek S, Kluckert M, Wellhäußer H, Eberle F, Nasterlack M, Leng G, Stenzl A, Brüning T; UroScreen Study Group. Performance of survivin mRNA as a biomarker for bladder cancer in the prospective study UroScreen. PLoS One. 2012;7(4):e35363. https://doi.org/10.1371/journal.pone.0035363. Epub 2012 Apr 16.

Kenney DM, Geschwindt RD, Kary MR, Linic JM, Sardesai NY, Li ZQ. Detection of newly diagnosed bladder cancer, bladder cancer recurrence and bladder cancer in patients with hematuria using quantitative rt-PCR of urinary survivin. Tumour Biol. 2007;28(2):57–62.

Kollarik B, Zvarik M, Bujdak P, Weibl P, Rybar L, Sikurova L, Hunakova L. Urinary fluorescence analysis in diagnosis of bladder cancer. Neoplasma. 2018;65(2):234–41.

Larré S, Catto JW, Cookson MS, Messing EM, Shariat SF, Soloway MS, Svatek RS, Lotan Y, Zlotta AR, Grossman HB. Screening for bladder cancer: rationale, limitations, whom to target, and perspective. Eur Urol. 2013;63(6):1049–58.

Letašiová S, Medve'ová A, Šovčíková A, Dušinská M, Volkovová K, Mosoiu C, Bartonová A. Bladder cancer, a review of the environmental risk factors. Environ Health. 2012;11(Suppl. 1):S11.

Li S, Li L, Zeng Q, Zhang Y, Guo Z, Liu Z, Jin M, Su C, Lin L, Xu J, Liu S. Characterization and noninvasive diagnosis of bladder cancer with serum surface enhanced Raman spectroscopy and genetic algorithms. Sci Rep. 2015;5:9582.

Liang LG, Sheng YF, Zhou S, Inci F, Li L, Demirci U, Wang S. An integrated double-filtration microfluidic device for detection of extracellular vesicles from urine for bladder cancer diagnosis. Methods Mol Biol. 2017;1660:355–64.

Llewellyn MA, Gordon NS, Abbotts B, James ND, Zeegers MP, Cheng KK, Macdonald A, Roberts S, Parish JL, Ward DG, Bryan RT. Defining the frequency of human papillomavirus and polyomavirus infection in urothelial bladder tumours. Sci Rep. 2018;8(1):11290.

Maas M, Walz S, Stühler V, Aufderklamm S, Rausch S, Bedke J, Stenzl A, Todenhöfer T. Molecular markers in disease detection and follow-up of patients with non-muscle invasive bladder cancer. Expert Rev Mol Diagn. 2018;18(5):443–55.

Mäkelä VJ, Kotsar A, Tammela TL, Murtola TJ. Bladder cancer survival in men using 5-alpha-reductase inhibitors. J Urol. 2018;(18)43085–6. pii:S0022–5347.

Malats N, Real FX. Epidemiology of bladder cancer. Hematol Oncol Clin North Am. 2015;29(2):177–89, vii.

Martini T, Mayr R, Lodde M, Seitz C, Trenti E, Comploj E, Palermo S, Pycha A, Mian C, Zywica M, Weidner W, Lüdecke G. Validation of RiskCheck Bladder Cancer©, version 5.0 for risk-adapted screening of bladder cancer. Urol Int. 2013;91(2):175–81.

Messing EM, Madeb R, Young T, Gilchrist KW, Bram L, Greenberg EB, Wegenke JD, et al. Long-term outcome of hematuria home screening for bladder cancer in men. Cancer. 2006;107(9):2173–9.

Orywal K, Jelski W, Werel T, Szmitkowski M. The diagnostic significance of serum alcohol dehydrogenase isoenzymes and aldehyde dehydrogenase activity in urinary bladder cancer patients. Anticancer Res. 2017;37(7):3537–41.

Pashos CL, Botteman MF, Laskin BL, Redaelli A. Bladder cancer: epidemiology, diagnosis, and management. Cancer Pract. 2002;10(6):311–22.

Pedersen M, Stafoggia M, Weinmayr G, Andersen ZJ, Galassi C, Sommar J, Forsberg B, Olsson D, Oftedal B, Krog NH, Aamodt G, Pyko A, Pershagen G, Korek M, De Faire U, Pedersen NL, Östenson CG, Fratiglioni L, Sørensen M, Eriksen KT, Tjønneland A, Peeters PH, Bueno-de-Mesquita B, Vermeulen R, Eeftens M, Plusquin M, Key TJ, Jaensch A, Nagel G, Concin H, Wang M, Tsai MY, Grioni S, Marcon A, Krogh V, Ricceri F, Sacerdote C, Ranzi A, Cesaroni G, Forastiere F, Tamayo I, Amiano P, Dorronsoro M, Stayner LT, Kogevinas M, Nieuwenhuijsen MJ, Sokhi R, de Hoogh K, Beelen R, Vineis P, Brunekreef B, Hoek G, Raaschou-Nielsen O. Is there an association between ambient air pollution and bladder cancer incidence? Analysis of 15 European Cohorts. Eur Urol Focus. 2018;4(1):113–20.

Pesch B, Nasterlack M, Eberle F, Bonberg N, Taeger D, Leng G, Feil G, Johnen G, Ickstadt K, Kluckert M, Wellhäusser H, Stenzl A, Brüning T; UroScreen Group. The role of haematuria in bladder cancer screening among men with former occupational exposure to aromatic amines. BJU Int. 2011;108(4):546–52.

Pospisilova S, Pazourkova E, Horinek A, Brisuda A, Svobodova I, Soukup V, Hrbacek J, Capoun O, Hanus T, Mares J, Korabecna M, Babjuk M. MicroRNAs in urine supernatant as potential non-invasive markers for bladder cancer detection. Neoplasma. 2016;63(5).799–808.

Ratert N, Meyer HA, Jung M, Lioudmer P, Mollenkopf HJ, Wagner I, Miller K, Kilic E, Erbersdobler A, Weikert S, Jung K. miRNA profiling identifies candidate mirnas for bladder cancer diagnosis and clinical outcome. J Mol Diagn. 2013;15(5):695–705.

Rybotycka Z, Długosz A. Diagnostic significance of protein NMP22 in bladder cancer. Pol Merkur Lekarski. 2015;38(228):309.

Sanchini MA, Gunelli R, Nanni O, Bravaccini S, Fabbri C, Sermasi A, Bercovich E, Ravaioli A, Amadori D, Calistri D. Relevance of urine telomerase in the diagnosis of bladder cancer. JAMA. 2005.

Schiffer E, Vlahou A, Petrolekas A, Stravodimos K, Tauber R, Geschwend JE, Neuhaus J, Stolzenburg JU, Conaway MR, Mischak H, Theodorescu D. Prediction of muscle-invasive bladder cancer using urinary proteomics. Clin Cancer Res. 2009;15(15):4935–43.

Schmitz-Dräger BJ, Droller M, Lokeshwar VB, Lotan Y, Hudson MA, van Rhijn BW, Marberger MJ, Fradet Y, Hemstreet GP, Malmstrom PU, Ogawa O, Karakiewicz PI, Shariat SF. Molecular markers for bladder cancer screening, early diagnosis, and surveillance: the WHO/ICUD consensus. Urol Int. 2015;94(1):1–24.

Schmitz-Dräger BJ, Todenhöfer T, van Rhijn B, Pesch B, Hudson MA, Chandra A, Ingersoll MA, Kassouf W, Palou J, Taylor J, Vlahou A, Behrens T, Critelli R, Grossman HB, Sanchez-Carbayo M, Kamat A. Considerations on the use of urine markers in the **management** of patients with low-/intermediate-risk non-muscle invasive bladder cancer. Urol Oncol. 2014;32(7):1061–8.

Shimizu Y, Furuya H, Bryant Greenwood P, Chan O, Dai Y, Thornquist MD, Goodison S, Rosser CJ. A multiplex immunoassay for the non-invasive detection of bladder cancer. J Transl Med. 2016;14:31.

Simonis K, Shariat SF, Rink M. Smoking and smoking cessation effects on oncological outcomes in nonmuscle invasive bladder cancer. Curr Opin Urol. 2014;24(5):492–9.

Soukup V, Kalousová M, Capoun O, Sobotka R, Breyl Z, Pešl M, Zima T, Hanuš T. Panel of urinary diagnostic markers for non-invasive detection of primary and recurrent urothelial urinary bladder carcinoma. Urol Int. 2015;95(1):56–64.

Starke N, Singla N, Haddad A, Lotan Y. Long-term outcomes in a high-risk bladder cancer screening cohort. BJU Int. 2016;117(4):611–9.

Szygula M, Wojciechowski B, Adamek M, Pietrusa A, Kawczyk-Krupka A, Cebula W, Zieleznik W, Biniszkiewicz T, Duda W, Sieroń A. Fluorescent diagnosis of urinary bladder cancer-a comparison of two diagnostic modalities. Photodiagnosis Photodyn Ther. 2004;1(1):23–6.

Tan WS, Rodney S, Lamb B, Feneley M, Kelly J. Management of non muscle invasive bladder cancer: a comprehensive analysis of guidelines from the United States, Europe and Asia. Cancer Treat Rev. 2016;47:22–31.

Teleka S, Häggström C, Nagel G, Bjørge T, Manjer J, Ulmer H, Liedberg F, Ghaderi S, Lang A, Jonsson H, Jahnson S, Orho-Melander M, Tretli S, Stattin P, Stocks T. Risk of bladder cancer by disease severity in relation to metabolic factors and smoking; a prospective pooled cohort study of 800,000 men and women. Int J Cancer. 2018.

Turco P, Houssami N, Bulgaresi P, Troni GM, Galanti L, Cariaggi MP, Cifarelli P, Crocetti E, Ciatto S. Is conventional urinary cytology still reliable for diagnosis of primary bladder carcinoma? Accuracy based on data linkage of a consecutive clinical series and cancer registry. Acta Cytol. 2011;55(2):193–6.

van Osch FHM, Jochems SHJ, Reulen RC, Pirrie SJ, Nekeman D, Wesselius A, James ND, et al. The association between smoking cessation before and after diagnosis and non muscle-invasive bladder cancer recurrence: a prospective cohort study. Cancer Causes Control. 2018;29(7):675–83.

Vickers AJ, Bennette C, Kibel AS, Black A, Izmirlian G, Stephenson AJ, Bochner B. Who should be included in a clinical trial of screening for bladder cancer? A decision analysis of data from the Prostate, Lung, Colorectal and Ovarian Cancer Screening Trial. Cancer. 2013;119(1):143–9.

Wach S, Weigelt K, Michalke B, Lieb V, Stoehr R, Keck B, Hartmann A, et al. Diagnostic potential of major and trace elements in the serum of bladder cancer patients. J Trace Elem Med Biol. 2018;46:150–55.

Whelan P, Britton JP, Dowell AC. Three-year follow-up of bladder tumours found on screening. Br J Urol. 1993;72(6):893–6.

Xylinas E, Kluth LA, Rieken M, Karakiewicz PI, Lotan Y, Shariat SF. Urine markers for detection and surveillance of bladder cancer. Urol Oncol. 2014;32(3):222–9.

Yeung C, Dinh T, Lee J. The health economics of bladder cancer: an updated review of the published literature. Pharmacoeconomics. 2014;32(11):1093–104.

Zlotta AR, Roumeguere T, Kuk C, Alkhateeb S, Rorive S, Lemy A, van der Kwast TH, Fleshner NE, Jewett MA, Finelli A, Schulman C, Lotan Y, Shariat SF, Nortier J. Select screening in a specific high-risk population of patients suggests a stage migration toward detection of non-muscle-invasive bladder cancer. Eur Urol. 2011;59(6):1026–31.

Chapter 15
Bladder Cancer Screening Systematic Review Conclusion

Bladder cancer (BCa) is the fourth most common cancer in men (Larré et al. 2013). Survival from the disease has not improved over 25 years. Population-based screening theoretically provides the best opportunity to improve the outcomes of aggressive BCa (Larré et al. 2013). Any patient with haematuria is screened in the UK. Potential tests include urine cytology, haematuria on dipstick, flexible cystoscopy and upper tract imaging, USS KUB or CT Urogram (Pashos et al. 2002). Cystoscopy, commonly accepted as a gold standard for the detection of bladder cancer, is invasive and relatively expensive, while urine cytology is of limited value specifically in low-grade disease (Schmitz-Dräger et al. 2015).

Bladder cancer continues to be one of the most common and expensive malignancies (Yeung et al. 2014). Ten years ago, urinary markers held the potential to lower treatment costs of bladder cancer/Adjunct cytology remains a part of diagnostic standard of care, but recent research suggests that it is not cost effective due to its low diagnostic yield (Yeung et al. 2014). Analysis of intravesical chemotherapy after transurethral resection of bladder tumor (TURBT), neo-adjuvant therapy for cystectomy, and robot-assisted laparoscopic cystectomy suggests that these technologies are cost effective and should be implemented more widely for appropriate patients.

Because of its relatively low incidence, bladder cancer screening might have a better ratio of benefits to harms if it is restricted to a high-risk population (Vickers et al. 2013). The 5-year probability of being diagnosed with invasive bladder cancer was 0.24% (Vickers et al. 2013). In a typical scenario, a risk score >6 would result in approximately 25% of the population being screened to prevent 57 invasive or high-grade bladder cancers per 100,000 population (Vickers et al. 2013). Screening for bladder cancer can be optimized by restricting it to a subgroup of patients considered to be at elevated risk. Different eligibility criteria for a screening trial can be compared rationally using decision-analytic techniques.

More than 25% of bladder cancer (BC) cases are still muscle-invasive at first diagnosis (Zlotta et al. 2011). Screening is unproven to enable the detection of more non-muscle-invasive tumors (Zlotta et al. 2011). BC association with

© Springer Nature Switzerland AG 2020
S. S. Goonewardene et al., *Management of Non-Muscle Invasive Bladder Cancer*,
https://doi.org/10.1007/978-3-030-28646-0_15

aristolochic acid nephropathy (AAN) was reported after intake of slimming pills containing Chinese herbs (Zlotta et al. 2011). Zlotta et al. evaluated whether a BC screening protocol in a high-risk and unique patient population had an impact on the stage of tumor presentation.

BC was diagnosed in 25 patients (52%) (Zlotta et al. 2011). Among 43 patients who underwent screening cystoscopies (Zlotta et al. 2011). This demonstrated BC screening in high-risk groups may allow identification of tumors before muscle invasion (Zlotta et al. 2011). The optimal screening schedule and the relevance of the present findings in smoking-related BC remain to be defined.

Cassidy et al. identify significant predictors of initial and repeated adherence with bladder cancer screening in a high-risk occupationally exposed cohort (Cassidy et al. 2011). The study analyzed longitudinal (13 years) health survey data and a cross-sectional behavioral health survey from the Drake Health Registry Study (Cassidy et al. 2011). Construct validity of the behavioral health survey scales was evaluated using factor analysis. Initial compliance and repeated adherence were examined in separate logistic regression models (Cassidy et al. 2011). "Barriers to screening" and "social influence" were associated with initial participation. Lower or no alcohol consumption, comorbidities, worry that screening would find bladder cancer, and ease of arranging schedules were associated with continued adherence (Cassidy et al. 2011). Factors affecting adherence with bladder cancer screening change for initial participation and for continued adherence. To enhance overall adherence, specific strategies should be implemented when initiating a screening program and revised accordingly over time.

To assess the positive predictive value (PPV) of microhaematuria (μH) and visible haematuria (GH) in bladder cancer screening and the influence of haematuria on tumour tests in a prospective study (Pesch et al. 2011). While the PPV of μH for bladder cancer was low, there was a strong influence of haematuria and leukocytes on the protein-based tumour test NMP22® (Pesch et al. 2011). Erythrocytes and leukocytes should be determined at least semi-quantitatively for the interpretation of positive NMP22 test results (Pesch et al. 2011). In addition, a panel of tumour tests that includes methods not affected by the presence of erythrocytes or leukocytes such as cytology and UroVysion(TM) would improve bladder cancer screening (Pesch et al. 2011).

Bonberg et al. explore changes at chromosomes 3, 7, 17 and 9p21 in order to assess associations with bladder cancer for possible improvements of the UroVysion™ assay regarding screening (Bonberg et al. 2013). The UroVysion assay showed a reasonable performance in detecting bladder cancer in the present study population and shared positive test results with cytology, which is much cheaper (Bonberg et al. 2013). A simpler, faster and cheaper version of the UroVysion assay might rely on the very strong correlations between gains at chromosomes 3, 7 and 17, resulting in a similar performance in detecting bladder cancer with single-probe PIs compared with the full set of these probes (Bonberg et al. 2013). Loss of 9p21 was less predictive for developing bladder cancer in UroScreen (Bonberg et al. 2013).

Bladder cancer is 1 of the 10 most frequently diagnosed types of cancer. Screening could identify high-grade bladder cancer at earlier stages, when it may be more easily and effectively treated. Chou et al. (2010), updated the 2004 U.S. Preventive Services Task Force evidence review on screening for bladder cancer in adults in primary care settings (Chou et al. 2010). No randomized trials or high-quality controlled observational studies evaluated clinical outcomes associated with screening compared with no screening or treatment of screen-detected bladder cancer compared with no treatment (Chou et al. 2010). No study evaluated the sensitivity or specificity of tests for hematuria, urinary cytology, or other urinary biomarkers for bladder cancer in asymptomatic persons without a history of bladder cancer (Chou et al. 2010). The positive predictive value of screening is less than 10% in asymptomatic persons, including higher-risk populations (Chou et al. 2010). No study evaluated harms associated with treatment of screen-detected bladder cancer compared with no treatment (Chou et al. 2010).

References

Bonberg N, Taeger D, Gawrych K, Johnen G, Banek S, Schwentner C, Sievert KD, Wellhäußer H, Kluckert M, Leng G, Nasterlack M, Stenzl A, Behrens T, Brüning T, Pesch B, UroScreen Study Group. Chromosomal instability and bladder cancer: the UroVysion(TM) test in the UroScreen study. BJU Int. 2013;112(4):E372–82.

Cassidy LD, Marsh GM, Talbott EO, Kelsey SF. Initial and continued adherence with bladder cancer screening in an occupationally exposed cohort. J Occup Environ Med. 2011;53(4):455–6.

Chou R, Dana T. Screening adults for bladder cancer: a review of the evidence for the U.S. preventive services task force. Ann Intern Med. 2010;153(7):461–8.

Lané S, Catto JW, Cookson MS, Messing EM, Shariat SF, Soloway MS, Svatek RS, Lotan Y, Zlotta AR, Grossman HB. Screening for bladder cancer: rationale, limitations, whom to target, and perspectives. Eur Urol. 2013;63(6):1049–58.

Pashos CL, Botteman MF, Laskin BL, Redaelli A. Bladder cancer: epidemiology, diagnosis, and management. Cancer Pract. 2002;10(6):311–22.

Pesch B, Nasterlack M, Eberle F, Bonberg N, Taeger D, Leng G, Feil G, Johnen G, Ickstadt K, Kluckert M, Wellhäusser H, Stenzl A, Brüning T, UroScreen Group. The role of haematuria in bladder cancer screening among men with former occupational exposure to aromatic amines. BJU Int. 2011;108(4):546–52.

Schmitz-Dräger BJ, Droller M, Lokeshwar VB, Lotan Y, Hudson MA, van Rhijn BW, Marberger MJ, Fradet Y, Hemstreet GP, Malmstrom PU, Ogawa O, Karakiewicz PI, Shariat SF. Molecular markers for bladder cancer screening, early diagnosis, and surveillance: the WHO/ICUD consensus. Urol Int. 2015;94(1):1–24. https://doi.org/10.1159/000369357 Epub 2014 Dec 10.

Vickers AJ, Bennette C, Kibel AS, Black A, Izmirlian G, Stephenson AJ, Bochner B. Who should be included in a clinical trial of screening for bladder cancer?: a decision analysis of data from the Prostate, Lung, Colorectal and Ovarian Cancer Screening Trial. Cancer. 2013;119(1):143–9.

Yeung C, Dinh T, Lee J. The health economics of bladder cancer: an updated review of the published literature. Pharmacoeconomics. 2014;32(11):1093–104.

Zlotta AR, Roumeguere T, Kuk C, Alkhateeb S, Rorive S, Lemy A, van der Kwast TH, Fleshner NE, Jewett MA, Finelli A, Schulman C, Lotan Y, Shariat SF, Nortier J. Select screening in a specific high-risk population of patients suggests a stage migration toward detection of non-muscle-invasive bladder cancer. Eur Urol. 2011;59(6):1026–31.

Chapter 16
Statement of Main Findings and Specific Areas of Unmet Needs Arising from Systematic Review on Bladder Cancer Screening

This review depicts the role of screening in bladder cancer, with a focus on current screening and molecular based tests. What is clearly apparent are the lack of clinical guidelines incorporating molecular testing, despite their being a number of good quality studies present. This is something that clearly needs to be addressed further and the role in replacement of cystoscopy has yet to be determine. Research focused on improving the specificity of this marker seems to a critical focus of research in all areas, and also allows correlation to the clinical world.

Bladder cancer screening was the focus of research in all studies. This is a very sizable group, not just in the UK but through the world (Figs. 16.1 and 16.2).

Fig. 16.1 Themes identified, based on the systematic review

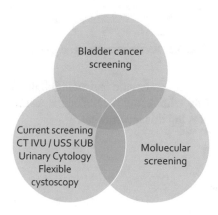

© Springer Nature Switzerland AG 2020
S. S. Goonewardene et al., *Management of Non-Muscle Invasive Bladder Cancer*,
https://doi.org/10.1007/978-3-030-28646-0_16

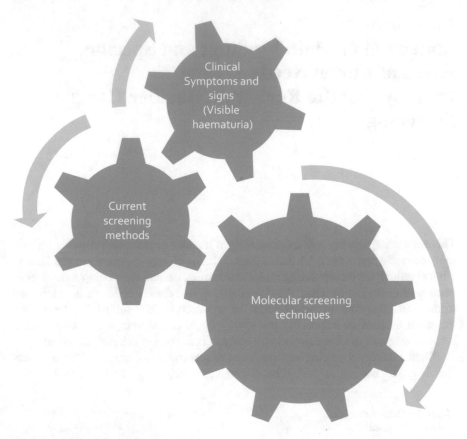

Fig. 16.2 Screening pathway components

The systematic review highlighted the requirement for a current screening pathway with a role for molecular testing. This requires further input into research to develop this area further.

Chapter 17
Usefulness of Screening in Bladder Cancer

The 2nd International Consultation on Bladder Cancer presented recommendations on the screening, diagnosis, and markers of bladder cancer (Kamat et al. 2013). This demonstrated cystoscopy alone is the most cost-effective method to detect recurrence of bladder cancer (Kamat et al. 2013). White-light cystoscopy is the gold standard for evaluation of the lower urinary tract. But to support this, technology like fluorescence-aided cystoscopy and narrow-band imaging can aid in improving evaluations (Kamat et al. 2013). Urine cytology is useful for the diagnosis of high-grade tumor recurrence (Kamat et al. 2013). Molecular medicine holds the promise that clinical outcomes will be improved by directing therapy toward the mechanisms and targets associated with the growth of an individual patient's tumor (Kamat et al. 2013).

Larré et al. reviewed the current literature regarding the usefulness and feasibility of screening for bladder cancer. There was no level 1 evidence (obtained from a randomised controlled trial [RCT]) addressing the impact of screening on survival or tumour downstaging (Larré et al. 2013). No study assessed the diagnostic performance of urinary markers in the context of screening (Larré et al. 2013). Screening is likely to be of benefit in high-risk populations using cost-efficient high-performing urinary biomarkers (Larré et al. 2013). This demonstrated screening is feasible in a high-risk population.

Bladder cancer (BC) screening is not accepted in part owing to low overall incidence (Krabbe et al. 2015).

Incidence rates were significantly higher in men than in women (Krabbe et al. 2015). Men older than 60 years with a smoking history of >30 pack years had incidence rates of more than 2/1,000 person-years, which could serve as an excellent population for screening trials (Krabbe et al. 2015). Sex differences in the incidence of Bladder Cancer cannot be readily explained by the differences in exposure to tobacco, as sex disparity persisted regardless of smoking intensity (Krabbe et al. 2015).

© Springer Nature Switzerland AG 2020
S. S. Goonewardene et al., *Management of Non-Muscle Invasive Bladder Cancer*,
https://doi.org/10.1007/978-3-030-28646-0_17

Taiwo et al., presented results of a bladder cancer screening program conducted in 18 aluminum smelters (Taiwo et al. 2015). ImmunoCyt/uCyt+ and cytology in combination demonstrated a sensitivity of 62.30%, a specificity of 92.60%, a negative predictive value of 99.90%, and a positive predictive value of 2.96% (Taiwo et al. 2015). Fourteen cases of bladder cancer were detected, and the standardized incidence ratio of bladder cancer was 1.18 (95% confidence interval, 0.65 to 1.99) (Taiwo et al. 2015). Individuals who tested positive on either test who were later determined to be cancer free had undergone expensive and invasive tests.

The prognosis of bladder cancer (BC) depends on histology, grade, and stage (Roobol et al. 2010). Patients with NMI bladder cancer (70% of the urothelial carcinomas) have a relatively good prognosis. Yet invasive, high grade bladder cancer has a poor prognosis. Patients will not survive their disease in many cases due to their metastases, despite the current available treatment options. Early detection can only be beneficial regarding mortality if the high-risk cancers are recognized and treated at a localized stage (Roobol et al. 2010).

The recently initiated [Bladder Cancer Urine Marker Project (BLU-P) evaluated a screening algorithm using next to hematuria testing, sensitive specific urine markers for bladder cancer (NMP22, FGFR3, MA analyses and MLPa) in an attempt to circumvent the high number of cystoscopies (Roobol et al. 2010). Out of 1611 patients, 23.5% tested positive for hematuria (11.6% had one or more true positive test results). The additional molecular-based screening tests before referring to cystoscopy resulted in a decrease in cystoscopies from 378 to 66 (82.5%). So far only 1 bladder cancer case was detected (Roobol et al. 2010). Further research is needed to evaluate whether this extremely low detection rate is caused by, e.g., a healthy screening bias or whether using the molecular urine tests is too strict and diagnoses are missed (Roobol et al. 2010).

Whether or not to screen also depends on exposure to risk factors. The risk level for a professional group and the latency period were selected to define a targeted screening protocol (Clin et al. 2014). The NMP22BC test, exclusive hematuria testing, and combinations of urine cytology with NMP22BC test or hematuria testing revealed a high proportion of false positive results (Clin et al. 2014).

Urine cytology is the test that offers the best specificity (Clin et al. 2014). Although poor for all bladder cancer stages and grades combined, its sensitivity is better for high grades, which require early diagnosis since late-stage cancers are of very poor prognosis (Clin et al. 2014). These results suggest that urine cytology is currently the only technique suitable for proposal within the context of a first line targeted screening strategy for occupational bladder cancer (Clin et al. 2014).

References

Clin B, "RecoCancerProf" Working Group, Pairon JC. Medical follow-up for workers exposed to bladder carcinogens: the French evidence-based and pragmatic statement. BMC Public Health. 2014;14:1155.

Kamat AM, Hegarty PK, Gee JR, Clark PE, Svatek RS, Hegarty N, Shariat SF, Xylinas E, Schmitz-Dräger BJ, Lotan Y, Jenkins LC, Droller M, van Rhijn BW, Karakiewicz PI. International consultation on urologic disease-European association of urology consultation on bladder cancer 2012. ICUD-EAU international consultation on bladder cancer 2012: screening, diagnosis, and molecular markers. Eur Urol. 2013;63(1):4–15.

Krabbe LM, Svatek RS, Shariat SF, Messing E, Lotan Y. Bladder cancer risk: use of the PLCO and NLST to identify a suitable screening cohort. Urol Oncol. 2015;33(2):65.e19–25.

Larré S, Catto JW, Cookson MS, Messing EM, Shariat SF, Soloway MS, Svatek RS, Lotan Y, Zlotta AR, Grossman HB. Screening for bladder cancer: rationale, limitations, whom to target, and perspectives. Eur Urol. 2013;63(6):1049–58.

Roobol MJ, Bangma CH, el Bouazzaoui S, Franken-Raab CG, Zwarthoff EC. Feasibility study of screening for bladder cancer with urinary molecular markers (the BLU-P project). Urol Oncol. 2010;28(6):686–90.

Taiwo OA, Slade MD, Cantley LF, Tessier-Sherman B, Galusha D, Kirsche SR, Donoghue AM, Cullen MR. Bladder cancer screening in aluminum smelter workers. J Occup Environ Med. 2015;57(4):421–7.

Part V
Techniques in Endoscopic Resection

Chapter 18
Management of Non Muscle Invasive Bladder Cancer

Bladder cancer is the 8th most common cancer with 74,000 new cases in the United States (Tan et al. 2016). Transurethral resection and intravesical treatments remain the main treatment modality. Up to 31–78% of cases recur, hightlighting the need for intensive treatment and surveillance protocols (Tan et al. 2016). This makes bladder cancer one of the most expensive cancers to manage (Tan et al. 2016).

Burger et al. (2012) presented a review summary of the Second International Consultation on Bladder Cancer recommendations on NMIBC. This highlighted urothelial cancer of the bladder staged Ta, T1, and carcinoma in situ (CIS), (NMIBC), poses demanding challenges in diagnostics and treatment. This was split into 2 groups. On the one hand, the high recurrence rate and low progression rate with Ta low-grade disease requires risk-adapted treatment and surveillance to provide care while minimizing treatment-related burden. But, the propensity of Ta high-grade, T1, and CIS to progress demands intense care and timely consideration of radical cystectomy.

The European Association of Urology (EAU) panel on Non-muscle-invasive Bladder Cancer (NMIBC) released an updated version of the guidelines on Non-muscle-invasive Bladder Cancer (Babjuk et al. 2017). Tumours staged as TaT1 or carcinoma in situ (CIS) are grouped as NMIBC (Babjuk et al. 2017). Diagnosis depends on cystoscopy and histologic evaluation of the tissue obtained by transurethral resection of the bladder (TURBT) in papillary tumours or by multiple bladder biopsies in CIS (Babjuk et al. 2017). In papillary lesions, a complete TURBT is essential for the patient's prognosis. If the initial resection is incomplete, there is no muscle in the specimen, or a high-grade or T1 tumour is detected, a second TURBT should be performed within 2–6 wk (Babjuk et al. 2017).

For patients with a low-risk tumour and intermediate-risk patients at a lower risk of recurrence, one immediate instillation of chemotherapy is recommended (Babjuk et al. 2017). Patients with an intermediate-risk tumour should receive 1 yr of full-dose bacillus Calmette-Guérin (BCG) intravesical immunotherapy

© Springer Nature Switzerland AG 2020
S. S. Goonewardene et al., *Management of Non-Muscle Invasive Bladder Cancer*,
https://doi.org/10.1007/978-3-030-28646-0_18

or instillations of chemotherapy for a maximum of 1 yr (Babjuk et al. 2017). In patients with high-risk tumours, full-dose intravesical BCG for 1–3 yr is indicated (Babjuk et al. 2017).

Non-muscle invasive bladder cancer (NMIBC) represents a considerably diverse patient group and the management of this complex disease is debatable (Power et al. 2016). Power et al. (2016), compared the NMIBC guideline recommendations from the EAU (Europe), CUA (Canada), NCCN (United States), AUA (United States), and NICE (United Kingdom). Despite a paucity of high level evidence regarding the majority of management topics in NMIBC, there was general agreement among the various guideline panels.

Although associated with an overall favorable survival rate, the heterogeneity of non-muscle invasive bladder cancer (NMIBC) affects patients' rates of recurrence and progression (Chang et al. 2016). Risk stratification should influence evaluation, treatment and surveillance (Chang et al. 2016). This guideline attempts to provide a clinical framework for the management of NMIBC (Chang et al. 2016). The intensity and scope of care for NMIBC should focus on patient, disease, and treatment response characteristics (Chang et al. 2016). This guideline attempts to improve a clinician's ability to evaluate and treat each patient, but higher quality evidence in future trials will be essential to improve level of care for these patients (Chang et al. 2016).

Treatment of these tumors has three objectives: (1) to eradicate existing disease, (2) to provide prophylaxis against tumor recurrence, and (3) to avoid deep invasion into the muscle layers of the bladder (Lum et al. 1991). Transurethral resection is the primary treatment to eradicate NMI bladder tumors, but 40–80% of these tumors recur (Lum et al. 1991). Randomized trials have shown that recurrence rates are decreased by adjuvant intravesicular pharmacotherapy with a number of drugs: bacillus Calmette-Guérin vaccine (BCG), doxorubicin, mitomycin that adjuvant intravesicular pharmacotherapy can prevent progression to invasive bladder cancer in the high-risk patient with NMI bladder cancer (Lum et al. 1991).

Bladder cancer is a complex and aggressive disease for which treatment strategies have had limited success (Apolo et al. 2015). Improvements in detection, treatment, and outcomes in bladder cancer will require the integration of multiple new approaches, including genomic profiling, immunotherapeutics, and large randomized clinical trials (Apolo et al. 2015). Efforts are underway to develop better noninvasive urine biomarkers for use in primary or secondary detection of NMIBC, exploiting our genomic knowledge of mutations in genes such as RAS, FGFR3, PIK3CA, and TP53 and methylation pathways alone or in combination (Apolo et al. 2015).

The diagnosis and the follow-up of non-muscle invasive bladder are based on flexible cystoscopy associated with urinary cytology (Pignot et al. 2011). At present time, no molecular marker, and no imaging allows to reduce the rhythm and the modalities of surveillance such as defined by the guidelines (Pignot et al. 2011). Early cystectomy is the current option for BCG-refractory high risk bladder tumor (Pignot et al. 2011).

Although the management of non invasive bladder tumours (NMIBC) has significantly improved the last years, it remains difficult to predict the heterogeneous outcome of such tumours, especially the high grade NMIBC (Wallerand 2010). Obviously, the fluorescence cystoscopy allows the detection of tumours such as carcinoma in situ more efficiently than the white light cystoscopy (Wallerand 2010). The role of prognostic markers within bladder cancer has not yet been determined, either by research or by clinical guidelines. As yet, this area in bladder cancer diagnostics remains unaddressed.

Recurrence, despite resection, of high grade NMIBC can occur. Rodriguez Faba et al. (2013), established the optimal current approach for the early diagnosis and management of non-muscle-invasive bladder cancer (NMIBC) (Rodriguez Faba et al. 2013). Good quality of TUR and the implementation of photodynamic diagnosis in selected cases provide a more accurate diagnosis and reduce the risk of residual tumor in bladder cancer. Although insufficient evidence is available to warrant the use of new urinary molecular markers in isolation, their use in conjunction with cytology and cystoscopy can improve early diagnosis and follow-up (Rodriguez Faba et al. 2013). BCG plus maintenance for at least one year remains the standard adjuvant treatment in high-risk BC.

References

Apolo AB, Vogelzang NJ, Theodorescu D. New and promising strategies in the management of bladder cancer. Am Soc Clin Oncol Educ Book. 2015:105–12.

Babjuk M, Böhle A, Burger M, Capoun O, Cohen D, Compérat EM, Hernández V, Kaasinen E, Palou J, Rouprêt M, van Rhijn BW, Shariat SF, Soukup V, Sylvester RJ, Zigeuner R. EAU guidelines on non-muscle-invasive urothelial carcinoma of the bladder: update 2016. Eur Urol. 2017;71(3):447–61.

Burger M, Oosterlinck W, Konety B, Chang S, Gudjonsson S, Pruthi R, Soloway M, Solsona E, Sved P, Babjuk M, Brausi MA, Cheng C, Comperat E, Dinney C, Otto W, Shah J, Thürof J, Witjes JA. International consultation on urologic disease-European association of urology consultation on bladder cancer 2012. ICUD-EAU International consultation on bladder cancer 2012: non-muscle-invasive urothelial carcinoma of the bladder. Eur Urol. 2013;63(1):36–44.

Chang SS, Boorjian SA, Chou R, Clark PE, Daneshmand S, Konety BR, Pruthi R, et al. Diagnosis and treatment of non-muscle invasive bladder cancer: Aua/Suo guideline. J Urol. 2016;196(4):1021–9.

Lum BL, Torti FM. Adjuvant intravesicular pharmacotherapy for NMI bladder cancer. J Natl Cancer Inst. 1991;83(10):682–94.

Pignot G, Irani J, Bastide C, Ravery V. New concepts in management of NMIBC in 2010. Prog Urol. 2011;21(Suppl. 2):S34–7.

Power NE, Izawa J. Comparison of guidelines on non-muscle invasive bladder cancer (EAU, CUA, AUA, NCCN, NICE). Bladder Cancer. 2016;2(1):27–36.

Rodriguez Faba O, Gaya JM, López JM, Capell M, De Gracia-Nieto AE, Gómez Correa E, Breda A, Palou J. Current management of non-muscle-invasive bladder cancer. Minerva Med. 2013;104(3):273–86.

Tan WS, Rodney S, Lamb B, Feneley M, Kelly J. Management of non-muscle invasive bladder cancer: a comprehensive analysis of guidelines from the United States, Europe and Asia. Cancer Treat Rev. 2016;47:22–31.

Wallerand H. Management of non invasive bladder tumours (NMIBC). Bull Cancer. 2010;97 (Suppl. Cancer de la vessie):11–7.

Chapter 19
A New Technique—En Bloc Resection of Bladder Tumours

Currently, transurethral resection of a bladder tumor (TUR) is the gold standard treatment for non-muscle invasive bladder cancer (NMIBC) (Alyaev et al. 2018). The standard non-muscle invasive bladder cancer (NMIBC) endoscopic diagnosis suffers from the frequently unsatisfactory white light evaluation accuracy leading to residual lesions being left behind (Geavlete et al. 2013).

Monopolar transurethral resection of bladder tumors (TURBT) is marked by a substantial morbidity rate. Standard TURBT for a bladder wall tumor has a high recurrence rate, which is caused mainly by malignant cell implantation during the surgery (Alyaev et al. 2018). The non-conformity of the standard TURBT with the established oncological principle of dissecting through normal tissue prompted a review of optimal surgical modality (Alyaev et al. 2018).

Small size tumors (under 1 cm) are feasible for "en bloc" resection (Geavlete et al. 2013). Bipolar TURBT has challenged the gold-standard status of monopolar resection due to the reduced complication rates, and a lower rate of TURBT syndrome. En-bloc resection of the bladder wall tumor has been proposed as an alternative method for surgical management of NMIBC.

The en-bloc technique involves the resection of bladder tumor through the underlying muscle layer as a single piece thus providing high quality material for subsequent morphological study and reducing the risk of metastasizing by implantation of malignant cells (Alyaev et al. 2018). The overall conclusion is that en-bloc resection provides an adequate tissue specimen for pathology, including the detrusor muscle for accurate staging and grading.

The "en bloc" resection of small size or thin pedicle tumors provides the conditions for avoiding tumoral tissue scattering and smashing (Geavlete et al. 2013). In contrast, bipolar resection is characterized by decreased perioperative bleeding risks and faster patient recovery. Having in mind the various modalities of ameliorating the bladder cancer diagnostic and treatment, NMIBC management should be tailored in accordance with the particularities of each case.

© Springer Nature Switzerland AG 2020
S. S. Goonewardene et al., *Management of Non-Muscle Invasive Bladder Cancer*,
https://doi.org/10.1007/978-3-030-28646-0_19

References

Alyaev YG, Rapoport LM, Vinarov AZ, Sorokin NI, Dymov AM, Kislyakov DA, Afanasyevskaya EV, Lekarev VY. En-bloc laser resection of the urinary bladder tumor. Urologiia. 2018;2:147–53.

Geavlete B, Stănescu F, Moldoveanu C, Jecu M, Adou L, Bulai C, Ene C, Geavlete P. NBI cystoscopy and bipolar electrosurgery in NMIBC management-an overview of daily practice. J Med Life. 2013;6(2):140–5.

Chapter 20
Prognostic Factors for Endoscopic Resection in NMIBC

Adjuvant diagnostic and therapeutic procedures reduce the risk of recurrence and progression in high-risk non-muscle-invasive bladder cancer (NMIBC) (Poletajew et al. 2018). However indications and oncological outcomes are varied. Poletajew et al. (2018), reviewed therapeutic decisions in primary high-risk NMIBC and adherence to clinical guidelines in this field. The strongest predictive factor for restaging TURBT was G3 or high-grade cancer (RR 1.68, $p < 0.01$), if recieving BCG therapy it was carcinoma in situ (RR 3.20, $p = 0.01$), for immediate cystectomy it was stage T1 tumor (RR 3.71, $p < 0.01$), for no additional procedures it was G2 or low-grade cancer (RR 2.18, $p < 0.01$). Clinical management of patients with high-risk NMIBC is suboptimal and not standardized. Standardisation will enable the field to evolve and develop and also further patient care.

On average 20–30% of patients with non muscle-invasive bladder cancer will subsequently develop muscle-invasive disease with approximately 50% of the patients already bearing occult regional or distant metastases at that time (Merseburger et al. 2008). Few interdisciplinary centres are demonstrating multimodality bladder sparing approaches as equally effective when compared with radical cystectomy for muscle-invasive bladder cancer. So far no investigation could demonstrate prospective controlled data on long-term oncologic and functional outcomes comparing bladder-conserving strategies with radical cystectomy. Without prospective controlled trials evaluating the long-term oncological results and the health-related quality of life for the multimodality treatment regimen for muscle-invasive bladder cancer, the radical surgical approach should still be considered as the standard treatment (Merseburger et al. 2008). Multimodality bladder preserving strategies might be a therapeutic option for carefully selected patients.

© Springer Nature Switzerland AG 2020
S. S. Goonewardene et al., *Management of Non-Muscle Invasive Bladder Cancer*,
https://doi.org/10.1007/978-3-030-28646-0_20

References

Merseburger AS, Matuschek I, Kuczyk MA. Bladder preserving strategies for muscle-invasive bladder cancer. Curr Opin Urol. 2008;18(5):513–8.

Poletajew S, Biernacki R, Buraczynski P, Chojnacki J, Czarniecki S, Gajewska D, Pohaba T, Sondka-Migdalska J, Skrzypczyk M, Suchojad T, Wojtkowiak D, Zaforemski B, Zapala L, Zemla A, Radziszewski P. Predictors and prognostic implications of clinical decisions in patients with primary high-risk non-muscle-invasive bladder cancer–results of a cross country retrospective study. Neoplasma. 2018;65(1):147–52.

Chapter 21
NMIBC and Oncological Outcomes from Endoscopic Resection

Leliveld et al. evaluated high risk non muscle invasive bladder cancer (NMIBC) and assessed factors associated with treatment, recurrence and progression free survival rates (Leliveld et al. 2011). 74/412 (18%) patients with high risk NMIBC underwent a transurethral resection (TURBT). Adjuvant treatment after TURBT was performed in 90.7% in teaching hospitals versus 71.8% in non-teaching hospitals ($p<0.001$) (Leliveld et al. 2011). Recurrence occurred in 191/392 (49%). Progression occured in 84/392 (21.4%) of patients. The mean 5-years progression free survival was 71.6% (95% CI 65.5–76.8). In this pattern of care study in high risk NMIBC, 18% of the patients were treated with TURBT as single treatment (Leliveld et al. 2011). Age and treatment in non-teaching hospitals were associated with less adjuvant treatment post op. None of the variables sex, age, comorbidity, hospital type, stage and year of treatment was associated with 5-year recurrence or progression rates.

On average 20–30% of patients with non muscle-invasive bladder cancer will develop muscle-invasive disease with approximately 50% already having regional or distant metastases (Merseburger et al. 2008). Few interdisciplinary centres are demonstrating multimodality bladder sparing approaches as equally effective when compared with radical cystectomy for muscle-invasive bladder cancer (Merseburger et al. 2008). Multimodality treatment regimens including a thoroughly performed en-bloc resection of the bladder tumour, external beam radiation therapy, and chemotherapy. Whilst more expensive, in appropriately selected patients this can lead to curative oncological outcomes. Without prospective controlled trials evaluating the long-term oncological results and the health-related quality of life for the multimodality treatment regimen for muscle-invasive bladder cancer, the radical surgical approach should still be considered as the standard treatment (Merseburger et al. 2008). Multimodality bladder preserving strategies might be a therapeutic option for carefully selected patients, who are not fit for radical therapies.

© Springer Nature Switzerland AG 2020

S. S. Goonewardene et al., *Management of Non-Muscle Invasive Bladder Cancer*,
https://doi.org/10.1007/978-3-030-28646-0_21

References

Leliveld AM, Bastiaannet E, Doornweerd BH, Schaapveld M, de Jong IJ. High risk bladder cancer: current management and survival. Int Braz J Urol. 2011;37(2):203–10.

Merseburger AS, Matuschek I, Kuczyk MA. Bladder preserving strategies for muscle-invasive bladder cancer. Curr Opin Urol. 2008;18(5):513–8.

Chapter 22
Recurrence in NMIBC

European Association of Urology (EAU) guidelines recommend a follow-up transurethral resection of bladder tumors (reTUR-B) for intermediate and high-risk non-muscle invasive bladder cancer (NMIBC) 2–6 weeks after the initial resection (Merseburger et al. 2008). Management of high-risk non-muscle invasive bladder cancer (NMIBC) is challenging. It is vital to detect recurrences early and predict which tumors are likely to progress (Merseburger et al. 2008). Merseburger reviewed was risk factors for recurrence and progression and approaches including pathological aspects of NMIBC, methods for tumor visualization, urine cytology, urinary molecular markers, scoring systems and nomograms (Merseburger et al. 2008). Clinical and pathological factors are predictive of recurrence and progression. However, genomic information such as molecular subtyping may improve understanding of prognosis (Merseburger et al. 2008). White light cystoscopy is still a dominant approach but enhanced cystoscopy is likely superior for detection of cancer especially carcinoma in situ (Merseburger et al. 2008). Urinary biomarkers are evolving; however, they are not ready to replace cystoscopy and trials are still necessary to determine optimal clinical utility (Merseburger et al. 2008). Prognostic scoring systems and nomograms are available for counseling the patients but there is room to improve predictive accuracy.

Luján et al. (2014) studied new mathematical models for NMIBC—biological characteristics enabling accurate risk estimation of multiple recurrence and tumor progression. 468 (48.8%) patients developed at least one tumor recurrence and tumor progression was reported in 52 (5.4%) patients (Luján et al. 2014). Variables for multiple-recurrence risk awere found to be: age, grade, number, size, treatment and the number of prior recurrences. All these together with age, stage and grade are the variables for progression risk. The high concordance reported besides to the validation process in external source, allow accurate multi-recurrence/progression risk estimation.

Hartinger et al. reviewed parameters for residual tumor in re-resection TURBT and evaluated the prognostic value (Hartinger et al. 2013). A total number of 555

© Springer Nature Switzerland AG 2020   121
S. S. Goonewardene et al., *Management of Non-Muscle Invasive Bladder Cancer*,
https://doi.org/10.1007/978-3-030-28646-0_22

operations were carried out and 179 patients received re-resection TURBT as per EAU guidelines. Age ($p=0.8$), sex ($p=0.7$), initial staging ($p=0.2$), initial grading ($p=0.3$) and surgeon's level of training ($p=0.7$) did not have an impact on the rate of residual tumor (Hartinger et al. 2013). Tumors categorized as high risk according to the EAU risk score in initial TURBT ($p<0.01$) and multifocality ($p=0.01$) were associated with significantly higher rates of residual tumor (Hartinger et al. 2013). Re-resection is strongly indicated in high risk bladder tumors as well as multifocal tumors showing a significantly increased residual tumor rate (Hartinger et al. 2013).

Busato Júnior et al. (2016) evaluated the validation of European Organization for Research and Treatment of Cancer (EORTC) risk tables to predict progression in non-muscle-invasive bladder cancer (NMIBC). Progression to muscle-invasive disease occurred in 42 patients (20.5%) (Busato Júnior et al. 2016). Significant characteristics related to progression were male gender, pT1 stage, lesion size ≥3 cm, high grade of disease, and no combined intravesical therapy (Busato Júnior et al. 2016). 1- and 5-year progression rates were lower than the values predicted by EORTC risk tables, mainly in high-risk groups.

References

Busato Júnior WF, Almeida GL, Ribas CA, Ribas Filho JM, De Cobelli O. EORTC risk model to predict progression in patients with non-muscle-invasive bladder cancer: is it safe to use in clinical practice? Clin Genitourin Cancer. 2016;14(2):176–82.

Hartinger J, Häußermann R, Olbert P, Hofmann R, Hegele A. Predictors for presence of residual tumor in follow-up transurethral resection of bladder tumors: single center results. Urologe A. 2013;52(4):557–61.

Luján S, Santamaría C, Pontones JL, Ruiz-Cerdá JL, Trassierra M, Vera-Donoso CD, Solsona E, Jiménez-Cruz F. Risk estimation of multiple recurrence and progression of non muscle invasive bladder carcinoma using new mathematical models. Actas Urol Esp. 2014;38(10):647–54.

Merseburger AS, Matuschek I, Kuczyk MA. Bladder preserving strategies for muscle-invasive bladder cancer. Curr Opin Urol. 2008;18(5):513–8.

Chapter 23
Definitive Treatment in NMIBC

Despite the good quality of treatment expected with optimized transurethral resection (TUR) and adjuvant Bacillus Calmette-Guérin (BCG) regimen, many high-risk non-muscle invasive bladder cancer (NMIBC) patients recur and progress (Colombo et al. 2013). According to the EORTC Tables of risk, cases with a score of 10–17 and those with a score of 7–23 are at high risk of recurrence and progression. AUA consider all T1 stage tumors, high grade Ta and CIS at high risk of recurrence and progression. Long-term follow-up demonstrates T1, G3 patients treated with BCG have up to 45% and 17% rate of recurrence and progression, respectively (Colombo et al. 2013). Consequently, EAU, AUA and NCCN Guidelines for bladder cancer recommend radical cystectomy as a first treatment option for those patients who failed after two cycles of adjuvant BCG. Yet there is no an early radical cystectomy is better than any additional salvage strategy, in terms of oncologic outcome. On the other hand, it is well accepted that radical cystectomy is burdened with consistent reduction of overall post-operative quality of life (Colombo et al. 2013). The reluctance to accept extirpative surgery may explain the reduced disease-free survival rate, when radical cystectomy has been extremely delayed (Colombo et al. 2013).

Recently, clinical, laboratory and pathologic acquisitions allowed the development of more accurate predictive factors for tumor progression in NMIBC (Colombo et al. 2013). Among these factors, clinical type of BCG-failure, morphology and tumor growth patterns, pathologic sub-staging is an aid in treatment decision making.

The optimal time of cystectomy for non-muscle invasive bladder cancer (NMIBC) is controversial. Ali- El-Dein compared cancer-specific survival in primary versus deferred cystectomy for T1 bladder cancer (Ali-El-Dein et al. 2011). Primary cystectomy at the diagnosis of NMIBC was performed in 134 patients (group 1) and deferred cystectomy was done after failed conservative treatment in 70 (group 2). Although the 3-year (84% in group 1 vs. 79% in group 2), 5-year (78% vs. 71%) and 10-year (69% vs. 64%) cancer-specific survival rates were

© Springer Nature Switzerland AG 2020
S. S. Goonewardene et al., *Management of Non-Muscle Invasive Bladder Cancer*,
https://doi.org/10.1007/978-3-030-28646-0_23

lower in the deferred cystectomy group. This was not statistically significant. In group 2, survival was significantly lower in cases undergoing >3 TURBTs than in cases with fewer TURBTs (Ali-El-Dein et al. 2011). Cancer-specific survival is statistically comparable for primary and deferred cystectomy in T1 bladder cancer, although there is a non-significant difference in favor of primary cystectomy.

Non-muscle invasive bladder cancer (NMIBC) comprises about 70% of all newly diagnosed bladder cancer, and includes tumors with stage Ta, T1 and carcinoma in situ (CIS.) Since, NMIBC patients with progression to muscle-invasive disease tend to have worse prognosis than with patients with primary muscle-invasive disease, there is a need to significantly improve risk stratification and earlier definitive treatment for high-risk NMIBC. The most important prognostic factor for progression is grade of tumor. T category, tumor size, number of tumors, concurrent CIS, intravesical therapy, response to bacillus Calmette-Guerin at 3- or 6-month follow-up, prior recurrence rate, age, gender, lymphovascular invasion and depth of lamina propria invasion are other important clinical and pathological parameters to predict recurrence and progression in patients with NMIBC (Isharwal and Konety 2015). The European Organization for Research and Treatment of Cancer (EORTC) risk tables is the best-established predictive models for recurrence and progression risk calculation (Isharwal and Konety 2015). Molecular biomarkers such as Ki-67, FGFR3 and p53 appear to be promising in predicting recurrence and progression but need further validation prior to using them in clinical practice. Future research should focus on enhancing the predictive accuracy of risk assessment tools by incorporating additional prognostic factors such as depth of lamina propria invasion and molecular biomarkers after rigorous validation in multi-institutional cohorts.

References

Ali-El-Dein B, Al-Marhoon MS, Abdel-Latif M, Mesbah A, Shaaban AA, Nabeeh A, Ibrahiem el-HI. Survival after primary and deferred cystectomy for stage T1 transitional cell carcinoma of the bladder. Urol Ann. 2011;3(3):127–32.

Colombo R, Maccagnano C, Rocchini L, Pellucchi F. When the conservative treatment in high-risk non-muscle invasive bladder cancer patients should be abandoned. Urologia. 2013;80(Suppl. 21):48–52.

Isharwal S, Konety B. Non-muscle invasive bladder cancer risk stratification. Indian J Urol. 2015;31(4):289–96.

Chapter 24
A Systematic Review of En-Bloc Resection

A systematic review relating to bladder cancer and en-bloc resection was conducted. This was to identify references relating to bladder cancer and en-bloc resection. The search strategy aimed to identify all references related to bladder cancer AND En-bloc resection. Search terms used were as follows: (Bladder cancer) AND (en-bloc). The following databases were screened from 1989 to June 2019:

- CINAHL
- MEDLINE (NHS Evidence)
- Cochrane
- AMed
- EMBASE
- PsychINFO
- SCOPUS
- Web of Science.

In addition, searches using Medical Subject Headings (MeSH) and keywords were conducted using Cochrane databases. Two UK-based experts in bladder cancer were consulted to identify any additional studies.

Studies were eligible for inclusion if they reported primary research focusing on bladder cancer and en- bloc resection. Papers were included if published after 1984 and had to be in English. Studies that did not conform to this were excluded. Only primary research was included. The overall aim was to identify the role of en-bloc resection in bladder tumour resection.

Abstracts were independently screened for eligibility by two reviewers and disagreements resolved through discussion or third party opinion. Agreement level was calculated using Cohen's Kappa to test the intercoder reliability of this screening process. Cohen's Kappa allows comparison of inter-rater reliability between papers using relative observed agreement. This also takes account of

© Springer Nature Switzerland AG 2020   125
S. S. Goonewardene et al., *Management of Non-Muscle Invasive Bladder Cancer*,
https://doi.org/10.1007/978-3-030-28646-0_24

the comparison occurring by chance. The first reviewer agreed all 24 papers to be included, the second, agreed on 24.

Data extraction was piloted by the researcher and amended in consultation with the research team (author and two academic supervisors). Data collected included authors, year and country of publication, study aims, setting, intervention aims, number of participants, study design, intervention components and delivery methods, comparison groups and outcome measures, notes and follow-up questions for the authors. Studies were quality assessed using the PRISMA criteria for randomised controlled trials, Mays et al. (Moher et al. 2009; Moher, Liberati et al. 2009, 154, 153; Mays et al. 2005) for the action research and qualitative studies and the Critical Skills Appraisal programme for cohort studies. This was also applied to randomised controlled trials and qualitative studies.

The search identified 24 papers (Fig. 24.1). All 24 mapped to the search terms and eligibility criteria. The current systematic reviews were examined to gain further knowledge about the subject. 366 papers were excluded due to not conforming to eligibility criteria or adding to the evidence for bladder cancer screening. Of the 366 papers left, relevant abstracts were identified and the full papers obtained (all of which were in English), to quality assure against criteria. There was one case report, 22 cohort studies and one prospective clinical trial. There was considerable heterogeneity of design among the included studies therefore a narrative review of the evidence was undertaken. There was significant heterogeneity within studies, including clinical topic, numbers, outcomes, as a results a narrative review was thought to be best.

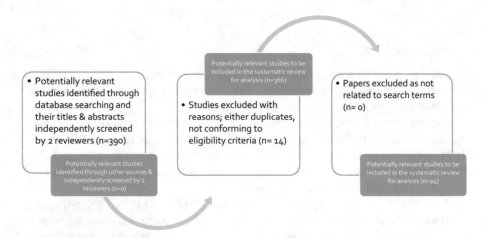

Fig. 24.1 Flow chart of studies identified through the systematic review (adapted from PRISMA)

References

Mays N, Pope C, Popay J. Systematically reviewing qualitative and quantitative evidence to inform management and policy-making in the health field. J Health Serv Res Policy. 2005;10(Suppl. 1):6–20.

Moher D, Liberati A, Tetzlaff J, Altman DG. Preferred Reporting Items for systematic reviews and meta-analyses: the prisma statement. BMJ (Online). 2009;339(7716):332–36.

Chapter 25
Systematic Review—Results from En-Bloc Resection of Bladder Cancer

25.1 Technique of En-Bloc Resection

Bladder cancer is the second most common malignancy of the urinary tract and the 9th worldwide. Seventy-five percent are non-muscle invasive and 25% are muscle invasive (Islas-García et al. 2016). Islas-García et al. (2016) describe enbloc resection with a Hybrid Knife(®) as an alternative treatment for nonmuscle invasive bladder tumours (Islas-García et al. 2016). This procedure minimises bleeding, gives surgical vision and minimises the risk of bladder perforation and tumour implants (Islas-García et al. 2016). It also allows determination of margin status, vascular infiltration and bladder muscle invasion in the histopathology assessment (Islas-García et al. 2016).

Zhang evaluated the safety of retrograde en bloc resection of bladder tumor (RERBT) compared with conventional monopolar resection for NMI bladder tumors (Zhang et al. 2017a, b). In the RERBT group, the tumors were en bloc removed retrogradely using a conventional monopolar electrode. Of the 90 patients, 40 underwent RERBT and 50 underwent TURBT. The cumulative recurrence rates were similar. Detrusor muscle could be identified pathologically in 100% of RERBT tumor specimens and the biopsy of tumor bases, but only in 54% and 70%, respectively, of TURBT samples ($p<0.01$) (Zhang et al. 2017a, b). The RERBT technique is feasible and safe for NMI bladder tumors using conventional monopolar resection setting, with the advantages of adequate tumor resection and the ability to collect good quality tumor specimens for pathological diagnosis and staging compared to conventional TURBT.

Lodde evaluated the feasibility and safety of transurethral en bloc resection of bladder tumors using a flat loop (Lodde et al. 2003). In 37 patients, 62 lesions were removed using a flat loop to perform the en bloc technique. This method was found to be safe to perform in the case of papillary tumors with a diameter of up to 25 mm and that are found in specific areas of the bladder (Lodde et al. 2003).

© Springer Nature Switzerland AG 2020   129
S. S. Goonewardene et al., *Management of Non-Muscle Invasive Bladder Cancer*,
https://doi.org/10.1007/978-3-030-28646-0_25

Excellent pathologic evaluation of the grade and stage of the removed specimen is possible (Lodde et al. 2003).

25.2 Conventional Versus En-Bloc Resection in Non-Muscle Invasive Bladder Cancer

Conventional, transurethral resection of bladder tumor (TURBT) encompasses systematic resection of the tumor but has a very high recurrence rate (Sureka et al. 2014). Part of this maybe due to pathology of disease. Sureka evaluated the outcome of en-bloc TURBT (ET) in comparison with conventional TURBT (CT) in non-muscle invasive bladder carcinoma in terms of recurrence and progression (Sureka et al. 2014). A total of 21 patients of ET were compared with 24 patients of CT. There was a significant reduction in the recurrence rate and time to recurrence with ET. Rate of progression was also relatively less with ET, though not statistically significant (Sureka et al. 2014). This highlights the impact of en-bloc resection in NMIBC.

25.3 En-Bloc Resection and Oncological Outcomes

Transurethral resection of bladder tumor (TURBT) using a wire loop is considered the gold standard for staging and treating non-muscle invasive bladder cancer (NMIBC). Zhang et al. (2018) evaluated the safety and efficacy of the bipolar button electrode for en bloc resection of NMIBC (2018). A total of 118 neoplasms were removed en bloc from 82 patients. No complications were encountered. The bladder detrusor muscle layer was provided in all cases (Zhang et al. 2018). The 18-month recurrence-free survival was 88.5% (23/26) and 74.5% (38/51) for Ta and T1 patients, respectively. The current results demonstrated that transurethral en bloc resection with bipolar button electrode is an effective, feasible, and safe treatment for NMIBC.

Hurle, described an "en bloc" technique, assessed the quality of resection, and reported oncological outcomes (Hurle et al. 2016). Of 87 enrolled patients, 2 were nonurothelial carcinoma and 11 were muscle invasive bladder carcinoma at the definitive pathology (Hurle et al. 2016). The study cohort consisted of 74 transitional cell carcinoma NMIBC cases. The 2-year recurrence-free survival was 85.59%. All resections had muscle. The recurrence rate at the first follow-up cystoscopy (3 months) was 5.4% (4/74) (Hurle et al. 2016). An extraperitoneal perforation occurred in one case. At multivariable analysis, only gender and the presence of carcinoma in situ were independent predictors of recurrence. The mid-term follow-up and the absence of a control group are the main limitations (Hurle et al. 2016). This demonstrated the feasibility and safety of en bloc resection of bladder tumor, with a recurrence-free survival of 85% after 2 years.

25.4 Pathological Staging and En-Bloc Resection

Detrusor muscle in primary transurethral resection of the bladder tumor (TURBT) may not be found in up to 50% of the cases (Upadhyay et al. 2012). Upadhyay et al. (2012) assessed detrusor muscle on en-bloc TURBT using a conventional electrocautery loop (Upadhyay et al. 2012). 2–4 cm en-bloc TURBT, were compared with conventional resection for presence of muscle (Upadhyay et al. 2012). The conventional electrocautery loop was bent to 45° and the whole tumor was resected en bloc (Upadhyay et al. 2012). There were no perforations. Twenty of 21 (94.4%) en-bloc resections had detrusor muscle compared to 15 of 25 (60%) in the control arm (p 0.001) (Upadhyay et al. 2012). This demonstrates En-bloc TURBT is safe and gives well-controlled resection of the whole tumor (Upadhyay et al. 2012). Yield of detrusor muscle present in the specimen is significantly better with en-bloc TURBT (Upadhyay et al. 2012).

Ukai et al. (2010) demonstrated the usefulness of transurethral resection in one piece as an accurate pathological staging tool for bladder tumour (Ukai et al. 2010). Portions of muscularis propria were identified beneath the tumor base in the specimens of 80 (82%) patients (Ukai et al. 2010). In seven (7%) patients, the tumours had a deep resection margin positive for carcinoma and were ambiguously staged as "pT1 or higher" or "pT2 or higher". Thus, definite pathological staging of specimens was possible in 90 (93%) patients (pTa, 30; pT1, 58; pT2, 2) (Ukai et al. 2010). An accurate pathological stage can be assigned to the specimen when resected in one piece in most bladder cancer patients.

Naselli et al. assessed safety and efficacy, pathological assessment and recurrence rate, of en bloc transurethral resection (EBTUR) (Naselli and Puppo 2017). Overall, 895 patients underwent EBTUR, accounting for 1191 lesions. Forty complications (4%) were recorded. Only 10 (1%) were grade III, mostly bladder perforation or bleeding (Naselli and Puppo 2017). Fifty-nine conversions (6.5%) to conventional transurethral resection (TUR) have been reported because of difficult locations of tumors or failure to extract the specimen (Naselli and Puppo 2017). Overall, 731 (96%) cases with detrusor muscle were computed (Naselli and Puppo 2017). Recurrence rate varied from 6 to 55%. Most of the recurrence occurred outside primary tumor site. Mean weighted follow-up across all series was 20 months, whereas overall recurrence rate was 23% (Naselli and Puppo 2017). Irrespective of the technique adopted, EBTUR is a safe procedure. The presence of detrusor muscle in the specimen is high if compared with historical series of conventional TUR (Naselli and Puppo 2017). Indeed, recurrence rate is comparable.

25.5 The Vela Laser and En-Bloc Resection

Xu evaluated the safety and efficacy of 1.9 μm Vela laser in treatment of primary non-muscle-invasive bladder cancer (Xu et al. 2018). En bloc transurethral resection with 1.9 μm Vela laser ($n = 26$) or conventional transurethral resection ($n = 44$)

were analyzed retrospectively. The 1.9 μm Vela laser obtained a higher rate of specimens meeting pathologic assessment requirements for staging compared with
conventional transurethral resection of bladder tumor (Xu et al. 2018). No obturator nerve reflex and bladder perforation occurred during surgery in the 1.9 μm
Vela laser group. However, 7 in the conventional transurethral resection of bladder
tumor group encountered obturator nerve reflex, and 3 of these encountered bladder
perforation ($p < 0.05$) (Xu et al. 2018). There was no significant difference in the
overall recurrence rate between the 2 groups. En bloc transurethral resection with
1.9 μm Vela laser highlights a reduction in intraoperative complications, improving
the quality of the specimens admitted for pathologic assessment, and shortening the
duration of postoperative continuous bladder irrigation (Xu et al. 2018).

Zhang et al. evaluated the safety and efficacy of the Vela laser for en bloc resection of papillary bladder tumors (Zhang et al. 2017a, b). 38 patients underwent
en bloc resection with the Vela laser and a 26F continuous flow resectoscope or
18F flexible cystoscope. The en bloc resection of all tumors was successful, with
2 cases located at the bladder dome requiring the use of a flexible cystoscope for
better management (Zhang et al. 2017a, b). No complications were encountered.
All resected tumors were intact with the detrusor muscle layer and architecture
available for pathologic evaluation. One patient with stage T2b tumor underwent
laparoscopic cystectomy 1 week after the initial surgery. At a median follow-up
period of 21.8 months, the recurrence rate at 12 months was 21.6% (8 of 37). This
demonstrated the Vela laser is an effective, feasible, and safe thulium laser for en
bloc bladder tumor resection (Zhang et al. 2017a, b). It was associated with negligible complications and allows accurate pathologic evaluation. The Vela laser can
serve as an alternative treatment method for nonmuscle-invasive bladder cancer or
infiltrating tumor.

25.6   Holmium Laser and En-Bloc Resection

D'Souza and D'Souza (2016), compared the safety and efficiency of conventional
monopolar and holmium laser *en bloc* transurethral resection of bladder tumor
(CM-TURBT and HoL-EBRBT) while managing primary nonmuscle-invasive
bladder cancer (D'Souza and D'Souza 2016). Patient demographics and tumor
characteristics in both groups were compared before surgery. There was no significant difference in operative duration among the groups. Compared with the
CM-TURBT group, HoL-EBRBT group had less intraoperative and postoperative complications, including obturator nerve reflex ($p < 0.01$), bladder perforation ($p < 0.01$), as well as bleeding and postoperative bladder irritation ($p < 0.01$)
(D'Souza and D'Souza 2016). There were no significant differences among the
two groups in the transfusion rate and occurrence of urethral strictures. Patients
in the HoL-EBRBT group had less catheterization and hospitalization time than
those in the CM-TURBT group ($p < 0.01$), and there were no significant differences in each risk subgroup as well as the overall recurrence rate among the

CM-TURBT and HoL-EBRBT groups (D'Souza and D'Souza 2016). HoL-EBRBT might prove to be preferable alternatives to CM-TURBT management of nonmuscle-invasive bladder cancer. HoL-EBRBT however did not demonstrate an obvious advantage over CM-TURBT in tumor recurrence rate.

Transurethral en bloc resection of bladder tumors is desirable for evaluating the pathological depth of bladder tumors in resected specimens (Saito 2001). The safety, technique and effectiveness of en bloc resection of bladder tumors was investigated using a holmium laser or knife electrode (Saito 2001). A total of 35 patients with transitional cell carcinoma of various sizes underwent transurethral en bloc resection with the muscle layer by holmium laser or knife electrode. The holmium laser was used for tumors at the bladder neck, as in prostate resection, while tumors at the bladder wall were treated with a knife electrode (Saito 2001). A circular incision was made around the tumor, followed by level incisions beneath it with subsequent tumor retrieval. The circular incision connected marks made about 10 mm. away from the tumor edge and continued until the NMI muscle layer was visualized (Saito 2001). The resected 1 piece specimen was grasped with a loop electrode and retrieved. This technique has been used in 35 consecutive patients (50 lesions). Tissue slides crossing the center of the tumor correctly determined the depth of cancer invasion as stages pTa to pT2. No uncontrollable bleeding, perforation or other serious complications occurred. Transurethral en bloc resection is a safe and useful technique that also provides sufficient material for pathological evaluation (Saito 2001).

25.7   En-Bloc Resection Using an Endoscopic Snare Resection

Transurethral resection of bladder tumor (TURBT) is the standard of care for initial bladder tumor management (Maurice et al. 2012). Maurice et al. (2012) reviewed the endoscopic snare resection of bladder tumor (ESRBT). Eleven tumors managed by ESRBT were reviewed retrospectively. Via cystoscopy, tumors were resected en bloc with an electrosurgical polypectomy snare and retrieved transurethrally (Maurice et al. 2012). There were no intraoperative or postoperative complications (mean follow-up: 17 mos; range 10–25 mos). ESRBT is a feasible technique for the resection of pedunculated bladder tumors (Maurice et al. 2012). It offers evident and theoretical advantages over TURBT and may augment bladder tumor management. Further study is needed.

25.8   Thuliam Laser and En-Bloc Resection

Migliari et al. (2015), evaluated if thulium laser enucleation of bladder tumor (ThuLEBT) allows improvements over monopolar resection (Migliari et al. 2015). Mean tumor diameter in the ThuLEBT group was 2.5 cm (range 0.5–4.5).

Re-resection and cold cup biopsy (in 90 days) were negative for bladder cancer (BC) persistence or recurrence with ThuLEBT. In the monopolar group seven patients were found with disease persistence (Migliari et al. 2015). No patient in the laser group experienced obturator nerve kick and no bladder perforation occurred; when involved, ureteral meatus was sharply excised without distortion (Migliari et al. 2015). ThuLEBT may represent a potential alternative to TURB-T, which nowadays is considered the standard for diagnosis and treatment of NMIBC. ThuLEBT allowed accurate reporting of neoplastic depth invasion, suggesting the possibility to avoid a second-look (Migliari et al. 2015).

Muto et al. (2014) determined whether thulium-yttrium-aluminum-garnet laser resection of bladder tumor (TmLRBT) may offer advantages over classic resection (Muto et al. 2014). Pathology reported urothelial carcinoma with Ta low grade in 31 patients (56.4%), T1 high grade in 18 (32.7%), and T2 high grade in 6 (10.9%). Detrusor was present in all (Muto et al. 2014). In a case of T1 G3, endoscopic re-evaluation showed a focal infiltration of the bladder detrusor, so the patient underwent radical cystectomy. The recurrence rate with NMI disease is 14.5%. All recurrences were outside the site of first resection, and there was no progression in tumor grade (Muto et al. 2014). TmLRBT is a simple method that seems to overcome the "incise and scatter" problem associated with traditional transurethral resection of bladder tumor (Muto et al. 2014).

Exact pathological staging of bladder cancer is crucial for further treatment (Wolters et al. 2011). One rate limiting factor is the 'incise and scatter' effect with conventional TURBT that can impact on tumour recurrence (Wolters et al. 2011). En bloc resection techniques are en emerging issue. Wolters presented initial results with Thulium:YAG (Tm:YAG) en bloc resection of bladder tumours for treatment and accurate staging (Wolters et al. 2011). Pathological evaluation revealed 1 patient with pTa G1, 2 patients with pTa G2 and 3 patients with pT1 G3. All of the resected specimens provided detrusor muscle, and all biopsies were positive for muscle cells (Wolters et al. 2011). No intra-, peri- or post-operative complications were observed. Bladder irrigation was mandatory in only 50% of the patients. All patients were negative for residual TCC in re-resection 6 weeks after initial treatment (Wolters et al. 2011). TmLRBT has been proven safe and effective for both, treatment and pathological staging of primary TCC of the bladder. Tm: YAG en bloc resection therefore could be an appropriate tool for accurate staging with possibly lower scattering potential for the assessment and treatment of patients with TCC (Wolters et al. 2011).

25.9   Green Light Laster and En-Bloc Resection

Chen et al. evaluated the safety and efficacy of LBO laser en bloc resection compared with transurethral resection (TURBT) (Chen et al. 2016). A total of 158 patients (83 underwent laser resection and 75 TURBT) were included. The LBO laser group was also associated with less hemoglobin loss compared with TURBT group $(0.87 \pm 0.28 \, g/mL$ vs. $1.00 \pm 0.33 \, g/mL$, $p = 0.009$). Obturator nerve kick was absent during laser resection, but present in nine patients during TURBT ($p = 0.001$), with two bladder perforations. The recurrence-free survival rate did not differ significantly between two groups (Chen et al. 2016). The results have shown that LBO laser en bloc resection is feasible, safe, and effective alternative for the treatment of primary non-muscle-invasive bladder tumors. Besides, it can provide intact specimen for the pathologic diagnosis.

Laser therapy provides an alternative option for treating non-muscle-invasive bladder cancer (NMIBC) (Chen et al. 2017). Chen et al. (2017) investigated the efficacy and safety of the 120-W front-firing KTP laser for the treatment of NMIBC (Chen et al. 2017). A total of 64 patients with NMIBC treated with either a 120-W front-firing KTP-photoselective vapo-enucleation (PVEBT, $n = 34$) or transurethral resection (TURBT, $n = 30$) (Chen et al. 2017). En bloc resection was applied to the patients in PVEBT group. There was no significant difference in pathologic type, and T stage ($p = 0.870$) between the two groups. Compared with the TURBT group, patients treated with PVEBT had a shorter hospitalization stay ($p = 0.044$), a shorter operation time ($p = 0.008$), and high rate of detrusor muscle ($p = 0.044$) (Chen et al. 2017). PVEBT is superior to TURBT in terms of the rate of 1-year recurrence ($p = 0.015$) and tumor grade progression rate ($p = 0.019$). The 120-W front-firing KTP laser en bloc enucleation technique is a safe and feasible procedure for treating patients with NMIBC (Chen et al. 2017).

The standard procedure for staging and treating nonmuscle-invasive bladder cancer (NMIBC) is still TURBT. Recently, lasers have been explored as treatment tools for bladder tumors (He et al. 2014). En bloc enucleation using a front-firing green-light potassium-titanyl-phosphate laser and outcomes were reported (He et al. 2014). All patients successfully went through a session of treatment with front-firing green-light laser enucleation of the bladder tumor. Complications such as bladder hemorrhage, vesicle perforation, and obturator nerve reflex were not present. No tumor recurrence was observed at the initial 6-month follow-up (He et al. 2014). The modified technique using a front-firing green-light laser to en bloc enucleate bladder tumors is effective and safe for treatment of NMIBC.

25.10   Hybrid Therapy—Water-Jet and Hybrid Knife En-Bloc Dissection

Fritsche, conducted the first prospective clinical trial on the application of a combined water-jet dissector and needle-knife (HybridKnife) in transurethral dissection (TUD) of urothelial carcinoma of the bladder (UCB) (Fritsche et al. 2011). Thirty separate urothelial tumors of the bladder were dissected with the HybridKnife. The goal was to determine the safety, effectiveness of resection, and overall applicability of the HybridKnife (Fritsche et al. 2011). No perforation or other complication was seen. All tumors could be dissected from the bladder wall en bloc. The application of the HybridKnife appears to be a feasibly safe and applicable for en-bloc dissection (Fritsche et al. 2011) and allows for histopathologic assessment. A possibly improved oncologic outcome has to be addressed in further studies (Fritsche et al. 2011).

TURBT is the standard approach to bladder tumors but has disadvantages. Nagele et al. demonstrate the feasibility and applicability of waterjet hydrodissection for removing papillary NMI bladder tumors (Nagele et al. 2011). In five patients diagnosed with NMI papillary bladder tumor, transurethral submucosal dissection was conducted using the T-type I-Jet HybridKnife (Nagele et al. 2011). All tumors could be resected en bloc, and the lamina propria was intact in all specimens, allowing the pathologist to distinguish between NMI and invasive tumors. Pathological analysis confirmed R0 resection in all samples (Nagele et al. 2011). These initial results prove the feasibility of waterjet hydrodissection for removing bladder tumors. In contrast to conventional TURB, this new technique allows the pathologist to assess the entire lamina propria and the resection edges due to the en-bloc resection and to determine invasiveness as well as R0 versus R1 resection (Nagele et al. 2011). These first results are promising, long-term oncological follow-up, and prospective randomized surveys investigating the recurrence rate have to be evaluated.

25.11 Literature on En-Bloc Resection

Bladder cancer (BC) is an increasing problem worldwide (Kramer et al. 2015). With an older population, new strategies for the transurethral management of BC are required (Kramer et al. 2015). Laser devices used for en bloc resection provide an alternative to more invasive techniques. A systematic review identified eighteen publications in English, including 800 patients (Ho:YAG = 652 patients and Tm:YAG = 148 patients). Tumor vaporization seems to be an alternative for the treatment of recurrent tumors in selected patients (Kramer et al. 2015). The principle of en bloc resection should provide accurate staging but further studies are needed. Peri- and postoperative complications are scarce (Kramer et al. 2015). Due to the nature of the energy source, bladder perforation caused by obturator nerve reflex is unlikely when using lasers (Kramer et al. 2015). There is a trend toward decreased recurrence rates (Kramer et al. 2015). Lasers are potentially useful alternatives to conventional TURBT, but well-designed RCTs are needed to make results comparable.

Bladder cancer of the urothelium is the second most common malignancy among urological tumors. In terms of increased incidence rates are associated with higher age, new treatment challenges appear (Kramer et al. 2012). The standard treatment for non-muscle invasive bladder cancer (NMIBC) is monopolar transurethral resection using resection loops (TURB). Different concepts of en bloc resection of bladder tumors using alternative energy resources (e.g. holmium laser, thulium laser and the water-jet HybridKnife) have been developed

(Kramer et al. 2012). Goals of new treatment modalities are reduction of perioperative and postoperative comorbidities, better pathological work-up of the specimens and increased recurrence-free survival (Kramer et al. 2012). Postulated advantages using laser devices are a more precise cutting line as well as better hemostasis. The evidential value of this review is limited due to the lack of randomized, prospective studies. However, there is a tendency towards a limitation of perioperative and postoperative morbidities as well as higher chance of well-preserved tissues for better pathohistological evaluation using en bloc resection methods (Kramer et al. 2012). More studies with long-term follow-up periods and better randomization are needed to clarify whether en bloc strategies provide better long-term oncological survival.

Wu et al. (2016), conducted a meta-analysis was to compare the feasibility of en bloc transurethral resection of bladder tumor (ETURBT) versus conventional transurethral resection of bladder tumor (CTURBT) (Wu et al. 2016). Seven trials with 886 participants were included, 438 underwent ETURBT and 448 underwent CTURBT. There was no significant difference in operation time between 2 groups ($p = 0.38$) (Wu et al. 2016). There was significant difference in 24-month recurrence rate (24-month RR) (odds ratio [OR] 0.66, 95% CI 0.47–0.92, $p = 0.02$) (Wu et al. 2016). The rate of complication with respect to bladder perforation ($p = 0.004$), bladder irritation ($p < 0.01$), and obturator nerve reflex ($p < 0.01$) was lower in ETURBT (Wu et al. 2016). The postoperative adjuvant intravesical chemotherapy was evaluated by subgroup analysis, and 24-month RR in CTURBT is higher than that in ETURBT in mitomycin intravesical irrigation group ($p = 0.02$) (Wu et al. 2016). The first meta-analysis indicates that ETURBT might prove to be preferable alternative to CTURBT management of nonmuscle invasive bladder carcinoma. ETURBT is associated with shorter HT and CT, less complication rate, and lower recurrence-free rate. Moreover, it can provide high-qualified specimen for the pathologic diagnosis. Well designed randomized controlled trials are needed to make results comparable.

25.12 Systematic Review Conclusions from En-Bloc Resection of Bladder Cancer

Currently, transurethral resection of a bladder tumor (TUR) is the gold standart treatment for non-muscle invasive bladder cancer (NMIBC) (Alyaev et al. 2018). Standard TUR for a bladder wall tumor has a high recurrence rate, which is caused mainly by malignant cell implantation during the surgery or inadequate resection. Besides, specimens obtained with conventional TUR are insufficient for accurate pathological staging (Alyaev et al. 2018). The non-conformity of the standard TUR with the established oncological principle of dissecting through normal tissue prompted a search for the optimal surgical modality. En-bloc resection of the bladder wall tumor has been proposed as an alternative method for surgical management of NMIBC) (Alyaev et al. 2018). This technique involves the resection of bladder tumor through the underlying muscle layer as a single piece thus providing high quality material for subsequent morphological study and reducing the risk of metastasizing by implantation of malignant cells. This paper presents an analysis of relevant research literature published in the last twenty years, describes all currently existing techniques of the bladder tumor resection using a variety of energy sources, including laser) (Alyaev et al. 2018).

References

Alyaev YG, Rapoport LM, Vinarov AZ, Sorokin NI, Dymov AM, Kislyakov DA, Afanasyevskaya EV, Lekarev VY. En-bloc laser resection of the urinary bladder tumor. Urologiia. 2018;2:147–53.

Chen J, Zhao Y, Wang S, Jin X, Sun P, Zhang L, Wang M. Green-light laser en bloc resection for primary non-muscle-invasive bladder tumor versus transurethral electroresection: a prospective, nonrandomized two-center trial with 36-month follow-up. Lasers Surg Med. 2016;48(9):859–65.

Cheng B, Qiu X, Li H, Yang G. The safety and efficacy of front-firing green-light laser endoscopic en bloc photoselective vapo-enucleation of non-muscle-invasive bladder cancer. Ther Clin Risk Manag. 2017;11(13):983–8.

D'Souza N, D'Souza VA. Holmium laser transurethral resection of bladder tumor: our experience [in English]. Urol Ann. 2016;8(4):439–443.

Fritsche HM, Otto W, Eder F, Hofstädter F, Denzinger S, Chaussy CG, Stief C, Wieland WF, Burger M. Water-jet-aided transurethral dissection of urothelial carcinoma: a prospective clinical study. J Endourol. 2011;25(10):1599–603.

He D, Fan J, Wu K, Wang X, Wu D, Li L, Li X, Liu L, Cao P, Cao J, Chang LS. Novel green-light KTP laser en bloc enucleation for nonmuscle-invasive bladder cancer: technique and initial clinical experience. J Endourol. 2014;28(8):975–9.

Hurle R, Lazzeri M, Colombo P, Buffi N, Morenghi E, Peschechera R, Castaldo L, Pasini L, Casale P, Seveso M, Zandegiacomo S, Taverna G, Benetti A, Lughezzani G, Fiorini G, Guazzoni G. "En bloc" resection of nonmuscle invasive bladder cancer: a prospective single-center study. Urology. 2016;90:126–30.

Islas-García JJ, Campos-Salcedo JG, López-Benjume BI, Torres-Gómez JJ, Aguilar-Colmenero J, Martínez-Alonso IA, Gil-Villa SA. Surgical technique for en bloc transurethral resection of bladder tumour with a Hybrid Knife(®). Actas Urol Esp. 2016;40(4):263–7.

Kramer MW, Wolters M, Abdelkawi IF, Merseburger AS, Nagele U, Gross A, Bach T, Kuczyk MA, Herrmann TR. Transurethral en bloc resection of non-muscle invasive bladder cancer. What is the state of the art? Urologe A. 2012;51(6):798–804. https://doi.org/10.1007/s00120-012-2876-8.

Kramer MW, Wolters M, Cash H, Jutzi S, Imkamp F, Kuczyk MA, Merseburger AS, Herrmann TR. Current evidence of transurethral Ho:YAG and Tm:YAG treatment of bladder cancer: update 2014. World J Urol. 2015;33(4):571–9.

Lodde M, Lusuardi L, Palermo S, Signorello D, Maier K, Hohenfellner R, Pycha A. En bloc transurethral resection of bladder tumors: use and limits. Urology. 2003;62(6):1089–91.

Maurice MJ, Vricella GJ, MacLennan G, Buehner P, Ponsky LE. Endoscopic snare resection of bladder tumors: evaluation of an alternative technique for bladder tumor resection. J Endourol. 2012;26(6):614–7.

Migliari R, Buffardi A, Ghabin H. Thulium laser endoscopic en bloc enucleation of nonmuscle-invasive bladder cancer. J Endourol. 2015;29(11):1258–62.

Muto G, Collura D, Giacobbe A, D'Urso L, Muto GL, Demarchi A, Coverlizza S, Castelli E. Thulium:yttrium-aluminum-garnet laser for en bloc resection of bladder cancer: clinical and histopathologic advantages. Urology. 2014;83(4):851–5.

Nagele U, Kugler M, Nicklas A, Merseburger AS, Walcher U, Mikuz G, Herrmann TR. Waterjet hydrodissection: first experiences and short-term outcomes of a novel approach to bladder tumor resection. World J Urol. 2011;29(4):423–7.

Naselli A, Puppo P. En Bloc transurethral resection of bladder tumors: a new standard? J Endourol. 2017;31(S1):S20–4.

Saito S. Transurethral en bloc resection of bladder tumors. J Urol. 2001;166(6):2148–50.

Sureka SK, Agarwal V, Agnihotri S, Kapoor R, Srivastava A, Mandhani A. Is en-bloc transurethral resection of bladder tumor for non-muscle invasive bladder carcinoma better than conventional technique in terms of recurrence and progression? A prospective study. Indian J Urol. 2014;30(2):144–9.

Ukai R, Hashimoto K, Iwasa T, Nakayama H. Transurethral resection in one piece (TURBO) is an accurate tool for pathological staging of bladder tumor. Int J Urol. 2010;17(8):708–14.

Upadhyay R, Kapoor R, Srivastava A, Krishnani N, Mandhani A. Does En-bloc transurethral resection of bladder tumor give a better yield in terms of presence of detrusor muscle in the biopsy specimen? Indian J Urol. 2012;28(3):275–9.

Wolters M, Kramer MW, Becker JU, Christgen M, Nagele U, Imkamp F, Burchardt M, Merseburger AS, Kuczyk MA, Bach T, Gross AJ, Herrmann TR. Tm:YAG laser en bloc mucosectomy for accurate staging of primary bladder cancer: early experience. World J Urol. 2011;29(4):429–32.

Wu YP, Lin TT, Chen SH, Xu N, Wei Y, Huang JB, Sun XL, Zheng QS, Xue XY, Li XD. Comparison of the efficacy and feasibility of en bloc transurethral resection of bladder tumor versus conventional transurethral resection of bladder tumor: a meta-analysis. Medicine (Baltimore). 2016;95(45):5372.

Xu H, Ma J, Chen Z, Yang J, Yuan H, Wang T, Liu J, Yang W, Ye Z. Safety and efficacy of en bloc transurethral resection with 1.9 μm vela laser for treatment of non-muscle invasive bladder cancer. Urology. 2018;113:246–50.

Zhang KY, Xing JC, Li W, Wu Z, Chen B, Bai DY. A novel transurethral resection technique for NMI bladder tumor: retrograde en bloc resection. World J Surg Oncol. 2017a;15(1):125.

Zhang Z, Zeng S, Zhao J, Lu X, Xu W, Ma C, Wang Y, Chen X, Jia G, Zhou T, Sun Y, Xu C. A pilot study of vela laser for en bloc resection of papillary bladder cancer. Clin Genitourin Cancer. 2017b;15(3):e311–4.

Zhang J, Wang L, Mao S, Liu M, Zhang W, Zhang Z, Guo Y, Huang B, Yan Y, Huang Y, Yao X. Transurethral en bloc resection with bipolar button electrode for non-muscle invasive bladder cancer. Int Urol Nephrol. 2018;50(4):619–23.

Part VI
Management of Low and Intermediate Risk Bladder Cancer

Chapter 26
NMIBC—Fulguration in Low Risk Disease

Low risk non muscle invasive disease, may be common but low risk. Al Hussein et al. (2015) reviewed endoscopic treatment of low-risk non-muscle-invasive bladder cancer (NMIBC) via office-based fulguration versus operating room-based transurethral resection of the bladder (TURB) (Al Hussein et al. 2015).

A Markov state-transition model was created to compare the economic burden of managing patients with office-based fulguration versus TURB (Al Hussein et al. 2015). Patients were modeled as being followed up routinely with flexible cystoscopy, whereas tumor recurrences were treated with either fulguration or TURB (Al Hussein et al. 2015). This study demonstrated office-based cystoscopy and fulguration was more cost-effective than TURB for treating recurrent low-risk NMIBC (Al Hussein et al. 2015).

The management of recurrent nonmuscle invasive bladder cancer (NMIBC) post-transurethral resection has been based around electrocautery techniques, either under local or general anesthetic. Syed et al. determined the long-term outcome of the management of NMIBC recurrences treated with Holmium:Yttrium Aluminum Garnet (Ho:YAG) laser ablation under local anesthetic with a flexible cystoscope (Syed et al. 2013). Local, on-site recurrence rates after first treatment for all NMIBC disease were 10% (Syed et al. 2013). In patients with low risk NMIBC (G1/2, Ta), this reduced to around 4% post laser treatment. Higher recurrence rates (14%) were seen in those with high-grade (G3, T1) disease. Treatment was more successful with disease around the trigone, posterior and lateral bladder walls, with a significantly higher risk of recurrence for tumor around the ureteric orifice (Syed et al. 2013). The median time to local recurrence was 12 months and off-site recurrence was 25 months.

© Springer Nature Switzerland AG 2020
S. S. Goonewardene et al., *Management of Non-Muscle Invasive Bladder Cancer*,
https://doi.org/10.1007/978-3-030-28646-0_26

References

Al Hussein, Al Awamlh B, Lee R, Chughtai B, Donat SM, Sandhu JS, Herr HW. A cost-effective-ness analysis of management of low-risk non-muscle-invasive bladder cancer using office-based fulguration. Urology. 2015;85(2):381–6.

Syed HA, Talbot N, Abbas A, MacDonald D, Jones R, Marr TJ, Rukin NJ. Flexible cystoscopy and Holmium:Yttrium aluminum garnet laser ablation for recurrent nonmuscle invasive blad-der carcinoma under local anesthesia. J Endourol. 2013;27(7):886–91.

Chapter 27
Active Surveillance in Non-Muscle Invasive Bladder Cancer

27.1 Systematic Review Methods—Active Surveillance in Non-Muscle Invasive Bladder Cancer

A systematic review relating to bladder cancer and en-bloc resection was conducted. This was to identify references relating to active surveillance in non-muscle invasive bladder cancer was conducted. The search strategy aimed to identify all references related to bladder cancer AND screening. Search terms used were as follows: (Bladder cancer) AND (low risk) AND (Active Surveillance). The following databases were screened from 1989 to June 2019:

- CINAHL
- MEDLINE (NHS Evidence)
- Cochrane
- AMed
- EMBASE
- PsychINFO
- SCOPUS
- Web of Science.

In addition, searches using Medical Subject Headings (MeSH) and keywords were conducted using Cochrane databases. Two UK-based experts in bladder cancer were consulted to identify any additional studies.

Studies were eligible for inclusion if they reported primary research focusing on bladder cancer and en-bloc resection. Papers were included if published after 1984 and had to be in English. Studies that did not conform to this were excluded. Only primary research was included. The overall aim was to identify the role of en-bloc resection in bladder tumour resection. The search identified 30 papers.

© Springer Nature Switzerland AG 2020
S. S. Goonewardene et al., *Management of Non-Muscle Invasive Bladder Cancer*,
https://doi.org/10.1007/978-3-030-28646-0_27

Abstracts were independently screened for eligibility by two reviewers and dis-agreements resolved through discussion or third party opinion. Agreement level was calculated using Cohen's Kappa to test the intercoder reliability of this screen-ing process. Cohens' Kappa allows comparison of inter-rater reliability between papers using relative observed agreement. This also takes account of the compari-son occurring by chance. The first reviewer agreed all 8 papers to be included, the second, agreed on 8.

Data extraction was piloted by the researcher and amended in consultation with the research team (author and two academic supervisors). Data collected included authors, year and country of publication, study aims, setting, intervention aims, number of participants, study design, intervention components and delivery meth-ods, comparison groups and outcome measures, notes and follow-up questions for the authors. Studies were quality assessed using the PRISMA criteria for ran-domised controlled trials, Mays et al. (Moher et al. 2009; Moher, Liberati et al. 2009, 154, 153; Mays et al. 2005) for the action research and qualitative studies and the Critical Skills Appraisal programme for cohort studies. This was also applied to randomised controlled trials and qualitative studies.

The search identified 8 papers (Fig. 27.1). All 8 mapped to the search terms and eligibility criteria. The current systematic reviews were examined to gain further knowledge about the subject. 22 papers were excluded due to not conforming to eligibility criteria or adding to the evidence for bladder cancer screening. Of the 8 papers left, relevant abstracts were identified and the full papers obtained (all of which were in English), to quality assure against criteria. All studies in this SR were cohort studies, of moderate quality. There was considerable heterogeneity of design among the included studies therefore a narrative review of the evidence was undertaken. There was significant heterogeneity within studies, including clinical topic, numbers, outcomes, as a results a narrative review was thought to be best.

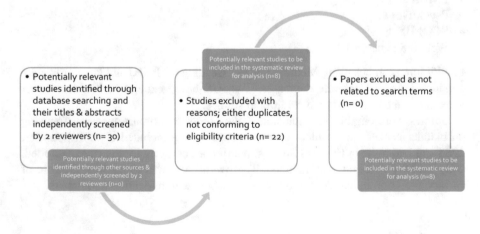

Fig. 27.1 Flow chart of studies identified through the systematic review (adapted from PRISMA)

27.2   Short Term Oncological Outcomes for Active Surveillance and Low Risk Bladder Cancer

Hurle et al. investigated predictive factors of active surveillance for nonmuscle invasive bladder cancer (Hurle et al. 2018). On univariate analysis time from the first resection to start of active surveillance was inversely associated with recurrence-free survival (HR 0.99, 95% CI 0.98–1.00, $p=0.027$) (Hurle et al. 2018). Multivariate analysis demonstrated an association with age at active surveillance start (HR 0.97, 95% CI 0.94–1.00, $p=0.031$) and the size of the lesion at the first transurethral resection (HR 1.55, 95% CI 1.06–2.27, $p=0.025$) (Hurle et al. 2018). Active surveillance is a potential short-term strategy for unfit patients with small, low grade pTa/pT1a recurrent papillary bladder tumors who are not fit for major surgery.

Hurle et al. (2016) reported the oncological outcomes and progression risk for non-muscle-invasive bladder cancer (NMIBC) included in an active surveillance (AS) programme after recurrence (Hurle et al. 2016). Hurle conducted a prospective study with low grade pTa-pT1a NMIBC tumour recurrence. There was disease progression in 28 patients (51%). In all, 15 patients (27.3%) had an increase in the number and/or size of the tumour, nine (16.4%) had haematuria, and four (7.3%) had a positive cytology. Only five (9%) patients progressed to a high-grade tumour (Grade 3) or presented with associated CIS. The overall adherence to the follow-up schedule was 95%. An active surveillance protocol for NMIBC is an option for small, recurrent cancers in unfit patients but must be closely monitored.

pT1 has a high risk of disease recurrence and progression (Hurle et al. 2016). Induction and maintenance intravesical Bacillus Calmette-Guerin (BCG) has been proven to reduce tumour progression. The conventional clinicopathological factors in the EORTC model are relevant for outcomes of pT1 stage bladder tumors and BCG immunotherapy (Hurle et al. 2016). To perform a cystectomy depends on a number of clinicopathologic parameters, but none are able to sufficiently identify patients for the appropriate therapeutic modality (Hurle et al. 2016). However the EORTC model may allow for a degree of prediction in which patients are suitable for active surveillance.

Haukaas determined the natural history of bladder transitional cell carcinoma (TCC) in NMI disease (Haukaas et al. 1999). The disease progressed in 42 of 231 (18%) patients. Differences in the progression-free interval between patients with G1 and G3 tumours, and with pTa and pT1 disease, were statistically significant (Haukaas et al. 1999). There were no deaths among patients with initial pTaG1 tumours. The long-term prognosis is good for patients with p TaG1 tumours which potentially make them candidates for active surveillance but under strict regulations.

Low-grade Ta papillary tumors are categorized as low-risk NMIBC because of their favorable prognosis (Miyake et al. 2016). A new evolution in thinking and management has meant overdiagnosis and overtreatment should be avoided considering the patients quality of life (Miyake et al. 2016). There are specifics to manage if active surveillance is an standard option in selected patients (Miyake et al. 2016). A specific follow-up protocol specifying intervals of cystoscopy, urine cytology, urine markers, and imaging need to be optimized and validated (Miyake et al. 2016).

27.3 Long Term Oncological Outcomes for Active Surveillance and Low Risk Bladder Cancer

Hernández reviewed the long term oncological long-term safety of AS and determined variables associated with progression. In all, 252 AS patients were studied, with a median follow-up of 6 years (Hernández et al. 2016). 203 (80.6%) underwent active treatment. After remaining under observation, 86.4% had not progressed in stage, and 79.3% in grade. Of these patients, 4 experienced progression to T2; all of them were previously T1G2 (Hernández et al. 2016). This demonstrates AS in a high-selectivity group of patients with recurrent non-muscle-invasive bladder tumor is feasible and oncologically safe but must be closely monitored. Patients with previous history of T1 should not be included in AS protocols even when very small recurrences are diagnosed (Hernández et al. 2016). The simple fact bladder cancer has recurred means it is by definition higher risk disease.

27.4 Active Surveillance in Recurrent Low Grade Bladder Cancer

Gofrit evaluated the safety of an active surveillance program, without resection of the tumor, in patients with recurrent low grade bladder cancer (Gofrit and Shapiro 2008). Active surveillance was offered to patients with small (<10 mm) papillary tumors who had previous resections of NMI (Ta) low-grade (G1-2) bladder tumors (Gofrit and Shapiro 2008). The surveillance protocol included cystoscopy and urinary cytology every 3 months for 2 years and then every 6 months. Surveillance was stopped and TURBT conducted for symptoms, positive cytology, or significant alteration in tumor morphology, size or on patient choice (Gofrit and Shapiro 2008). 43 active surveillance periods were documented in 31 patients (mean age 68 years). The main reasons for termination of surveillance were appearance of additional tumors (15 events), excessive tumor growth (12 events) and patient's request (7 events). All resected tumors were stage Ta except a single case of stage T1.

Hernández examined active surveillance, with low-risk tumors after the diagnosis of recurrence (Hernández et al. 2009). Hernández performed a prospective cohort (Hernández et al. 2009). The inclusion criteria were papillary tumors with negative cytology findings, previous nonmuscle-invasive tumor (Stage pTa, pT1a), grade 1–2, size <1 cm, and number of tumors <5. No symptomatic patients, carcinoma in situ or grade 3 tumors were included (Hernández et al. 2009). A retrospective analysis of a control group similar to those of the patients on active surveillance, but who underwent transurethral resection immediately after the recurrence was diagnosed was also performed (Hernández et al. 2009).

The data from 64 patients (70 observation events) were analyzed. The mean patient age was 66.7 years. The median follow-up was 38.6 months. The median time patients remained in observation was 10.3 months. After 10.3 months, 93.5% of the patients had not progressed in stage and 83.8% had not progressed in grade (Hernández et al. 2009). None of the patients experienced progression to muscle-invasive disease. A comparison between the rates of progression in the study and control groups showed no statistically significant difference.

Patients with recurrent, small (<1 cm), nonmuscle-invasive bladder tumors can be safely offered monitoring under an active surveillance protocol, with a minimal risk of progression in either grade or stage, thus reducing the amount of surgical intervention they might undergo throughout their life (Hernández et al. 2009).

27.5 Reviews on Low Risk Bladder Cancer and Active Surveillance

Low-grade Ta papillary tumors are low-risk NMIBC due to their favourable prognosis (Miyake et al. 2016). There are several issues when reviewing active surveillance as a standard option in selected patients (Miyake et al. 2016). A specific follow-up protocol including intervals of cystoscopy, urine cytology, urine markers, and imaging needs to be optimized and validated (Miyake et al. 2016). However, the pathology of disease must be taken into account, especially with a disease as aggressive as bladder cancer.

Tiu et al. reviewed the role of active surveillance for low risk bladder cancer (Tiu et al. 2014). Low-risk bladder cancer-defined as pTa low-grade papillary tumors–is the type of NMIBC with the most favorable oncologic outcome and which almost never progresses to muscle invasive disease or metastasizes (Tiu et al. 2014). Patients with low-grade bladder tumors often experience a recurrence after primary transurethral resection. Appropriately selected patients with recurrent low-risk bladder cancer could be managed with either office fulguration or cystoscopic surveillance. Active surveillance for patients with low-risk bladder cancer avoids or delays the surgical and anesthetic risks of a TURBT, thus optimizing quality of life without compromising the patient's risk of cancer progression (Tiu et al. 2014).

References

Gofrit ON, Shapiro A. Active surveillance of low grade bladder tumors. Arch Ital Urol Androl. 2008;80(4):132–5.
Haukaas S, Daehlin L, Maartmann-Moe H, Ulvik NM. The long-term outcome in patients with NMI transitional cell carcinoma of the bladder: a single-institutional experience. BJU Int. 1999;83(9):957–63.

Hernández V, Alvarez M, de la Peña E, Amaruch N, Martín MD, de la Morena JM, Gómez V, Llorente C. Safety of active surveillance program for recurrent nonmuscle-invasive bladder carcinoma. Urology. 2009;73(6):1306–10.

Hernández V, Llorente C, de la Peña E, Pérez-Fernández E, Guijarro A, Sola I. Long-term oncological outcomes of an active surveillance program in recurrent low grade Ta bladder cancer. Urol Oncol. 2016;34(4):165.e19–23.

Hurle R, Lazzeri M, Vanni E, Lughezzani G, Buffi N, Casale P, Saita A, et al. Active surveillance for low risk nonmuscle invasive bladder cancer: a confirmatory and resource consumption study from the bias project. J Urol. 2018;199(2):401–6.

Hurle R, Pasini L, Lazzeri M, Colombo P, Buffi N, Lughezzani G, Casale P, Morenghi E, Peschechera R, Zandegiacomo S, Benetti A, Saita A, Cardone P, Guazzoni G. Active surveillance for low-risk non-muscle-invasive bladder cancer: mid-term results from the bladder cancer Italian active surveillance (BIAS) project. BJU Int. 2016;118(6):935–9.

Mays N, Pope, C, Popay J. Systematically reviewing qualitative and quantitative evidence to inform management and policy-making in the health field. J Health Serv Res Policy. 2005;10(Suppl. 1): 6–20.

Miyake M, Fujimoto K, Hirao Y. Active surveillance for nonmuscle invasive bladder cancer. Investig Clin Urol. 2016;57(Suppl. 1):S4–13.

Moher D, Liberati A, Tetzlaff J, Altman DG. Preferred reporting items for systematic reviews and meta-analyses: the prisma statement. BMJ. 2009;339(7716):332–6.

Tiu A, Jenkins LC, Soloway MS. Active surveillance for low-risk bladder cancer. Urol Oncol. 2014;32(1):33.e7–10.

Chapter 28
Hyperthermic MMC—A Systematic Review

28.1 Hyperthermic MMC—Systematic Review Methodology

A systematic review relating to hyperthermic MMC was conducted. This was to identify the oncological outcomes from with hyperthermic mitomycin C for NMIBC. The search strategy aimed to identify all references related to this. Search terms used were as follows: (Bladder cancer) AND (hyperthermic) AND (Mitomycin). The following databases were screened from 1989 to June 2019:

- CINAHL
- MEDLINE (NHS Evidence)
- Cochrane
- AMed
- EMBASE
- PsychINFO
- SCOPUS
- Web of Science.

In addition, searches using Medical Subject Headings (MeSH) and keywords were conducted using Cochrane databases. Two UK-based experts in bladder cancer were consulted to identify any additional studies.

Studies were eligible for inclusion if they reported primary research focusing on bladder cancer and hyperthemic MMC. Papers were included if published after 1984 and had to be in English. Studies that did not conform to this were excluded. Only primary research was included. The overall aim was to identify outcomes from hyperthermic MMC in NMIBC.

Abstracts were independently screened for eligibility by two reviewers and disagreements resolved through discussion or third party opinion. Agreement level was calculated using Cohen's Kappa to test the intercoder reliability of this screening process. Cohens' Kappa allows comparison of inter-rater reliability between papers using relative observed agreement. This also takes account of the comparison occurring by chance. The first reviewer agreed all 21 papers to be included, the second, agreed on 21 (Fig. 28.1).

Data extraction was piloted by the researcher and amended in consultation with the research team (author and two academic supervisors). Data collected included authors, year and country of publication, study aims, setting, intervention aims, number of participants, study design, intervention components and delivery methods, comparison groups and outcome measures, notes and follow-up questions for the authors. Studies were quality assessed using the PRISMA criteria for randomised controlled trials, Mays et al. (Moher et al. 2009; Moher, Liberati et al. 2009, 154, 153; Mays et al. 2005) for the action research and qualitative studies and the Critical Skills Appraisal programme for cohort studies. This was also applied to randomised controlled trials and qualitative studies.

The search identified 21 papers (Fig. 28.1). All 21 mapped to the search terms and eligibility criteria. The current systematic reviews were examined to gain further knowledge about the subject. 127 papers were excluded due to not conforming to eligibility criteria or adding to the evidence for bladder cancer screening. Of the 21 papers left, relevant abstracts were identified and the full papers obtained (all of which were in English), to quality assure against criteria. There was considerable heterogeneity of design among the included studies therefore a narrative review of the evidence was undertaken. There was significant heterogeneity within studies, including clinical topic, numbers, outcomes, as a result a narrative review was thought to be best. All studies were cohort studies of moderate quality.

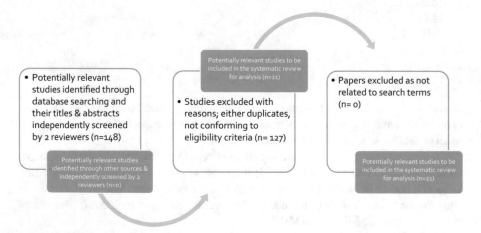

Fig. 28.1 Flow chart of studies identified through the systematic review (adapted from PRISMA)

28.2 What is Hyperthermic MMC?

Hyperthermia is the clinical application of heat, in which tumor temperatures are raised to 40–45 °C This proven radiation and chemosensitizer significantly improves clinical outcome for several tumor sites. Earlier studies of the use of pre-treatment planning for hyperthermia showed good qualitative but disappointing quantitative reliability.

Non-Muscle invasive bladder cancer (NMIBC) has a high tendency for recurrence and progression (Bahouth et al. 2016). Currently, all known intravesical agents are associated with adverse effects (AEs) and limited efficacy. The combination of hyperthermia (HT) with intravesical Mitomycin C (MMC) chemotherapy has been shown to improve outcomes. The added efficacy of HT to MMC was first shown in preclinical studies (Bahouth et al. 2016). The reports on patients with NMIBC have indicated that the treatment is safe and well tolerated. Several clinical studies reported the efficacy of radiofrequency-induced chemotherapy effect (RITE) in the treatment of patients with NMIBC. This modality was shown to be superior to MMC alone (Bahouth et al. 2016). RITE was effective also in patients with high-risk NMIBC, including those who failed Bacillus Calmette-Guérin (BCG).

28.3 Bioavailability of Hyperthermic MMC

Milia evaluated, for the first time, the mitomycin C (MMC) pharmacokinetics during intravesical hyperthermia treatment based on conductive heat and the stability and recovery of the drug at the end of the instillation period (Milia et al. 2014). Nine patients completed all the six planned cycles, whereas two patients missed the last cycle because of allergic reactions. No other systemic toxicity was observed, and the local toxicities were mild (Milia et al. 2014). MMC is stable during the instillation, and its absorption occurs mainly during the first minutes of the treatment. The plasmatic MMC concentration is always well below the threshold level for myelosuppression, as confirmed by the total lack of hematological toxicity evidenced by the patients (Milia et al. 2014). In order to evaluate the efficacy of the treatment performed with UniThermia ($^{®}$) in reducing the disease recurrence rate in short- and long-term follow-up (Milia et al. 2014).

Non-Muscle invasive bladder cancer (NMIBC) is a highly recurrent disease with potential progression to muscle invasive disease despite the standard bladder instillations with mitomycin C (MMC) or Bacille Calmette-Guérin immunotherapy (van Valenberg et al. 2016). Therefore, alternatives such as radiofrequency-induced chemohyperthermia (RF-CHT) with MMC are examined by van Valenberg et al. (2016).

Eleven patients were included of which six received RF-CHT. Ten patients had TaG2-LG/HG papillary tumours at pathology. One patient in the RF-CHT group appeared to be free of malignancy and was excluded from the analysis as no tumour biopsies were available (van Valenberg et al. 2016). The median MMC concentration in tumour tissue was higher in the RF-CHT group (median 665.00 ng/g vs. 63.75 ng/g, $U = 51.0$, $p = 0.018$). Moreover, in both techniques the MMC concentration was lower in normal tissue compared to tumour tissue (van Valenberg et al. 2016). Tissue MMC concentration measurements varied substantially within, and between, different patients from the same group (van Valenberg et al. 2016). Intravesical RF-CHT results in higher tumour MMC concentrations versus cold MMC instillation which contributes to its superior efficacy.

28.4 Predictive Factors for Hyperthermic MMC

Hyperthermic mitomycin (HM) is a novel treatment modality for selected patients with high-risk non-muscle invasive bladder cancer (NMIBC). Sooriakumaran sought to determine predictors of response to this therapy (Sooriakumaran et al. 2016) The presence of initial complete response (CR; no evidence of disease at first check video-cystoscopy and urine cytology) post-HM treatment was an independent predictor of good response to HM (Sooriakumaran et al. 2016). Female patients and those without carcinoma in situ (CIS) also appeared to respond better to the intervention. The overall bladder preservation rate at a median of 27 months was 81.4%; 17/97 (17.5%) patients died.

This paper demonstrated specific points (Sooriakumaran et al. 2016). High-risk NMIBC patients can be safely treated with HM and have good oncological outcome. However, those without an initial CR have a poor prognosis and should be counselled towards adopting other treatment methodologies such as cystectomy (Sooriakumaran et al. 2016). Female gender and lack of CIS may be good prognostic indicators for response to HM (Sooriakumaran et al. 2016).

28.5 Histopathological Changes from Hyperthermic Chemotherapy

Twelve patients suffering from NMI transitional cell carcinoma of the bladder underwent treatment combining simultaneous mitomycin C topical instillation and local endocavitary hyperthermia preoperatively (Rigatti et al. 1991). A specifically designed system to deliver and monito local bladder hyperthermia was used. The feasibility, the subjective tolerance and the side effects of the combined treatment were the main target of our investigation (Rigatti et al. 1991). Endoscopic and histologic features, assessed before, during and after this combined approach, showed selective damage to neoplastic areas with minimal changes in the normal urothelium (Rigatti et al. 1991). Local intravesical concurrent chemotherapy and hyperthermia administration is found to be a safe and well-tolerated approach for NMI bladder tumor treatment (Rigatti et al. 1991). The preliminary results encourage further studies to define the limits and prospects of this regimen, in both NMI bladder tumor ablation and prophylaxis of recurrences.

The role of a combined regimen of local hyperthermia and topical chemotherapy in patients with multifocal and recurrent NMI bladder tumors not curable by transurethral resection was evaluated in a neoadjuvant organ sparing clinical study (Colombo et al. 1998). After treatment transurethral resection appeared to be feasible and curative in 16 patients (84%). Histological study revealed complete and partial responses in 9 (47%) and 7 (37%) cases, respectively (Colombo et al. 1998). Due to extensive residual tumors radical cystectomy was performed in 3 patients (16%). At a median 33-month followup 8 NMI transitional tumor recurrences were documented and easily eradicated by transurethral resection or laser therapy in patients in whom the bladder had been saved (Colombo et al. 1998). Microwave induced hyperthermia combined with intravesical mitomycin C seems to be a feasible, safe and elective approach for conservative treatment of multifocal and recurrent NMI bladder tumors when other treatment strategies have failed (Colombo et al. 1998).

28.6   Assessment of Response to Hyperthermic MMC Using Urinary Cytokines

Arends investigated response of urinary cytokine and chemokine (CK) levels differed between cold mitomycin-C (cold-MMC)-treated patients and chemo-hyperthermia (C-HT)-treated patients, to shed light on the possible molecular mechanisms that might explain the superior outcome of C-HT (Arends et al. 2015). Furthermore, CK-differences were explored between C-HT responders and C-HT non-responders. Elevated urinary CK levels were observed in both groups after treatment. In general, CK-peaks were lower in the cold-MMC group in comparison with levels in the C-HT group. Significant higher MCP-1 and IL-6 levels were observed in C-HT-treated patients (Arends et al. 2015). Additionally, significant cumulative effects were observed for IP-10 and IL-2. However, IP-10 and IL-2 levels did not significantly differ between treatments. MDC levels after the first week of treatment were significantly higher in the C-HT responders compared with the non-responders (Arends et al. 2015).

MMC treatment leads to elevated urinary CK levels with significantly higher MCP-1 and IL-6 levels in C-HT-treated patients. Increased MDC levels after the first C-HT instillation appear to be related to good clinical outcome and might be of additional value to personalize treatment (Arends et al. 2015). Studies involving more patients and longer follow-up are needed to substantiate this observation.

28.7   Efficacy of Hyperthermic MMC Post Resection

Preventing the recurrence of non-muscle invasive bladder cancer (NMIBC) post-transurethral resection (TUR) remains challenging (Ba et al. 2017). Ba investigated the effectiveness and safety of bladder intracavitary hyperthermic perfusion chemotherapy (BHPC) for prevention of NMIBC post resection (Ba et al. 2017). 53 patients with NMIBC who underwent TUR were randomly assigned to receive BHPC (BHPC group, 28 patients) or intravesical chemotherapy alone (chemotherapy group, 25 patients) at the Intracelom Hyperthermic Perfusion Therapy Center of Guangzhou Medical University Cancer Hospital (Guangzhou, China). The tumor recurrence rate was significantly lower (10.7 vs. 28.0%; $p = 0.02$) and the DFS period was significantly longer (37 ± 1.2 vs. 19 ± 0.9 months; $p = 0.001$) in the BHPC group than in the chemotherapy group (Ba et al. 2017). This demonstrates that BHPC is safe and effective for preventing NMIBC recurrence post-TUR and prolongs DFS.

Malfezzini examined impact of intravesical chemotherapy and local microwave hyperthermia (ICLMH) and oncological outcomes. Treatment was completed as planned by 32 patients (76.2%). The percentage of disease-free patients the year before study was 14.9% (95% CI 5.5–28.8) versus 88.8% (95% CI 73.7–94.8) after ICLMH ($p < 0.0001$). Patient EORTC scores, multifocality, and tumour stage were all associated significantly and independently with a higher risk of recurrence after ICLMH treatment with HR of 41.1 ($p = 0.01$), 17.7 ($p = 0.02$), and 8.5 ($p = 0.02$), respectively. After a median follow-up of 38 months, 24 patients (57.1%) did not show evidence of disease, whereas 13 patients (30.9%) underwent disease recurrence and 5 patients (11.9%) showed also stage progression. Toxicity consisted in grades 1 and 2 frequency, non-infectious cystitis, and haematuria. This demonstrates ICLMH significantly increases the DFI of NMIBC patients with high EORTC score for recurrence and progression.

Geijsen examined the safety and feasibility of this treatment combination for intermediate and high risk nonmuscle invasive bladder cancer (Geijesen et al. 2015). The records of 18 of 20 patients could be analysed (Geijesen et al. 2015). Four patients (22%) discontinued treatment because of physical complaints without exceeding grade 2 toxicity (Geijesen et al. 2015). Toxicity scored according to CTC 3.0 was limited to grade 1 in 43% of cases and grade 2 in 14%. The 24-month recurrence-free survival rate was 78% (Geijesen et al. 2015). Treatment with regional hyperthermia combined with mitomycin C in patients with intermediate and high risk nonmuscle invasive bladder cancer is feasible with low toxicity and excellent bladder temperatures.

Despite an initial adequate response many patients with nonmuscle invasive urothelial cell carcinoma of the bladder eventually have recurrence after intravesical bacillus Calmette-Guerin treatments (Nativ et al. 2009). Nativ, assessed efficacy of combined bladder wall hyperthermia and intravesical mitomycin C instillation (thermo-chemotherapy) THE Kaplan-Meier estimated disease-free survival rate was 85% and 56% after 1 and 2 years, respectively (Nativ et al. 2009).

No maintenance treatment was associated with decreased efficacy, that is the recurrence rate was 61% at 2 years versus 39% in those with maintenance treatments ($p = 0.01$). The progression rate was 3% (Nativ et al. 2009). Thermo-chemotherapy may be effective for papillary nonmuscle invasive urothelial cell carcinoma of the bladder that recurs after BCG treatment without increasing the risk of tumor progression. Maintenance therapy is important and improves the outcome (Nativ et al. 2009).

Non-muscle invasive bladder cancer (NMIBC) is a highly recurrent disease with potential progression to muscle invasive disease despite the standard bladder instillations with mitomycin C (MMC) or Bacille Calmette-Guérin immunotherapy (van Valenberg et al. 2016). Therefore, alternatives such as radiofrequency-induced chemohyperthermia (RF-CHT) with MMC are examined by (van Valenberg et al. 2016). Eleven patients were included of which six received RF-CHT. Ten patients had TaG2-LG/HG papillary tumours at pathology. One patient in the RF-CHT group appeared to be free of malignancy and was excluded from the analysis as no tumour biopsies were available (van Valenberg et al. 2016). The median MMC concentration in tumour tissue was higher in the RF-CHT group (median 665.00 ng/g vs. 63.75 ng/g, $U = 51.0$, $p = 0.018$). Moreover, in both techniques the MMC concentration was lower in normal tissue compared to tumour tissue (van Valenberg et al. 2016). Tissue MMC concentration measurements varied substantially within, and between, different patients from the same group (van Valenberg et al. 2016). Intravesical RF-CHT results in higher tumour MMC concentrations versus cold MMC instillation which contributes to its superior efficacy

28.8 Hyperthermic MMC and Intermediate Risk Disease

Sousa examine the effectiveness of hyperthermic intravesical chemotherapy (HIVEC™) with mitomycin-C (MMC) for patients with intermediate-high-risk non-muscle invasive bladder cancer (NMIBC) (D'Souza and Verma 2016). 40 patients with intermediate-high-risk NMIBC received HIVEC™ treatment with a Combat BRS system. A total of 40 patients completed the induction therapy: 24 patients received the Neoadjuvant HIVEC™ treatment. Of these patients, 15 (62.5%) showed a complete response. Eight patients (33.3%) showed a partial response, and one patient (4.1%) showed no response at all. The 4-year cumulative incidence of recurrence was 20.8%. The adjuvant HIVEC™ treatment was given to 16 patients. The 2-year cumulative incidence of recurrence was 12.5% for this group. The recirculation of hyperthermic MMC using Combat's HIVEC™ treatment is safe and effective and is capable of achieving good success rates in both neoadjuvant and adjuvant settings (Sousa et al. 2016). This treatment seems to be appropriate for NMIBC intermediate-high-risk patients who cannot tolerate or have contraindications for standard BCG therapy or in cases in which there are supply issues or shortages of BCG.

Moskovitz evaluated the efficacy of combined local hyperthermia and intra-vesical mitomycin-C (MMC) in a selected group of patients with intermediate or high-risk recurrent transitional cell carcinoma (TCC) of bladder (Moskovitz et al. 2005). Thirty-two patients were eligible for analysis. The prophylactic protocol was administered to 22 patients. After a mean follow-up of 289 days, 20 patients (91%) were recurrence free. Two patients (9%) had tumour recurrence after a mean period of 431 days. The ablative protocol was administered to 10 patients. Complete tumour ablation was achieved in eight patients (80%) after a mean follow up of 104.5 days (Moskovitz et al. 2005). The efficacy and safety results confirm those reported in previously published studies, suggesting the promis-ing value of this combined treatment modality for both prophylactic and ablative patients (Moskovitz et al. 2005).

28.9   Hyperthermic MMC and High-Risk Disease

Gofrit evaluated the effectiveness of combined local bladder hyperthermia and intravesical chemotherapy for the treatment of patients with high-grade (G3) NMI bladder cancer (Gofrit et al. 2004). Combined chemo-thermotherapy was admin-istered to 52 patients with high-grade NMI bladder cancer (40 patients with Stage T1 tumor, 11 with Ta, and 3 with concomitant or isolated carcinoma in situ) . After a mean follow-up of 35.3 months, 15 patients (62.5%) were recurrence free. The bladder preservation rate was 95.8% (Gofrit et al. 2004). The ablative protocol was administered to 28 patients. Complete ablation of the tumor was accomplished in 21 patients (75%). After a mean follow-up of 20 months, 80.9% of these patients were recurrence free (Gofrit et al. 2004). The bladder preservation rate for the ablative group was 78.6% (Gofrit et al. 2004). Combined local bladder hyperther-mia and intravesical chemotherapy has a beneficial prophylactic effect in patients with G3 NMI bladder cancer. Ablation of high-grade bladder tumors is feasible, achieving a complete response in about three quarters of the patients.

Non-muscle invasive bladder cancer (NMIBC) classified as T1G3 represents one of the most challenging issues in urologic oncology—this is highrisk dis-ease (Halachmi et al. 2011). Halachmi et al. (2011) retrospectively evaluated the clinical data of patients with T1G3 NMIBC who underwent TURBT followed by thermochemotherapy (TCT) treatment (Halachmi et al. 2011). A total 51 patients were available for analysis. Median follow-up time of tumor-free patients was 18 months (average 20, range 2–49 months). Seventeen patients (33.3%) had tumor recurrence and 4 of them progressed to muscle invasive disease (Halachmi et al. 2011). The median time to recurrence was 9 months (average 11, range 2–31 months). The Kaplan-Meier estimated recurrence rate for this group is: 42.9% at 2 years, 51.0% at 4 years. Hyperthermic MMC can be an effective adju-vant treatment option after TURBT to prevent recurrence in patients with T1G3 NMIBC (Halachmi et al. 2011). Progression rate after this treatment was low (7.9%). This treatment was well tolerated.

Ekin examined the effectiveness of mitomycin-C and chemo-hyperthermia in combination for patients with high-risk non-muscle-invasive bladder cancer (Ekin et al. 2015). A total of 40 patients completed induction therapy. Thirteen (32.5%) were diagnosed with tumor recurrence. Median follow-up was 30 months (range 9–39). The Kaplan-Meier-estimated recurrence-free rates for the entire group at 12 and 24 months were 82% and 61% (Ekin et al. 2015). There was no statistically significant difference between patient subgroups. Adverse effects were seen in 53% of patients and these were frequently grades 1 and 2 (Ekin et al. 2015). Intravesical therapy with combination of mitomycin-C and chemohyperthermia seems to be appropriate in high-risk patients with non-muscle-invasive bladder cancer who cannot tolerate or have contraindications for standard BCG therapy.

Gözen, evaluated the efficacy of combined local bladder hyperthermia and intravesical mitomycin-C (MMC) instillation in patients with high-risk recurrent NMIBC (Gözen et al. 2017). Mean age was 72 (32–87) years. 10 patients had multifocal disease, 9 had CIS, 6 had recurrent disease and 2 had highly recurrent disease (>3 recurrences in a 24 months period). 6 patients underwent previous intravesical chemotherapy with MMC (Gözen et al. 2017). The average number of maintenance sessions per patient was 7.6. After a mean follow-up of 433 days, 15 patients (83.3%) were recurrence-free. 3 patients had tumour recurrence after a mean period of 248 days without progression. Side effects were limited to grade 1 in 2 patients and grade 2 in 1 patient (Gözen et al. 2017). BWT seems to be feasible and safe in high grade NMIBC. More studies are needed to identify the subgroup of patients who may benefit more from this treatment.

Di Stası performed a prospective study in patients with high risk NMI bladder cancer to assess the efficacy of intravesical electromotive versus passive MMC using bacillus Calmette-Guerin (BCG) as a comparative treatment (Di Stası et al. 2003). The complete response for electromotive versus passive MMC at 3 and 6 months was 53% versus 28% ($p = 0.036$) and 58% versus 31% ($p = 0.012$). For BCG the responses were 56 and 64% (Di Stası et al. 2003). Median time to recurrence was 35 versus 19.5 months ($p = 0.013$) and for BCG it was 26 months. Peak plasma MMC was significantly higher following electromotive MMC than after MMC (43 vs. 8 ng/ml), consistent with bladder content absorption (Di Stası et al. 2003). Intravesical electromotive administration increases bladder uptake of MMC, resulting in an improved response rate in cases of high risk NMI bladder cancer.

28.10 Delayed Cystectomy and Hyperthermic MMC

Non-muscle-invasive bladder cancer is characterized by a high recurrence rate after primary transurethral resection (Volpe et al. 2012). In case of bacillus Calmette-Guérin-refractory neoplasms, cystectomy is the gold standard. In this study the effects of thermochemotherapy with mitomycin C were evaluated in high-risk bladder cancer nonresponders to previous therapy (Volpe et al. 2012).

All the patients completed the study. The mean follow-up for all the patients enrolled was 14 months. Thirteen of 30 patients (43.30%) were disease free and 17 patients (56.70%) had recurrence (Volpe et al. 2012). In the prophylactic group, 7 of 16 patients (43.75%) were disease free and 9 patients (46.25%) had tumor recurrence; no progression was observed. In the ablative group, 3 patients (17, 64%) had progression to muscle-invasive disease. Side effects were generally mild (Volpe et al. 2012). Thermochemotherapy could be considered an additional tool in patients refractory to intravesical therapies before considering early cystectomy (Volpe et al. 2012).

28.11 Hyperthermic MMC for CIS

Witjes studied the results of chemotherapy combined with intravesical hyperthermia in patients with mainly BCG-failing carcinoma in situ (CIS) (Witjes et al. 2009). Fifty-one patients were treated between 1997 and 2005 from 15 European centers. Thirty-four were pre-treated with BCG. Mean age was 69.9 years (Witjes et al. 2009). Twenty-four patients had concomitant papillary tumors. The mean number of hyperthermia/MMC treatments per patient was 10.0. Of the 49 evaluable patients 45 had a biopsy and cytology proven complete response. In two patients CIS disappeared, but they had persistent papillary tumors (Witjes et al. 2009). Follow-up of 45 complete responders showed 22 recurrences after a mean of 27 months (median 22): T2 (4), T1 (4), T1/CIS (1), CIS (5), Ta/CIS (2), Ta (5) and Tx (1). Side effects (bladder complaints) were generally mild and transient (Witjes et al. 2009). In patients with primary or BCG-failing CIS, treatment with intravesical hyperthermia and MMC appears a safe and effective treatment (Witjes et al. 2009). The initial complete response rate is 92%, which remains approximately 50% after 2 years (Witjes et al. 2009).

28.12 Adjuvant Therapy

Colombo presented a long-term efficacy data of intravesical thermochemotherapy versus chemotherapy alone with mitomycin-C (MMC) randomly administered to patients with non-muscle-invasive bladder cancer (NMIBC) as an adjuvant treatment after complete transurethral resection (Colombo et al. 2011).

Data was gained for 65/75 (87%) of the original patientsThe 10-year disease-free survival rate for thermochemotherapy and chemotherapy alone were 53% and 15%, respectively ($p < 0.001$) (Colombo et al. 2011). An intent-to-treat analysis performed to overcome the potential bias introduced by the asymmetrical discontinuation rate still showed a significant advantage of the active treatment over the control treatment (Colombo et al. 2011). Bladder preservation rates for thermochemotherapy and chemotherapy alone were 86% and 79%, respectively.

This is the first analysis of long-term follow-up of patients treated with intravesical thermochemotherapy (Colombo et al. 2011). The high rate (53%) of patients who were tumour-free 10 years after treatment completion, as well as the high rate (86%) of bladder preservation, confirms the efficacy of this adjuvant approach for NMIBC at long-term follow-up, even in patients with multiple tumours (Colombo et al. 2011).

28.13   Adverse Effects with Hyperthermic MMC

Inman evaluated the safety and heating efficiency of external deep pelvic hyperthermia combined with intravesical mitomycin C (MMC) as a novel therapy for non-muscle-invasive bladder cancer (NMIBC) (Inman et al. 2014). Fifteen patients were enrolled on the clinical trial. The full treatment course was attained in 73% of subjects. Effective bladder heating was possible in all but one patient who could not tolerate the supine position due to lung disease (Inman et al. 2014). Adverse events were all minor (grade 2 or less) and no systemic toxicity was observed. The most common adverse effects were Foley catheter pain (40%), abdominal discomfort (33%), chemical cystitis symptoms (27%), and abdominal skin swelling (27%) (Inman et al. 2014). With a median follow-up of 3.18 years, 67% experienced another bladder cancer recurrence (none were muscle invasive) and 13% experienced an upper tract recurrence. External deep pelvic hyperthermia using the BSD-2000 device is a safe and reproducible method of heating the bladder in patients undergoing intravesical MMC. The efficacy of this treatment modality should be explored further in clinical trials.

Kiss prospectively evaluated the outcome of combined microwave-induced bladder wall hyperthermia and intravesical mitomycin C instillation (thermochemotherapy) in patients with recurrent non-muscle-invasive bladder cancer (Kiss et al. 2015). Adverse effects were frequent and severe: urinary urgency/frequency in 11 of 21 patients (52%), pain in eight of 21 patients (38%) and gross hematuria in five of 21 patients (24%). In eight of 21 patients (38%), thermochemotherapy had to be abandoned because of the severity of the adverse effects (pain in 3/8, severe bladder spasms in 2/8, allergic reaction in 2/8, urethral perforation in 1/8) (Kiss et al. 2015). Overall, six of 21 patients (29%) remained free of tumor after a median follow up of 50 months (range 1–120), six of 21 patients (29%) had to undergo cystectomy because of multifocal recurrences or cancer progression and seven of 21 patients (33%) died (2/7 of metastatic disease, 5/7 of non-cancer related causes) (Kiss et al. 2015). Given the high rate of severe side-effects leading to treatment discontinuation, as well as the limited tumor response, thermochemotherapy should be offered only in highly selected cases of recurrent non-muscle-invasive bladder cancer (Kiss et al. 2015).

The treatment of non muscle invasive bladder cancer (NMIBC) continues to be a challenge. Hyperthermia (HT) combined with intravesical chemotherapy is used to enhance the effects of chemotherapy (León-Mata et al. 2018). SYNERGO®:

The dropout rate varied between 3 and 40%, and the AE rate is up to 88%. The most common AEs were pain (2–40%), thermal reaction of the posterior wall (13–100%), bladder spasms (2–32%), dysuria (3–60%) and hematuria (2–62%) (León-Mata et al. 2018). COMBAT BRS®: The dropout rate is 3–11%. The AEs reported were CTCAE Grade 1–2: Pain 13–27%, bladder spasms 6–27% and hematuria 3–20% are the most relevant. In general, CTCAE grade 3–4 toxicity is not reported. UNITHERMIA® (León-Mata et al. 2018): The dropout rate is 7–12%. The AEs described are: Pain 6–23%, bladder spasms 6–23%, hematuria 9–11, frequency 15–25% and allergy 6–11%. The majority of toxicities are CTCAE grade 1–2 (17–53%), with grade 3–4 in 9–15% and grade 5 in 0–2%. QHT adds little to the AEs of the treatment with MMC. QHT has proven to be a safe alternative for the treatment of intermediate and high risk NMIBC, with AE mainly grade 1–2 (León-Mata et al. 2018).

28.14 Combined Chemo Hyperthermia—Epirubicin and MMC

Nonmuscle invasive bladder cancer is characterized by a high recurrence rate. New adjuvant treatments are needed to decrease this high number of recurrences (Arends et al. 2014). Arends present the results of more than 10 years of experience with chemohyperthermia in patients with nonmuscle invasive bladder cancer (Arends et al. 2014). A total of 160 patients with nonmuscle invasive bladder cancer were included, including 20 (13%) treated with epirubicin and 129 (81%) previously treated with bacillus Calmette-Guérin. One and 2-year recurrence-free survival was 60% and 47%, respectively. Muscle invasive progression was seen in 4% of cases (Arends et al. 2014). Two-year recurrence-free survival in the epirubicin and mitomycin groups was 55% and 46%, respectively ($p = 0.30$). The highly recurrent nonmuscle invasive bladder cancer group had significant decreased recurrence-free survival compared to other groups ($p < 0.01$) (Arends et al. 2014). Patients treated with 2 or fewer versus greater than 2 transurethral bladder tumor resections before chemohyperthermia had higher recurrence-free survival ($p = 0.01$) (Arends et al. 2014). On multivariable analysis the highly recurrent cancer criteria remained independently associated with decreased recurrence-free survival (HR 2.40, 95% CI 1.30–4.43, $p = 0.01$) (Arends et al. 2014). Chemohyperthermia is an effective approach to nonmuscle invasive bladder cancer for which standard intravesical treatments fail. Patients with highly recurrent disease before chemohyperthermia have lower recurrence-free survival (Arends et al. 2014). Furthermore, recurrence-free survival appears to improve with earlier chemohyperthermia. No significant differences were observed between the 2 chemotherapy agents.

References

Alfred Witjes J, Hendricksen K, Gofrit O, Risi O, Nativ O. Intravesical hyperthermia and mitomycin-C for carcinoma in situ of the urinary bladder: experience of the European Synergo working party. World J Urol. 2009;27(3):319–24.

Arends TJ, van der Heijden AG, Witjes JA. Combined chemohyperthermia: 10-year single center experience in 160 patients with nonmuscle invasive bladder cancer. J Urol. 2014;192(3):708–13.

Arends TJ, Falke J, Lammers RJ, Somford DM, Hendriks JC, de Weijert MC, Arentsen HC, van der Heijden AG, Oosterwijk E, Alfred Witjes J. Urinary cytokines in patients treated with intravesical mitomycin-C with and without hyperthermia. World J Urol. 2015;33(10):1411–7.

Ba M, Cui S, Wang B, Long H, Yan Z, Wang S, Wu Y, Gong Y. Bladder intracavitary hyperthermic perfusion chemotherapy for the prevention of recurrence of non-muscle invasive bladder cancer after transurethral resection. Oncol Rep. 2017;37(5):2761–70.

Bahouth Z, Halachmi S, Moskovitz B, Nativ O. The role of hyperthermia as a treatment for non-muscle invasive bladder cancer. Expert Rev Anticancer Ther. 2016;16(2):189–98.

Colombo R, Da Pozzo LF, Lev A, Salonia A, Rigatti P, Leib Z, Servadio C, Caldarera E. Pavone-Macaluso M Local microwave hyperthermia and intravesical chemotherapy as bladder sparing treatment for select multifocal and unresectable NMI bladder tumors. J Urol. 1998;159(3):783–7.

Colombo R, Salonia A, Leib Z, Pavone-Macaluso M, Engelstein D. Long-term outcomes of a randomized controlled trial comparing thermochemotherapy with mitomycin-C alone as adjuvant treatment for non-muscle-invasive bladder cancer (NMIBC). BJU Int. 2011;107(6):912–8.

Di Stasi SM, Giannantoni A, Stephen RL, Capelli G, Navarra P, Massoud R, Vespasiani G. Intravesical electromotive mitomycin C versus passive transport mitomycin C for high risk NMI bladder cancer: a prospective randomized study. J Urol. 2003;170(3):777–82.

D'Souza N, Verma A. Holmium laser transurethral resection of bladder tumor: our experience. Urol Ann. 2016;8(4):439.

Ekin RG, Akarken I, Cakmak O, Tarhan H, Celik O, Ilbey YO, Divrik RT, Zorlu F. Results of Intravesical chemo-hyperthermia in high-risk non-muscle invasive bladder cancer. Asian Pac J Cancer Prev. 2015;16(8):3241–5.

Geijsen ED, de Reijke TM, Koning CC, Zum Vörde Sive Vörding PJ, de la Rosette JJ, Rasch CR, van Os RM, Crezee J. Combining mitomycin C and regional 70 MHz hyperthermia in patients with nonmuscle invasive bladder cancer: a Pilot study. J Urol. 2015;194(5):1202–8.

Gofrit ON, Shapiro A, Pode D, Sidi A, Nativ O, Leib Z, Witjes JA, van der Heijden AG, Naspro R, Colombo R. Combined local bladder hyperthermia and intravesical chemotherapy for the treatment of high-grade NMI bladder cancer. Urology. 2004;63(3):466–71.

Gözen AS, Umari P, Scheitlin W, Su FE, Akin Y, Rassweiler J. Effectivity of intravesical thermo-chemotherapy prophylaxis for patients with high recurrence and progression risk for non-muscle invasive bladder cancer. Arch Ital Urol Androl. 2017;89(2):102–5.

Halachmi S, Moskovitz B, Maffezzini M, Conti G, Verweij F, Kedar D, Sandri SD, Nativ O, Colombo R. Intravesical mitomycin C combined with hyperthermia for patients with T1G3 transitional cell carcinoma of the bladder. Urol Oncol. 2011;29(3):259–64.

Inman BA, Stauffer PR, Craciunescu OA, Maccarini PF, Dewhirst MW, Vujaskovic Z. A pilot clinical trial of intravesical mitomycin-C and external deep pelvic hyperthermia for non-muscle-invasive bladder cancer. Int J Hyperthermia. 2014;30(3):171–5.

Kiss B, Schneider S, Thalmann GN, Roth B. Is thermochemotherapy with the Synergo system a viable treatment option in patients with recurrent non-muscle-invasive bladder cancer? Int J Urol. 2015;22(2):158–62.

León-Mata J, Domínguez JL, Redorta JP, Sousa González D, Alvarez Casal M, Sousa Escandón A, Piñeiro Vázquez E. Analysis of tolerance and security of chemo hyperthermia with Mitomycin C for the treatment of non-muscle invasive bladder cancer. Arch Esp Urol. 2018;71(4):426–37.

Mays N, Pope C, Popay J. Systematically reviewing qualitative and quantitative evidence to inform management and policy-making in the health field. J Health Serv Res Policy. 2005;10(Suppl. 1):6–20.

Milla P, Fiorito C, Soria F, Arpicco S, Cattel L, Gontero P. Intravesical thermo-chemotherapy based on conductive heat: a first pharmacokinetic study with mitomycin C in NMI transitional cell carcinoma patients. Cancer Chemother Pharmacol. 2014;73(3):503–9.

Moher D, Liberati A, Tetzlaff J, Altman DG. Preferred reporting items for systematic reviews and meta-analyses: the prisma statement. BMJ. 2009;339(7716):332–6.

Moskovitz B, Meyer G, Kravtzov A, Gross M, Kastin A, Biton K, Nativ O. Thermo-chemotherapy for intermediate or high-risk recurrent NMI bladder cancer patients. Ann Oncol. 2005;16(4):585–9.

Nativ O, Witjes JA, Hendricksen K, Cohen M, Kedar D, Sidi A, Colombo R, Leibovitch I. Combined thermo-chemotherapy for recurrent bladder cancer after bacillus Calmette-Guerin. J Urol. 2009;182(4):1313–7.

Rigatti P, Lev A, Colombo R. Combined intravesical chemotherapy with mitomycin C and local bladder microwave-induced hyperthermia as a preoperative therapy for NMI bladder tumors. A preliminary clinical study. Eur Urol. 1991;20(3):204–10.

Sooriakumaran P, Chiocchia V, Dutton S, Pai A, Ayres BE, Le Roux P, Swinn M, Bailey M, Perry MJ, Issa R. Predictive factors for time to progression after hyperthermic mitomycin C treatment for high-risk non-muscle invasive urothelial carcinoma of the bladder: an observational cohort study of 97 patients. Urol Int. 2016;96(1):83–90.

Sousa A, Piñeiro I, Rodríguez S, Aparici V, Monserrat V, Neira P, Carro E, Murias C, Uribarri C. Recirculant hyperthermic IntraVEsical chemotherapy (HIVEC) in intermediate-high-risk non-muscle-invasive bladder cancer. Int J Hyperthermia. 2016;32(4):374–80.

van Valenberg H, Colombo R, Witjes F. Intravesical radiofrequency-induced hyperthermia combined with chemotherapy for non-muscle-invasive bladder cancer. Int J Hyperthermia. 2016;32(4):351–62.

Volpe A, Racioppi M, Bongiovanni L, D'Agostino D, Totaro A, D'Addessi A, Marangi F, Palermo G, Pinto F, Sacco E, Bassi PF. Thermochemotherapy for non-muscle-invasive bladder cancer: is there a chance to avoid early cystectomy? Urol Int. 2012;89(3):311–8.

Chapter 29
Literature Related to Hyperthermic MMC

The treatment of non muscle invasive bladder cancer (NMIBC) continues to be a challenge. Hyperthermia (HT) combined with intravesical chemotherapy is used to enhance the effects of chemotherapy (León-Mata et al. 2018). QHT has proven to be a safe alternative for the treatment of intermediate and high risk NMIBC, with AE mainly grade 1–2. The AEs reported have little variation with respect to the dose of MMC used, presenting different "profiles" related to the device used for its administration (León-Mata et al. 2018). The treatments with QHTMMC are well tolerated, without adding significantly more AE than the instillations of MMC alone and presenting a better toxicity profile than those reflected in the literature with respect to the treatment with BCG (León-Mata et al. 2018).

During the last 15 year, the combined regimen has been tested in different clinical settings (Lammers et al. 2011). A total of 22 studies met inclusion criteria and underwent data extraction. When possible, data were combined using random effects meta-analytic techniques. Recurrence was seen 59% less after C-HT than after MMC alone (Lammers et al. 2011). Due to short follow-up, no conclusions can be drawn about time to recurrence and progression. The overall bladder preservation rate after C-HT was 87.6%. This rate appeared higher than after MMC alone, but valid comparison studies were lacking. AEs were higher with C-HT than with MMC alone, but this difference was not statistically significant (Lammers et al. 2011). Published data suggest a 59% relative reduction in NMIBC recurrence when C-HT is compared with MMC alone. C-HT also appears to improve bladder preservation rate (Lammers et al. 2011).

© Springer Nature Switzerland AG 2020   165
S. S. Goonewardene et al., *Management of Non-Muscle Invasive Bladder Cancer*,
https://doi.org/10.1007/978-3-030-28646-0_29

References

Lammers RJ, Witjes JA, Inman BA, Leibovitch I, Laufer M, Nativ O, Colombo R. The role of a combined regimen with intravesical chemotherapy and hyperthermia in the management of non-muscle-invasive bladder cancer: a systematic review. Eur Urol. 2011;60(1):81–93.

León-Mata J, Domínguez JL, Redorta JP, Sousa González D, Alvarez Casal M, Sousa Escandón A, Piñeiro Vázquez E. Analysis of tolerance and security of chemo hyperthermia with mitomycin C for the treatment of non-muscle invasive bladder cancer. Arch Esp Urol. 2018;71(4):426–37.

Part VII
Management of High Risk Non-Muscle Invasive Bladder Cancer

Chapter 30
BCG—Patterns of Administration

Multiple clinical trials have demonstrated that intravesical Bacillus Calmette-Guérin (BCG) treatment reduces progression in non-muscle-invasive bladder cancer (NMIBC) (Ajili et al. 2012). However, patterns of administration vary. A focus group of specialized urologic oncologists (urologists, medical oncologists and radiation oncologists) reviewed the current guidelines and clinical evidence, discussed their experiences and formed a consensus regarding the optimal use of BCG (Ajili et al. 2012). The study concluded continuing therapy with 3-week BCG maintenance is superior to induction treatment only and a reliable alternative to radical cystectomy in truly BCG-refractory disease remains the subject of clinical trials (Ajili et al. 2012).

However, although BCG has been in use for almost 40 years, this agent is often underutilized (Kamat et al. 2015). This is caused by uncertainties about the optimal use of BCG, treatment schedules and patient selection (Kamat et al. 2015). When asked experts concluded that a reliable alternative to radical cystectomy in truly BCG-refractory disease remains the subject of clinical trials (Kamat et al. 2015).

Although bacillus Calmette-Guérin (BCG) has proven highly effective in non-muscle-invasive bladder cancer (NMIBC), but it can cause severe local and systemic side effects (Brausi et al. 2014). After transurethral resection, patients with intermediate- and high-risk NMIBC without carcinoma in situ were randomised to one-third dose or full dose BCG and 1 or 3 year of maintenance (Brausi et al. 2014). No significant differences in side effects were detected according to dose or duration of BCG treatment in the four arms (Brausi et al. 2014). Side effects requiring stoppage of treatment were seen more frequently in the first year, so not all patients are able to receive the 1–3 year of treatment recommended in current guidelines (Brausi et al. 2014).

© Springer Nature Switzerland AG 2020   169
S. S. Goonewardene et al., *Management of Non-Muscle Invasive Bladder Cancer*,
https://doi.org/10.1007/978-3-030-28646-0_30

References

Ajili F, Manai M, Darouiche A, Chebil M, Boubaker S. Tumor multiplicity is an independent prognostic factor of non-muscle-invasive bladder cancer treated with Bacillus Calmette-Guerin immunotherapy. Ultrastruct Pathol. 2012;36(5):320–4.

Brausi M, Oddens J, Sylvester R, Bono A, van de Beek C, van Andel G, Gontero P, Turkeri L, Marreaud S, Collette S, Oosterlinck W. Side effects of Bacillus Calmette-Guérin (BCG) in the treatment of intermediate- and high-risk Ta, T1 papillary carcinoma of the bladder: results of the EORTC genito-urinary cancers group randomised phase 3 study comparing one-third dose with full dose and 1 year with 3 years of maintenance BCG. Eur Urol. 2014;65(1):69–76.

Kamat AM, Flaig TW, Grossman HB, Konety B, Lamm D, O'Donnell MA, Uchio E, Efstathiou JA, Taylor JA 3rd. Expert consensus document: consensus statement on best practice management regarding the use of intravesical immunotherapy with BCG for bladder cancer. Nat Rev Urol. 2015;12(4):225–35.

Chapter 31
NMIBC—BCG Strain and Outcomes

BCG is an immunotherapy. There are at least 4 different strains, Connaught, Pasteur, Tice, RIVM Whether the commonly used Bacillus Calmette-Guérin (BCG) strains Connaught and Tice confer different treatment. This has been investigated by Rentsch et al., as a prospective randomized single-institution trial. This included 142 high-risk NMIBC patients with BCG Connaught or Tice. Treatment with BCG Connaught conferred significantly greater 5-year recurrence-free survival as opposed to BCG Tice ($p = 0.0108$) (Rentsch et al. 2014). Comparable numbers of patients experienced BCG therapy-related side effects in each treatment group ($p = 0.09$). This demonstrated BCG strain may have an impact on treatment outcome in NMIBC immunotherapy.

BCG RIVM strain was used in many treatment protocols for non-muscle invasive bladder cancer only as induction courses (Farah et al. 2014). Cho et al. (Anticancer Res 2012) compared BCG-RIVM induction and 'standard' maintenance (Lamm et al., J Urol. 2000) to mitomycin C. They found no statistically significant differences regarding disease recurrence and progression. This may indicate a lower level of treatment is required for induction than actually conducted.

Farah et al. (2014) determined the efficacy and tolerability of this specific BCG RIVM strain, using six-weekly, induction course and single monthly instillations as maintenance for one year, in high risk recurrent, multifocal low grade and multifocal high grade pTa/pT1, CIS transitional cell carcinoma of bladder (Farah et al. 2014). From 42 patients, recurrence occurred in 16 patients (26.7%) at a median follow-up of 24.2 months while progression occurred in five patients (8.3%) at a median follow-up of 33 months. Recurrence-free survival and progression-free survival rates were 73% and 92% respectively. Cystectomy was performed in seven patients (12%) with a cystectomy-free survival of 88%. There were no cancer specific deaths. Two patients died of other causes (3.3%). The overall survival rate was 97%. This protocol achieved equivalent recurrence-free, progression-free, disease specific survival and overall survival to the reported literature.

© Springer Nature Switzerland AG 2020   171
S. S. Goonewardene et al., *Management of Non-Muscle Invasive Bladder Cancer*,
https://doi.org/10.1007/978-3-030-28646-0_31

Increasing evidence suggests that there are marked differences in outcomes according to BCG substrains. BCG-Moreau was recently introduced to the European market to cover the issue of BCG shortage, but there are little data regarding the oncologic efficacy (Hofbauer et al. 2016). BCG-Moreau is an effective substrain for adjuvant instillation therapies of NMIBC, and outcomes appear to be comparable to series using other substrains (Hofbauer et al. 2016). During worldwide shortage of BCG-TICE, Connaught and RIVM, BCG-Moreau may serve as an equally effective alternative.

Potential differences in efficacy of different Bacillus Calmette-Guérin (BCG) strains are of importance for daily practice, especially in the era of BCG shortage (Witjes et al. 2016). Witjes et al. retrospectively, compared the outcome with BCG Connaught and BCG TICE in a large study cohort of pT1 high-grade non-muscle-invasive bladder cancer patients. Information on the BCG strain was available for 2099 patients: 957 on Connaught and 1142 on TICE (Witjes et al. 2016). Overall, 765 (36%) patients received some form of maintenance BCG, 560 (59%) on Connaught and 205 (18%) on TICE (Witjes et al. 2016). Connaught and TICE had a similar efficacy. Compared to no maintenance therapy, maintenance BCG significantly reduced the risk of recurrence, progression and death, both overall, and disease specific, for TICE, but not for Connaught (Witjes et al. 2016). BCG Connaught reduces the recurrence rate compared to BCG TICE when no maintenance is used, but the opposite is true when maintenance is given (Witjes et al. 2016).

References

Farah NB, Ghanem R, Amr M. Treatment efficacy and tolerability of intravesical Bacillus Calmette-Guerin (BCG)-RIVM strain: induction and maintenance protocol in high grade and recurrent low grade non-muscle invasive bladder cancer (NMIBC). BMC Urol. 2014;14:11.

Hofbauer SL, Shariat SF, Chade DC, Sarkis AS, Ribeiro-Filho LA, Nahas WC, Klatte T. The Moreau strain of Bacillus Calmette-Guerin (BCG) for high-risk non-muscle invasive bladder cancer: an alternative during worldwide BCG shortage? Urol Int. 2016;96(1):46–50.

Rentsch CA, Birkhauser FD, Biot C, Gsponer JR, Bisiaux A, Wetterauer C, Lagranderie M, et al. Bacillus Calmette-Guerin strain differences have an impact on clinical outcome in bladder cancer immunotherapy. Eur Urol. 2014;66(4):677–88.

Witjes JA, Dalbagni G, Karnes RJ, Shariat S, Joniau S, Palou J, Serretta V, Larré S, di Stasi S, Colombo R, Babjuk M, Malmström PU, Malats N, Irani J, Baniel J, Cai T, Cha E, Ardelt P, Varkarakis J, Bartoletti R, Spahn M, Pisano F, Gontero P, Sylvester R. The efficacy of BCG TICE and BCG Connaught in a cohort of 2,099 patients with T1G3 non-muscle-invasive bladder cancer. Urol Oncol. 2016;34(11):484.e19–25.

Chapter 32
Adverse Effects in BCG Therapy

Non-Muscle invasive urothelial carcinoma is a variable disease that needs a variety of surgical and non-surgical treatment strategies (Neuzillet et al. 2012). The disease course can range from recurrent low-grade papillary disease to aggressive disease concerning for progression from initial presentation (Neuzillet et al. 2012). For most patients some form of intravesical therapy will bridge the gap between transurethral resections (TUR) and radical surgery.

BCG therapy, which is the standard treatment for non-muscle invasive bladder tumours with high risk of recurrence and progression, has potential life-threatening adverse effects (AEs) (Neuzillet et al. 2013). Rapid deterioration of general condition in a patient with history of bladder tumour should question about an ongoing treatment with BCG and specify the date of the last instillation (Neuzillet et al. 2013). Trauma during catheterization and UTIS are risk factors of severe AEs (Neuzillet et al. 2013). In emergency, the diagnosis of severe AEs of BCG therapy is only based on the medical questioning with the notion of current BCG treatment and risk-bearing event upon instillation (Neuzillet et al. 2013). Management of AEs is related to their pathophysiological mechanisms and relies on a combination of antibiotics against BCG, the symptomatic treatment, and corticosteroid therapy which has shown to improve patient outcomes (Neuzillet et al. 2013).

Recent advances in the field continue to emphasize the importance of quality TUR and its strong impact on outcomes (Neuzillet et al. 2012). In addition, continued research to optimize intravesical therapies has provided more information about how, when, and in whom these agents should be utilized to enhance their efficacy (Neuzillet et al. 2012).

© Springer Nature Switzerland AG 2020
S. S. Goonewardene et al., *Management of Non-Muscle Invasive Bladder Cancer*,
https://doi.org/10.1007/978-3-030-28646-0_32

References

Neuzillet Y, Rouprêt M, Larré S, Irani J, Davin JL, Moreau JL, Pfister C. Diagnosis and management of severe adverse events occurring during BCG therapy for non-muscle invasive bladder cancer (NMIBC). Presse Med. 2013;42(7–8):1100–8.

Neuzillet Y, Rouprêt M, Wallerand H, Pignot G, Larré S, Irani J, Davin JL, Moreau JL, Soulié M, Pfister C, le comité de cancérologie de l'association française d'urologie. Diagnosis and management of adverse events occurring during BCG therapy for non-muscle invasive bladder cancer (NMIBC): review of the cancer committee of the French association of urology. Prog Urol. 2012;22(16):989–98.

Chapter 33
BCG and Elderly Patients

Although Bacillus Calmette-Guérin (BCG) is the recommended treatment in high-risk non-muscle-invasive bladder cancer (NMIBC), its efficacy in older patients is controversial (Oddens et al. 2014). Oddens et al. determined the effect of age on prognosis and treatment outcome in patients with stage Ta T1 NMIBC treated with maintenance BCG. With a median follow-up of 9.2 year, patients >70 year had a shorter time to progression ($p = 0.028$), overall survival ($p < 0.001$), and NMIBC-specific survival ($p = 0.049$) after adjustment for EORTC risk scores in the multivariate analysis (Oddens et al. 2014). The time to recurrence was similar compared with the younger patients. BCG was more effective than epirubicin for all four end points considered, and there was no evidence that BCG was any less effective compared with epirubicin in patients >70 year. In intermediate- and high-risk Ta T1 Urothelial cell carcinomapatients treated with BCG, patients >70 year of age have a worse long-term prognosis; however, BCG is more effective than epirubicin independent of patient age.

Bladder cancer is a disease of the elderly (Galsky 2015). There is a disconnect between the efficacy of treatments for patients with advanced disease, and their effectiveness, related to the advanced age at diagnosis (Galsky 2015). Standard treatments for patients with locally advanced or metastatic bladder cancer include radical cystectomy and/or cisplatin-based combination chemotherapy (Galsky 2015). However, there is significant potential for morbidity, and even mortality, with these treatments necessitating tools to risk stratify elderly patients to optimize the safety and benefit of treatments and alternative strategies in situations where the potential risks are likely to outweigh the potential benefits (Galsky 2015). This review considers the current standard treatments for advanced bladder cancer, approaches to risk stratify elderly patients, and highlights our relatively poor knowledge base regarding the optimal care of elderly patients with this disease.

Bladder cancer is diagnosed more often in the elderly (Ghebriou et al. 2014). The most effective treatment strategies are mostly very aggressive and not really applicable to an unfit patient population (Ghebriou et al. 2014). However, effective

© Springer Nature Switzerland AG 2020
S. S. Goonewardene et al., *Management of Non-Muscle Invasive Bladder Cancer*,
https://doi.org/10.1007/978-3-030-28646-0_33

options exist to treat the most vulnerable subjects. A multidisciplinary approach including a geriatric assessment is essential for optimal adaptation of treatment (Ghebriou et al. 2014). The Francilian Oncogeriatric Group (FROG) conducted a comprehensive literature search in order to review the applicable therapeutic options according to oncological and geriatric settings. International recommendations are essential to harmonize the management of elderly patients with bladder cancer (Ghebriou et al. 2014).

Urinary bladder cancer (UBC) is dominantly the cancer of the elderly occurring primarily in the 6th, 7th and 8th decade of life (Tadin et al. 2014). Tadin evaluated diagnostic accuracy of ultrasound T-staging (UTS) of bladder cancer. The best result was established for the stage T1, where the accuracy was 94.5%. In other stages the accuracy was between 84.9 and 91.8% (Tadin et al. 2014). The Youden's index for all the stages was over 0.6. UTS has a high diagnostic accuracy, especially for stages T1 and T2. It is extremely useful tool in differentiating the NMI UBC from the muscle-invasive one, being of significant importance in planning the further treatment of elderly patients and having important role in choosing appropriate surgical approach (Tadin et al. 2014). However, this is not the gold standard. CT Urogram is currently the gold standard for assessment of upper tracts and MRI pelvis with contrast is required for assessment of muscle invasive disease.

Bladder cancer (BC) predominantly affects the elderly and is often the cause of death among patients with muscle-invasive disease (Noon et al. 2013). Noon et al. determine the bladder cancer-specific mortality (CSM) rate and other-cause mortality (OCM) rate for patients with newly diagnosed BC.

The 5-year BC mortality rate varied between 1 and 59%, and OCM rate between 6 and 90%, depending primarily on the tumour type and patient age. Cancer-specific mortality was highest in the oldest patient groups (Noon et al. 2013). Few elderly patients received radical treatment for invasive cancer (52% vs. 12% for patients <60 years vs. >80 years, respectively). Female patients with high-risk non-muscle-invasive BC had worse CSM than equivalent males (Gray's $p<0.01$) (Noon et al. 2013). Bladder CSM is highest among the elderly. Female patients with high-risk tumours are more likely to die of their disease compared with male patients. Clinicians should consider offering more aggressive treatment interventions among older patients, if patients are fit.

The impact of bladder cancer diagnosis on health-related quality of life is poorly understood. Fung et al. compared health related quality of life before and after bladder cancer diagnosis (Fung et al. 2014). Future research into interventions to improve health related quality of life and methods to incorporate health related quality of life into decision making models are critical to improve outcomes in older patients with bladder cancer.

Bladder cancer is largely a disease of older adults, with nearly half of diagnoses occurring in those older than age 75 (Stensland et al. 2014). Extrapolating the available evidence to the population of older patients with bladder cancer requires careful assessment of an individual patient's functional status and comorbidities to estimate the likelihood of treatment-related harms (Stensland et al. 2014). This should be coupled with an understanding of an individual patient's goals of therapy, independence, estimated longevity, and social support to facilitate a shared medical decision regarding treatment (Stensland et al. 2014).

Bladder urothelial carcinoma is rare in young adults and occurs more commonly in older individuals (Telli et al. 2014). Telli et al. compared bladder cancer in young versus older adults. Young bladder cancer patients had smaller-sized tumors (less than 3 cm), less high-grade cancers, higher papillary urothelial neoplasms of low malignant potential, and low-grade tumors than patients older than 40 years. Telli et al. concluded that although the clinical stage distribution, natural history, and outcomes of bladder urothelial cancer in young adults are similar to those in their older counterparts, clinicians must be aware that patients over 40 years of age presented with higher-grade and larger (>3 cm) tumors and are more likely to experience tumor recurrence (Telli et al. 2014).

Bladder cancer is a disease of older patients who often have multiple comorbidities. Although cisplatin-based combination chemotherapy is the standard of care in the neoadjuvant and metastatic settings, outcomes remain poor, and approximately half of patients are ineligible for cisplatin where treatment options are severely limited (Milowsky and Kim 2014). Bladder cancer represents an ideal model to study the potential of targeted therapy in older patients who are too often unable to receive cisplatin-based therapy and where novel treatment strategies are desperately needed (Milowsky and Kim 2014).

Cancer is the leading cause of death among patients aged 65 years and older. In this population, the cancer diagnosis is often made at a more advanced stage and worse prognosis than in younger patients (Ploussard et al. 2014). Specific mortality in older patients is superior to that reported in their younger counterparts (Ploussard et al. 2014). Moreover, the impact of curative treatment that has proven benefit in overall population may be not well studied in the sub-group of older patients (Ploussard et al. 2014). Comorbidities increase the complexity of cancer management and affect survival.

In the elderly, an enhanced support including specific geriatric assessment and management optimizes the treatment course, including preoperative optimization, prevents treatment-related complications and loss of autonomy using or not geriatrics clinic or rehabilitation units, and limits the length of hospital stay and costs (Ploussard et al. 2014).

Leveridge et al. reviewed radical cystectomy (RC) outcomes and adjuvant chemotherapy (ACT) use in the elderly in routine practice (Leveridge et al. 2015). Bladder cancer occurs most commonly in the elderly. RC, standard treatment for muscle-invasive bladder cancer, presents challenges in older patients (Leveridge et al. 2015). Suboptimal evidence guides ACT use. Cystectomy carries a higher risk of postoperative mortality in elderly patients in routine clinical practice (Leveridge et al. 2015). ACT is used infrequently in older patients despite a substantial survival benefit observed across all age groups.

Coward et al. reported their experience with robotic radical cystectomy as applied to an older patient population with regard to perioperative measures and pathologic outcomes (Coward et al. 2011). A robotic approach to radical cystectomy for bladder cancer have recently been described, but its application in an older patient population, which is often the case in bladder cancer and cystectomy, has not yet been assessed (Coward et al. 2011). No differences were observed between the 2 groups in blood loss, time to discharge, or complication rate. Also, no significant differences were found in the surgical pathologic findings, including the organ-confined rate (62% vs. 71%) and lymph node yield (19.5 vs. 18.1) (Coward et al. 2011). Older patients do not appear to have any significant differences or compromises with regard to the perioperative and pathologic outcome.

Despite the fact that bladder cancer patients have the highest median age of any type of cancer, older patients with muscle invasion are often under-treated (VanderWalde et al. 2016).

Chronologic age should not exclude patients from curative-intent therapy. Functional age as determined by geriatric assessments and multidisciplinary evaluation can help clinicians decide on the best course of treatment for individual patients (VanderWalde et al. 2016). Cystectomy, perioperative chemotherapy, and curative-intent bladder preservation are reasonable options in healthy older adults (VanderWalde et al. 2016). Observation should be limited to patients with extremely poor performance status and very limited life expectancy.

California Cancer Registry data illustrate a peak in the incidence of bladder cancer in individuals 85 years or older (Schultzel et al. 2008). However, to our knowledge there is no known explanation for this late peak in bladder cancer (Schultzel et al. 2008). With the rate of bladder cancer in the population 85 years or older increasing at a rapid pace, it is critical to encourage investigators to include this age group as they continue to search for causative factors and genetic contributors to bladder cancer as well as effective treatments (Schultzel et al. 2008).

Bladder cancer is a disease of the elderly. Older patients might potentially be undertreated due to assumptions about benefit versus risk. Chau et al. determined outcomes in older patients receiving neoadjuvant chemotherapy for muscle-invasive bladder cancer (MIBC) (Chau et al. 2015). Elderly patients with good functional status and limited comorbidities diagnosed with MIBC receiving standard neoadjuvant chemotherapy followed by cystectomy or radiotherapy can have similar clinical outcomes as their younger counterparts (Chau et al. 2015).

References

Chau C, Wheater M, Geldart T, Crabb SJ. Clinical outcomes following neoadjuvant cisplatin-based chemotherapy for bladder cancer in elderly compared with younger patients. Eur J Cancer Care (Engl). 2015;24(2):155–62.

Coward RM, Smith A, Raynor M, Nielsen M, Wallen EM, Pruthi RS. Feasibility and outcomes of robotic-assisted laparoscopic radical cystectomy for bladder cancer in older patients. Urology. 2011;77(5):1111–4.

Fung C, Pandya C, Guancial E, Noyes K, Sahasrabudhe DM, Messing EM, Mohile SG. Impact of bladder cancer on health related quality of life in 1,476 older Americans: a cross-sectional study. J Urol. 2014;192(3):690–5.

Galsky MD. How I treat bladder cancer in elderly patients. J Geriatr Oncol. 2015;6(1):1–7.

Ghebriou D, Avenin D, Caillet P, Mongiat-Artus P, Durdux C, Massard C, Culine S. FRancilian Oncogeriatric Group (FROG)'s focus on management of elderly patients with bladder cancer. Bull Cancer. 2014;101(9):841–55.

Leveridge MJ, Siemens DR, Mackillop WJ, Peng Y, Tannock IF, Berman DM, Booth CM. Radical cystectomy and adjuvant chemotherapy for bladder cancer in the elderly: a population-based study. Urology. 2015;85(4):791–8.

Milowsky MI, Kim WY. The geriatrics and genetics behind bladder cancer. Am Soc Clin Oncol Educ Book. 2014:e192–5.

Noon AP, Albertsen PC, Thomas F, Rosario DJ, Catto JW. Competing mortality in patients diagnosed with bladder cancer: evidence of under treatment in the elderly and female patients. Br J Cancer. 2013;108(7):1534–40.

Oddens JR, Sylvester RJ, Brausi MA, Kirkels WJ, van de Beek C, van Andel G, de Reijke TM, Prescott S, Witjes JA, Oosterlinck W. The effect of age on the efficacy of maintenance Bacillus Calmette-Guérin relative to maintenance epirubicin in patients with stage Ta T1 urothelial bladder cancer: results from EORTC genito-urinary group study 30911. Eur Urol. 2014;66(4):694–701.

Ploussard G, Albrand G, Rozet F, Lang H, Paillaud E, Mongiat-Artus P. Challenging treatment decision-making in older urologic cancer patients. World J Urol. 2014;32(2):299–308.

Schultzel M, Saltzstein SL, Downs TM, Shimasaki S, Sanders C, Sadler GR. Late age (85 years or older) peak incidence of bladder cancer. J Urol. 2008;179(4):1302–5; discussion 1305–6.

Stensland KD, Galsky MD. Current approaches to the management of bladder cancer in older patients. Am Soc Clin Oncol Educ Book. 2014:e250–6.

Tadin T, Sotosek S, Rahelić D, Fuckar Z. Diagnostic accuracy of ultrasound T-staging of the urinary bladder cancer in comparison with histology in elderly patients. Coll Antropol. 2014;38(4):1123–6.

Telli O, Sarici H, Ozgur BC, Doluoglu OG, Sunay MM, Bozkurt S, Eroglu M. Urothelial cancer of bladder in young versus older adults: clinical and pathological characteristics and outcomes. Kaohsiung J Med Sci. 2014;30(9):466–70.

VanderWalde NA, Chi MT, Hurria A, Galsky MD, Nielsen ME. Treatment of muscle invasive bladder cancer in the elderly: navigating the trade offs of risk and benefit. World J Urol. 2016;34(1):3–11.

Chapter 34
A Systematic Review of NMIBC and Intravesical Chemotherapy

A systematic review relating to NMIBC and intravesical chemotherapy was conducted. This was to identify oncoloigcal outcomes from intravesical chemotherapy. The search strategy aimed to identify all references related to NMIBC AND Intravesical Chemotherapy. Search terms used were as follows: (NMIBC) AND (Intravesical Chemotherapy). The following databases were screened from 1989 to June 2019:

- CINAIIL
- MEDLINE (NHS Evidence)
- Cochrane
- AMed
- EMBASE
- PsychINFO
- SCOPUS
- Web of Science.

In addition, searches using Medical Subject Headings (MeSH) and keywords were conducted using Cochrane databases. Two UK-based experts in bladder cancer were consulted to identify any additional studies.

Studies were eligible for inclusion if they reported primary research focusing on bladder cancer and screening. Papers were included if published after 1984 and had to be in English. Studies that did not conform to this were excluded. Only primary research was included. The overall aim was to identify the role and components of bladder cancer screening.

Abstracts were independently screened for eligibility by two reviewers and disagreements resolved through discussion or third party opinion. Agreement level was calculated using Cohen's Kappa to test the intercoder reliability of this screening process. Cohens' Kappa allows comparison of inter-rater reliability between papers using relative observed agreement. This also takes account of

© Springer Nature Switzerland AG 2020
S. S. Goonewardene et al., *Management of Non-Muscle Invasive Bladder Cancer*,
https://doi.org/10.1007/978-3-030-28646-0_34

the comparison occurring by chance. The first reviewer agreed all 26 papers to be included, the second, agreed on 26 (Fig. 34.1).

Data extraction was piloted by the researcher and amended in consultation with the research team (author and two academic supervisors). Data collected included authors, year and country of publication, study aims, setting, intervention aims, number of participants, study design, intervention components and delivery methods, comparison groups and outcome measures, notes and follow-up questions for the authors. Studies were quality assessed using the PRISMA criteria for randomised controlled trials, Mays et al. (Moher et al. 2009; Moher, Liberati et al. 2009, 154, 153; Mays et al. 2005) for the action research and qualitative studies and the Critical Skills Appraisal programme for cohort studies. This was also applied to randomised controlled trials and qualitative studies.

The search identified 26 papers. All 26 mapped to the search terms and eligibility criteria. The current systematic reviews were examined to gain further knowledge about the subject. 282 papers were excluded due to not conforming to eligibility criteria or adding to the evidence. Of the 26 papers left, relevant abstracts were identified and the full papers obtained (all of which were in English), to quality assure against criteria. There was considerable heterogeneity of design among the included studies therefore a narrative review of the evidence was undertaken. There was significant heterogeneity within studies, including clinical topic, numbers, outcomes, as a results a narrative review was thought to be best. There were 25 cohort studies of moderate quality and one RCT of good quality.

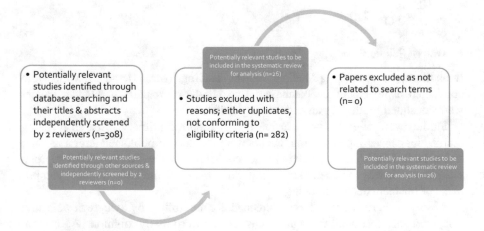

Fig. 34.1 Flow chart of studies identified through the systematic review (adapted from PRISMA)

References

Moher D, Liberati A, Tetzlaff J, Altman DG. Preferred reporting items for systematic reviews and meta-analyses: the prisma statement. BMJ. 2009;339(7716):332–6.

Mays N, Pope C, Popay J. systematically reviewing qualitative and quantitative evidence to inform management and policy-making in the health field. J Health Serv Res Policy. 2005;10(Suppl. 1):6–20.

Chapter 35
A Systematic Review of NMIBC and Intravesical Chemotherapy—Results

35.1 Intravesical Chemotherapy Post TURBT

Palou-Redorta, assessed immediate postoperative instillation of intravesical chemotherapy after transurethral resection of bladder tumour (TURBT) for non-muscle invasive bladder cancer (NMIBC) (Palou-Redorta et al. 2014). Urologists based in five European Union nations were asked to collect data from NMIBC-urothelial carcinoma after at least 1 TURBT. Overall, 771 patients received 954 TURBTs (mean-1.2/patient), of which 413 of the TURBTs (43.3%) were administered post operative chemotherapy (Palou-Redorta et al. 2014). Sixty-six of the 413 (16.0%) were for a recurrent tumour. Five of the tested variables were significantly associated with receiving post operative chemotherapy after TURBT. Country of origin affected whether intravesical chemotherapy was given, United Kingdom, patients most likely; France, least likely. In lower-risk conditions (no CIS, tumour <3 cm) or intermediate risk-more it was more likely to receive intravesical chemotherapy. This was also the case when a uro-oncology fellowship was completed. If the recurrence risk was assessed as a higher-risk condition ($\geq$T2, $\geq$3 cm, CIS, intravesical therapy was more likely or if a physician's NMIBC patients volume was high (Palou-Redorta et al. 2014). This study revealed wide practice variation and substantial noncompliance with European Association of Urology Guidelines on the use of chemotherapy after TURBT for NMIBC.

Post-operative single dose intravesical chemotherapy (PSDIVC) in non-muscle invasive bladder cancer reduces recurrence rates by up to 39%. However, some studies have suggested poor compliance stating logistical issues and reluctance to give chemotherapy prior to histological confirmation (Stroman et al. 2016). Stroman et al. (2016) examined an intervention bundle including pre-operative delivery of mitomycin C (MMC) to the theatre suite, proforma placed in the operative notes and designated roles for PSDIVC induction was introduced to improve instillation and documentation rates (Stroman et al. 2016). Sixty-four patients in

© Springer Nature Switzerland AG 2020

S. S. Goonewardene et al., *Management of Non-Muscle Invasive Bladder Cancer*,
https://doi.org/10.1007/978-3-030-28646-0_35

group A underwent TURBT prior to introduction of the intervention bundle. Fifty-four patients had non-muscle invasive bladder cancer (NMIBC), which would have been eligible for PSDIVC. Fifteen (28% of NMIBC) were administered PSDIVC. Twenty-three (36% of all patients) were either given PSDIVC or had a documented contraindication (Stroman et al. 2016). Thirty-one patients in group B underwent TURBT following induction of intervention bundle. Twelve (50% of NMIBC) patients were given PSDIVC. Twenty-eight (90% of all patients) were either given PSDIVC or had a documented contraindication.

The intervention bundle prompted increased administration of PSDIVC and documentation. Similar centres may benefit from an intervention to improve compliance.

Gudjonsson with an RCT assessed decrease recurrences in non-muscle-invasive bladder cancer (NMIBC). The European Association of Urology (EAU) guidelines recommend immediate, intravesical chemotherapy after transurethral resection (TUR) for all patients with Ta/T1 tumours (Gudjonsson et al. 2009). Gudjonsson studied the benefits of a single, early, intravesical instillation of epirubicin after TUR in patients with low- to intermediate-risk NMIBC (Gudjonsson et al. 2009) In this prospective randomised multicentre trial, 305 patients with primary as well as recurrent low- to intermediate-risk (Ta/T1, G1/G2) tumours were enrolled between 1997 and 2004. Patients were randomly allocated to receive 80 mg of epirubicin in 50 ml of saline intravesically within 24 h of TUR or no further treatment after TUR (Gudjonsson et al. 2009). A total of 219 patients remained for analysis after exclusions. The median follow-up time was 3.9 yr. During the study period, 62% (63 of 102) of the patients in the epirubicin group and 77% (90 of 117) in the control group experienced recurrence ($p = 0.016$) (Gudjonsson et al. 2009). A single, early instillation of epirubicin after TUR for NMIBC reduces the likelihood of tumour recurrence; however, the benefit seems to be minimal in patients at intermediate or high risk of recurrence (Gudjonsson et al. 2009).

35.2   NMIBC Intermediate and High-Risk Disease and BCG

Witjes examine the management of intermediate- and high-risk non-muscle-invasive bladder cancer (NMIBC), particularly with regard to the use of bacillus Calmette-Guérin (BCG) therapy, in North America and Europe (Witjes et al. 2013). In all, 971 patients (197 intermediate-risk; 774 high-risk) were included in the analysis; frequency counts and associated percentages were used to analyse treatment variables. In all, 47% of intermediate-risk patients received EAU or AUA guideline-recommended intravesical therapy: intravesical chemotherapy, BCG induction therapy or BCG induction plus maintenance (Witjes et al. 2013). Of the high-risk patients, 50% received maintenance BCG as recommended by the EAU and the AUA; although not recommended for high-risk NMIBC, 12.5% received intravesical chemotherapy. Of patients prescribed maintenance BCG, 93% were scheduled for at least 1 year of therapy. Notably, only 15% discontinued BCG maintenance and, of these discontinuations, 65% were due to reasons unrelated to BCG-associated adverse events (Witjes et al. 2013). There is significant non-adherence to EAU and AUA guideline recommendations for BCG use in intermediate- and high-risk NMIBC. However, most of those patients prescribed BCG maintenance therapy are scheduled for at least 1 year of therapy, as recommended by current guidelines for NMIBC management, and BCG maintenance discontinuation is low.

35.3   Adjuvant Therapy for NMIBC

Ofude et al. (2015) investigated whether the European Organization for Research and Treatment of Cancer (EORTC) scoring system can be used for the selection of adjuvant intravesical therapies for individual patients who undergo transurethral resection (TURB) for non-muscle-invasive bladder cancer (NMIBC) (Ofude et al. 2015). Ofude retrospectively analyzed the data of 469 TURB cases for NMIBC. The overall RFS rate at 1 and 3 years was 59.1 and 40.3%, respectively. Tumor number, size, and grade were significant predictors of time to recurrence. The EORTC score was a significant predictor of RFS according to multivariate analysis, and the hazard ratios increased according to each EORTC score in multivariate analysis of a combination of EORTC score and adjuvant therapies (Ofude et al. 2015). In groups with intermediate recurrence risk, the recurrence prevention effects in patients with an EORTC score of ≥ 5 were significantly greater with intravesical Bacillus Calmette-Guérin therapy than with weekly intravesical chemotherapy (Ofude et al. 2015). The EORTC scoring system provides useful information for the selection of adjuvant therapies for patients at intermediate risk of NMIBC recurrence.

The therapeutic strategy in intermediate risk (IR) non-muscle invasive bladder cancer (NMIBC) recurring after intravesical therapy (IT) is not well defined. Most patients are usually retreated by Bacillus Calmette-Guerin (BCG) (Serretta et al. 2015). Serretta evaluated the efficacy of intravesical chemotherapy given at recurrence after the first cycle of intravesical chemotherapy recurring 6 months or later (Serretta et al. 2015). The study included 179 patients. The first treatment was intravesical chemotherapy in 146 (81.6%) and BCG in 33 (18.4%), the redo intravescial therapy was given in 112 (62.6%) and BCG in 67 (37.4%) patients. Median time to recurrence was 18 and 16 months after first and second intravesical therapy ($p = 0.32$). At 3 years, 24 (35.8%) and 49 (43.8%) patients recurred after BCG and intravesical chemotherapy, respectively ($p = 0.90$). No difference in RFS was found between BCG and ICH given after a first cycle of intravesical chemotherapy ($p = 0.23$) (Serretta et al. 2015). Re-treatment with intravesical chemotherapy could represent an alternative to BCG in patients harboring intermediate risk—NMIBC recurring after TUR and previous intravesical chemotherapy, however, prospective trials are needed.

Seretta evaluated the efficacy of 1-year maintenance after a 6-week cycle of early intravesical chemotherapy, as the role of maintenance in intravesical chemotherapy is debated (Serretta et al. 2010). Between May 2002 and August 2003, 577 patients with non-muscle-invasive bladder cancer (NMIBC) underwent transurethral resection (TUR) and early intravesical chemotherapy (epirubicin, 80 mg/50 mL). They were randomized between a 6-week induction cycle and the induction cycle plus maintenance with 10 monthly instillations (Serretta et al. 2010). Treatment interruption for toxicity was required in 39 patients. One death due to toxicity of early instillation occurred. The median follow-up was 48 months. Ten patients (2.5%) progressed and 117 patients (29.6%) recurred. No statistically significant difference in the recurrence-free rate (RFS) was detected between the two arms ($p = 0.43$). An advantage in favour of the maintenance arm was evident only at 18 months after TUR ($p = 0.03$). A trend for a higher benefit from maintenance in primary and multiple tumours was detected (Serretta et al. 2010). In patients with intermediate risk NMIBC treated by TUR and early adjuvant chemotherapy, adding a maintenance regimen with monthly instillations for 1 year is of limited efficacy in preventing recurrence.

35.4   BCG and High Grade Non Muscle Invasive Bladder Cancer

Farah determined the efficacy and tolerability of this specific BCG RIVM strain, using six-weekly, induction course and single monthly instillations as maintenance for one year, in high risk recurrent, multifocal low grade and multifocal high grade pTa/pT1, CIS transitional cell carcinoma of bladder (Farah et al. 2014). Sixty evaluable patients–median age 63, median follow-up 3.98 years. Forty-two patients (70%) completed BCG-RIVM treatment as planned. BCG termination was necessary in 18 patients (30%). Recurrence occurred in 16 patients (26.7%) at a median follow-up of 24.2 months while progression occurred in five patients (8.3%) at a median follow-up of 33 months (Farah et al. 2014). Recurrence-free survival and progression-free survival rates were 73% and 92% respectively. Cystectomy was performed in seven patients (12%) with a cystectomy-free survival of 88%. There were no cancer specific deaths. Two patients died of other causes (3.3%). The overall survival rate was 97% (Farah et al. 2014).

35.5   NMIBC Intravesical Chemotherapy—Small Recurrent Tumours

The efficacy of intravesical chemotherapy in abolishing small papillary recurrences of non-muscle-invasive bladder cancer (NMIBC) was investigated (Decaestecker et al. 2016). 25 patients with 47 recurrence episodes were recruited from February 2003 until August 2011. The median follow-up was 35 months. After exclusion of 2 patients with intolerance to the instillations, 45 study episodes were analysed. All patients to whom this was proposed preferred the instillations over immediate TURB. Complete, partial and no response was seen in 23 (51%), 6 (13%) and 16 (36%) out of 45 episodes, respectively (Decaestecker et al. 2016). The median disease-free interval after complete remission was 16 months (95% confidence interval 9–24) . Small papillary recurrences of NMIBC completely disappear in about half of the cases receiving four weekly bladder instillations with MMC or ERC. This is followed by a disease-free interval. Intravesical chemotherapy was preferred by all patients over immediate TURB.

35.6 BCG or Intravesical Chemotherapy—For Intermediate Risk Bladder Cancer

Han evaluated the risk of recurrence in intermediate-risk non-muscle-invasive bladder cancer (NMIBC) after intravesical chemotherapy or Bacillus Calmette-Guérin (Han et al. 2015). A cohort of 746 patients with intermediate-risk NMIBC comprised the study group. In total, 507 patients (68.1%), 78 patients (10.5%), and 160 (21.4%) underwent TUR, TUR+BCG, or TUR+chemotherapy, respectively (Han et al. 2015). After a median follow-up period of 51.7 months, 286 patients (38.5%) developed tumor recurrence. The 5-yr recurrence rates for the TUR, chemotherapy, and BCG groups were 53.6%±2.7%, 30.8%±5.7%, and 33.6%+4.7%, respectively ($p < 0.001$). Chemotherapy and BCG treatment were found to be predictors of reduced recurrence (Han et al. 2015). Cox-regression analysis showed that TUR+BCG did not differ from TUR+chemotherapy in terms of recurrence risk. Adjuvant intravesical instillation is an effective prophylactic that prevents tumor recurrence in intermediate-risk NMIBC patients following TUR. In addition, both chemotherapeutic agents and BCG demonstrate comparable efficacies for preventing recurrence.

35.7 BCG and Risk Prediction

pT1 bladder urothelial carcinomas represent a heterogeneous group of tumours. Iidentifying the subset of tumors that carries a high risk of disease recurrence and progression is important (Ajili et al. 2013a). Induction and maintenance intravesical Bacillus Calmette-Guerin (BCG) has been proven to reduce tumour recurrence and progression. However, no markers are available to predict BCG response. Ajili evaluated the prognostic factors of stage in predicting recurrence after intravesical adjuvant BCG immunotherapy in patients with NMIBC (Ajili et al. 2013a). A significant concordance between the EORTCs predicted risks and the actuarial recurrence rate of NMIBC at one year was demonstrated (Ajili et al. 2013a). Management of pT1 bladder cancer patients remains one of the most difficult problems in urologic practice. At this time the decision to preserve the bladder or to perform a cystectomy depends on a number of clinicopathologic parameters, but none are able to sufficiently identify patients for the appropriate therapeutic modality (Ajili et al. 2013a). Additional studies using a more large scale of patients will be required to confirm this study.

35.8   NMIBC and MMC

Racioppi to verified the tolerability and the preliminary clinical results of intensive intravesical instillations of a mitomycin C (MMC) regimen (Racioppi et al. 2010). From September 2007 to November 2009, 40 consecutive evaluable patients with pathologically confirmed intermediate-risk non-muscle-invasive bladder cancer (NMIBC) were enrolled after complete TURBT. The mean age of the patients was 64.5 years. 40 mg MMC diluted in 50 ml of saline was instilled in the bladder three times a week for 2 weeks (Racioppi et al. 2010). The median follow-up was 9 months. All patients fulfilled the scheduled treatment. The local adverse events seen were negligible, while no significant deviation from normal values was observed in blood counts for each patient. Twenty-three of 40 patients (57.5%) showed negative at the cystoscopic control which was performed every 3 months with normal spontaneous and washing cytological exams (Racioppi et al. 2010). MMC is a well-known chemotherapeutic agent for the intravesical therapy of NMIBC. No significant local or systemic toxicity was reported. This demonstrates how intensive intravesical instillations of MMC might become a tool in the management of NMIBC.

Bosschieter investigated the timing of mitomycin C (on the day of resection or 1 day later) has an impact on time to recurrence of non-muscle-invasive bladder cancer (NMIBC) (Bosschieter et al. 2018a). All patients with NMIBC who were enrolled in a prospective trial between 1998 and 2003 and treated with an early mitomycin C instillation (on the day of TURBT or 1 day later), were selected. Administering an instillation of mitomycin C on the day of TURBT or 1 day later did not show a statistically significant difference in time to recurrence in a univariable model (log-rank $p = 0.99$). This does not support the theory that a very early instillation (on the day of TURBT) of mitomycin C decreases the risk of recurrence as compared with an early instillation (1 day after TURBT).

Bosschieter then compared the effect of a mitomycin C (MMC) instillation within 24 h to an instillation 2 wk after TURBT in patients with NMIBC with or without adjuvant instillations. 2844 NMIBC patients were randomised for immediate versus delayed MMC instillation after TURBT. Patients were categorised in low-risk (LOR), intermediate-risk (IMR), and high-risk (HIR) groups (Bosschieter et al. 2018b). A total of 2243 patients were eligible on an intention-to-treat basis. Recurrence risks were 43% and 46% in the LOR group (5-yr follow-up, $p = 0.11$), 20% and 32% in the IMR group (3-yr follow-up, $p = 0.037$), and 28% and 35% in the HIR group (3-yr follow-up, $p = 0.007$), for an immediate and a delayed instillation, respectively. For all patients, the recurrence risk was 27% (95% confidence interval [CI] , 24–30) in the immediate and 36% (95% CI, 33–39) in the delayed instillation group ($p < 0.001$) with a 27% reduction in relative recurrence risk (hazard ratio: 0.73, 95% CI, 0.63–0.85, $p < 0.001$) (Bosschieter et al. 2018b). The incidence of adverse events did not differ significantly between treatment groups (immediate instillation 25%, delayed instillation 22%, $p = 0.08$). An immediate, single instillation after TURBT reduces the recurrence risk in NMIBC patients, independent of the number of adjuvant installations.

De Nunzio studied the benefits of a single, early, intravesical instillation of mitomycin C(MMC) after transurethral bladder resection (TURB) in low-risk non-muscle-invasive bladder cancer (NMIBC) (De Nunzio et al. 2011). A total of 202 patients (97 in the MMC group and 105 in the control group) were assessed. Median age was 61 years (IQR 42–78), and median follow-up was 90 months (IQR 3–112). No significant differences for patients' characteristics were observed between the two groups (De Nunzio et al. 2011). During the study period, 10% (10/97) of the patients in the MMC group and 43% (46/105) in the control group experienced a recurrence ($p = 0.0001$). Four patients in the MMC group and 11 ($p = 0.008$) in the control group experienced an early recurrence (within 2 years). One patient in the control group presented a tumour progression (T2G3). MMC treatment was associated with a 31% absolute risk reduction of recurrence and a 3.26 numbers needed to treat to prevent one recurrence (De Nunzio et al. 2011). In this single-centre, long-term follow-up, experience a single, early instillation of MMC after TUR for low risk NMIBC is associated with a significant reduction in risk of early and late recurrences.

35.9 NMIBC and Keyhole Limpet Hemocyanin

Despite current treatment after transurethral resection of a bladder tumor, recurrences and progression remain a problem. Keyhole limpet hemocyanin (KLH) was beneficial in earlier studies. Lammers compared safety and efficacy of KLH to mitomycin (MM) (Lammers et al. 2012). Patients with intermediate—and high-risk non-muscle-invasive bladder cancer (NMIBC) without carcinoma in situ were enrolled in a randomized phase III trial. There were significantly more pT1 tumors in the MM group ($p = 0.01$). In a log-rank test, univariate and multivariate Cox regression analysis, KLH was less effective than MM regarding RFS (all $P < 0.001$) (Lammers et al. 2012). AEs were common but mild. Fever, flu-like symptoms, and fatigue occurred significantly more after KLH treatment. Allergic reactions and other skin disorders occurred significantly more after MM treatment. KLH had a different safety profile and was inferior to MM in preventing NMIBC recurrences. KLH tended to be more effective than MM in preventing progression. More research is needed to clarify the immunologic effects of KLH and the effects of KLH on progression.

35.10   Valrubicin and NMIBC

Cookson conducted a multicenter, retrospective study examining valrubicin for treatment of nonmuscle-invasive bladder cancer (NMIBC) (Cookson et al. 2014). The medical records of 113 patients met the inclusion criteria; 100 patients (88.5%) completed valrubicin treatment. The median age was 75 years (range 42–95 years). The median NMIBC duration was 31 months since diagnosis: 51.3% (58/113) had carcinoma in situ (CIS) alone, and 31.9% (36/113) had unspecified NMIBC (Cookson et al. 2014). Most patients, 94.7% (107/113), had more than three valrubicin instillations and 70.8% (80/113) completed a full course. The EFS rate (95% confidence interval) was 51.6% (40.9–61.3%), 30.4% (20.4–41.1%), and 16.4% (7.9–27.5%) at 3, 6, and 12 months, respectively. Median time to an event was 3.5 (2.5–4.0) months after the first valrubicin instillation (Cookson et al. 2014). Local adverse reactions (LARs) were experienced by 49.6% (56/113) of patients; most LARs were mild (93.6%). The most frequent LARs were hematuria, pollakiuria, micturition urgency, bladder spasm, and dysuria. In total, 4.4% (5/113) of patients discontinued valrubicin because of adverse events or LARs.

35.11   NMIBC—Blue Light Plus MMC

O'Brien determined if photodynamic 'blue-light'-assisted resection with single dose MMC leads to lower recurrence rates in newly presenting non-muscle-invasive bladder cancer (NMIBC) (O'Brien et al. 2013). Of the 249 patients, 209 (84%) had cancer and in 185 patients (89%) the cancer was diagnosed as NMIBC. There were no adverse events related to HAL. Single-shot intravesical mitomycin C was administered to 61/97 patients (63%) in the HAL-PDD arm compared with 68/88 patients (77%) in the white-light arm ($p = 0.04$) O'Brien et al. (2013). Intravesical HAL was an effective diagnostic tool for occult carcinoma in situ (CIS) . Secondary CIS was identified in 25/97 patients (26%) in the HAL-PDD arm compared with 12/88 patients (14%) in the white-light arm ($p = 0.04$). There was no significant difference in recurrence between the two arms at 3 or 12 months: in the HAL-PDD and the white-light arms recurrence was found in 17/86 and 14/82 patients (20 vs. 17%), respectively ($p = 0.7$) at 3 months, and in 10/63 and 15/67 patients (16 vs. 22%), respectively ($p = 0.4$) at 12 months (O'Brien et al. 2013). Despite HAL-PDD offering a more accurate diagnostic assessment of a bladder tumour, in this trial we did not show that this led to lower recurrence rates of newly presenting NMIBC compared with the best current standard of care (O'Brien et al. 2013).

35.12   BCG Activation by MMC in NMIBC

Svatek determined the safety and toxicities of sequential MMC (mitomycin C) + BCG (bacillus Calmette-Guérin) in patients with non-muscle-invasive bladder cancer (NMIBC) and explore evidence for potentiation of BCG activity by MMC (Svatek et al. 2015). Twelve patients completed therapy, including 3 patients receiving full doses. The regimen was well tolerated with no treatment-related dose-limiting toxicities. Urinary frequency and urgency, and fatigue were common (Svatek et al. 2015). Eleven (91.7%) patients were free of disease at a mean (range) follow-up of 21.4 (8.4–27.0) months. Median posttreatment urine concentrations of IL2, IL8, IL10, and TNFα increased over the 6-week treatment period. A greater increase in posttreatment urinary IL8 during the 6-week period was observed in patients receiving MMC + BCG compared with patients receiving BCG monotherapy. In mice, intravesical MMC + BCG skewed tumor-associated macrophages (TAM) toward a beneficial M1 phenotype (Svatek et al. 2015).

Intravesical bacillus Calmette-Guérin (BCG) is an effective therapy in non-muscle-invasive bladder cancer (NMIBC), but it has limitations in terms of recurrence and toxicity. Solsona et al. (2015) determine whether the sequential combination of mitomycin C (MMC) and BCG is superior to BCG alone in increasing a disease-free interval (DFI) (Solsona et al. 2015). Solsona conducted a prospective randomized trial including 407 patients with intermediate- to high-risk NMIBC and allocated 211 to the MMC and BCG arm and 196 to the BCG-alone arm (Solsona et al. 2015). In the intention-to-treat analysis at 5 yr, DFI was significantly improved by the sequential scheme (HR: 0.57; 95% confidence interval [CI], 0.39–0.83; $p = 0.003$), reducing the disease relapse rate from 33.9% to 20.6%. Higher toxicity was observed with the combination, even reducing the MMC dose, especially in G3 local toxicity compared with BCG with a difference of 17.4% (95% CI, 7.6–27.2; $p < 0.001$) (Solsona et al. 2015). In recurrent T1 tumors, the potential benefit of the sequential scheme was more evident than in the remaining subgroup (18.8% vs. 12.8%), with a number needed to treat of five versus eight to avoid an event and with similar toxicity. Although the sequential scheme is more effective than BCG alone in reducing disease relapse, due to higher toxicity it could be offered only to patients with a high likelihood of recurrence, such as those with recurrent T1 tumors.

Weiss sought to determine if the addition of perioperative mitomycin C (MMC) to treatment with bacillus Calmette-Guérin (BCG) after transurethral resection (TURBT) is superior to TURBT plus BCG alone in high grade non-muscle invasive bladder cancer (NMIBC) (Weiss et al. 2015). Of the 120 patients identified who received treatment for high grade NMIBC, 97 were treated with BCG alone and 23 received a single instillation of perioperative MMC in addition to BCG. There were no statistically significant differences noted in demographic or pathologic variables (Weiss et al. 2015). Patients were followed for a median of 4.5 years and a maximum of 21.8 years, with no differences demonstrated in recurrence-free survival ($p = 0.75$), overall survival ($p = 0.93$) or disease-free survival ($p = 0.76$). Both lack of lymphovascular invasion and BCG maintenance therapy reached significance as independent predictors of recurrence-free survival ($p = 0.19$ and $p = 0.28$) (Weiss et al. 2015). While our study indicates that perioperative MMC likely offers little benefit in regards to recurrence or survival in high grade NMIBC, at this point in time, a larger scale, randomized, controlled trial is needed to adequately address this question.

35.13 BCG Therapy, NMIBC and Elderly Patients

National guidelines recommend adjuvant intravesical Bacillus Calmette-Guérin (BCG) therapy for higher-risk non-muscle-invasive bladder cancer (NMIBC). Although a survival benefit has not been demonstrated, randomized trials have shown reduced recurrence and delayed progression after its use. (Spencer et al. 2013) investigated predictors of BCG receipt and its association with survival for older patients with NMIBC. Of 23,932 patients with NMIBC identified, 22% received adjuvant intravesical BCG. Predictors of receipt were stages Tis and T1, higher grade, and urban residence (Spencer et al. 2013). Age >80 years, fewer than two comorbidities, and not being married were associated with decreased use. In the survival analysis, BCG use was associated with better OS (hazard ratio [HR], 0.87; 95% CI, 0.83–0.92) in the entire cohort and BCSS among higher-grade cancers (poorly differentiated: HR, 0.78; 95% CI, 0.72–0.85; undifferentiated: HR, 0.66; 95% CI, 0.56–0.77) (Spencer et al. 2013).

Bladder cancer is a disease of older persons, the incidence of which is expected to increase as the population ages. Prognostic factors for local recurrence for patients with non-muscle invasive bladder cancer have not been fully established. Ajili et al. (2013b) determined the influence of age on the outcomes of non muscle invasive bladder (NMIBC) cancer treated with intravesical Bacillus Calmette-Guerin (BCG) therapy (Ajili et al. 2013b). Ajili retrospectively reviewed the clinical and pathologic data of primary NMIBC from 112 patients who were treated with transurethral resection followed by BCG-immunotherapy (Ajili et al. 2013b). Time follow-up was 30 months. Clinicopathologic characteristics and response to BCG therapy were correlated with age using univariate and multivariate methods of analysis. The results of our study have shown that aging has no impact on the outcomes of high-risk NMIBC treated by BCG immunotherapy.

References

Ajili F, Darouiche A, Chebil M, Boubaker S. The efficacy of intravesical bacillus Calmette-Guerin in the treatment of patients with pT1 stage non-muscle-invasive bladder cancer. Ultrastruct Pathol. 2013a;37(4):278–83.

Ajili F, Darouiche A, Chebil M, Boubaker S. The impact of age and clinical factors in non-muscle-invasive bladder cancer treated with Bacillus Calmette Guerin therapy. Ultrastruct Pathol. 2013b;37(3):191–5.

Bosschieter J, Nieuwenhuijzen JA, van Ginkel T, Vis AN, Witte B, Newling D, Beckers GMA, van Moorselaar RJA. Value of an immediate intravesical instillation of mitomycin C in patients with non-muscle-invasive bladder cancer: a prospective multicentre randomised study in 2243 patients. Eur Urol. 2018a;73(2):226–232.

Bosschieter J, van Moorselaar RJA, Vis AN, van Ginkel T, Lissenberg-Witte BI, Beckers GMA, Nieuwenhuijzen JA. The effect of timing of an immediate instillation of mitomycin C after transurethral resection in 941 patients with non-muscle-invasive bladder cancer. BJU Int. 2018b.

Cookson MS, Chang SS, Lihou C, Li T, Harper SQ, Lang Z, Tutrone RF. Use of intravesical valrubicin in clinical practice for treatment of nonmuscle-invasive bladder cancer, including carcinoma in situ of the bladder. Ther Adv Urol. 2014;6(5):181–91.

De Nunzio C, Carbone A, Albisinni S, Alpi G, Cantiani A, Liberti M, Tubaro A, Iori F. Long-term experience with early single mitomycin C instillations in patients with low-risk non-muscle-invasive bladder cancer: prospective, single-centre randomised trial. World J Urol. 2011;29(4):517–21.

Decaestecker K, Lumen N, Ringoir A, Oosterlinck W. Ablative intravesical chemotherapy for small recurrent non-muscle-invasive bladder cancer: a prospective study. Urol Int. 2016;96(1):14–9.

Farah NB, Ghanem R, Amr M. Treatment efficacy and tolerability of intravesical bacillus Calmette-Guerin (BCG)-RIVM strain: induction and maintenance protocol in high grade and recurrent low grade non-muscle invasive bladder cancer (NMIBC). BMC Urol. 2014;14:11. https://doi.org/10.1186/1471-2490-14-11.

Gudjónsson S, Adell L, Merdasa F, Olsson R, Larsson B, Davidsson T, Richthoff J, Hagberg G, Grabe M, Bendahl PO, Månsson W, Liedberg F. Should all patients with non-muscle-invasive bladder cancer receive early intravesical chemotherapy after transurethral resection? The results of a prospective randomised multicentre study. Eur Urol. 2009;55(4).773–80.

Han KS, You D, Jeong IG, Kwon T, Hong B, Hong JH, Ahn H, Ahn TY, Kim CS. Is intravesical Bacillus Calmette-Guérin therapy superior to chemotherapy for intermediate-risk non-muscle-invasive bladder cancer? An ongoing debate. J Korean Med Sci. 2015;30(3):252–8.

Lammers RJ, Witjes WP, Janzing-Pastors MH, Caris CT, Witjes JA. Intracutaneous and intravesical immunotherapy with keyhole limpet hemocyanin compared with intravesical mitomycin in patients with non-muscle-invasive bladder cancer: results from a prospective randomized phase III trial. J Clin Oncol. 2012;30(18):2273–9.

O'Brien T, Ray E, Chatterton K, Khan MS, Chandra A, Thomas K. Prospective randomized trial of hexylaminolevulinate photodynamic-assisted transurethral resection of bladder tumour (TURBT) plus single-shot intravesical mitomycin C vs conventional white-light TURBT plus mitomycin C in newly presenting non-muscle-invasive bladder cancer. BJU Int. 2013;112(8):1096–104.

Ofude M, Kitagawa Y, Yaegashi H, Izumi K, Ueno S, Kadono Y, Konaka H, Mizokami A, Namiki M. Selection of adjuvant intravesical therapies using the European Organization for Research and Treatment of Cancer scoring system in patients at intermediate risk of non-muscle-invasive bladder cancer. J Cancer Res Clin Oncol. 2015;141(1):161–8.

Palou-Redorta J, Rouprêt M, Gallagher JR, Heap K, Corbell C, Schwartz B. The use of immediate postoperative instillations of intravesical chemotherapy after TURBT of NMIBC among European countries. World J Urol. 2014;32(2):525–30.

Racioppi M, Volpe A, Cappa E, D'Agostino D, Pinto F, D'Addessi A, Sacco E, Bassi P. Intensive intravesical mitomycin C therapy in non-muscle-invasive bladder cancer: a dose intensity approach. Urol Int. 2010;85(3):266–9.

Serretta V, Morgia G, Altieri V, Di Lallo A, Ruggiero G, Salzano L, Battaglia M, Falsaperla M, Zito A, Sblendorio D, Melloni D, Allegro R, Members of Gruppo Studi Tumori Urologici

(GSTU) Foundation. A 1-year maintenance after early adjuvant intravesical chemotherapy has a limited efficacy in preventing recurrence of intermediate risk non-muscle-invasive bladder cancer. BJU Int. 2010;106(2):212–7.

Serretta V, Sommatino F, Gesolfo CS, Franco V, Cicero G, Allegro R. Intravesical chemotherapy for intermediate risk non-muscle invasive bladder cancer recurring after a first cycle of intravesical adjuvant therapy. Urol Ann. 2015;7(1):21–5.

Solsona E, Madero R, Chantada V, Fernandez JM, Zabala JA, Portillo JA, Alonso JM, Astobieta A, Unda M, Martinez-Piñeiro L, Rabadan M, Ojea A, Rodriguez-Molina J, Beardo P, Muntañola P, Gomez M, Montesinos M, Martinez Piñeiro JA, Members of Club Urológico Español de Tratamiento Oncológico. Sequential combination of mitomycin C plus bacillus Calmette-Guérin (BCG) is more effective but more toxic than BCG alone in patients with non-muscle-invasive bladder cancer in intermediate- and high-risk patients: final outcome of CUETO 93009, a randomized prospective trial. Eur Urol. 2015;67(3):508–16.

Spencer BA, McBride RB, Hershman DL, Buono D, Herr HW, Benson MC, Gupta-Mohile S, Neugut AI. Adjuvant intravesical bacillus calmette-guérin therapy and survival among elderly patients with non-muscle-invasive bladder cancer. J Oncol Pract. 2013;9(2):92–8.

Stroman L, Tschobotko B, Abboudi H, Ellis D, Mensah E, Kaneshayogan H, Mazaris E. Improving compliance with a single post-operative dose of intravesical chemotherapy after transurethral resection of bladder tumour. Nephrourol Mon. 2016;8(1):e29967.

Svatek RS, Zhao XR, Morales EE, Jha MK, Tseng TY, Hugen CM, Hurez V, Hernandez J, Curiel TJ. Sequential intravesical mitomycin plus Bacillus Calmette-Guérin for non-muscle-invasive urothelial bladder carcinoma: translational and phase I clinical trial. Clin Cancer Res. 2015;21(2):303–11.

Weiss BE, Pietzak EJ, Wein AJ, Malkowicz SB, Guzzo TJ. Single instillation of mitomycin C plus bacillus Calmette-Guérin (BCG) versus BCG alone in high grade non-muscle invasive bladder cancer. Can J Urol. 2015;22(4):7876–81.

Witjes JA, Palou J, Soloway M, Lamm D, Kamat AM, Brausi M, Persad R, Buckley R, Colombel M, Böhle A. Current clinical practice gaps in the treatment of intermediate- and high-risk non-muscle-invasive bladder cancer (NMIBC) with emphasis on the use of bacillus Calmette-Guérin (BCG): results of an international individual patient data survey (IPDS). JU Int. 2013;112(6):742–50.

Chapter 36
What the Literature Says Re BCG

The first European Association of Urology (EAU) guidelines on bladder cancer were published in 2002 [1]. Since then, the guidelines have been continuously updated (Babjuk et al. 2013). For patients with a low-risk tumour, one immediate instillation of chemotherapy is recommended. Patients with an intermediate-risk tumour should receive one immediate instillation of chemotherapy followed by 1 yr of full-dose bacillus Calmette-Guérin (BCG) intravesical immunotherapy or by further instillations of chemotherapy for a maximum of 1 yr. In patients with high-risk tumours, full-dose intravesical BCG for 1–3 yr is indicated.

Bacillus Calmette-Guérin (BCG) remains the most effective intravesical treatment for non-muscle-invasive bladder cancer (NMIBC), but the clinical development of BCG has been accompanied by controversy (Gontero et al. 2010). Recent publications have called into question a number of aspects related to its use. Gontero performed a systematic literature search of published articles in PubMed, Embase, and the Cochrane Central Register of Controlled Trials databases for the period from 1976 to November 2008 (Gontero et al. 2010). BCG is the most effective intravesical agent for preventing NMIBC recurrence, but its role in disease progression remains controversial. In intermediate-risk NMIBC, the superiority of BCG over chemotherapy is well established for disease recurrence but not for progression and needs to be balanced against higher toxicity (Gontero et al. 2010). With regard to high-risk NMIBC, there is sufficient evidence to show that BCG is the most effective treatment of carcinoma in situ for ablation, disease-free interval, and progression, but the impact of BCG on the natural history of T1G3 tumors relies on a low level of evidence. Maintenance remains crucial for efficacy. The dose can be safely and effectively reduced to decrease its toxicity, which is slightly greater than chemotherapy (Gontero et al. 2010). BCG should still be viewed as the most effective intravesical agent, but its role in the progression of papillary tumors needs to be clarified. BCG remains an alternative to intravesical chemotherapy in intermediate-risk NMIBC, and it is recommended as the standard of care for high-risk NMIBC.

© Springer Nature Switzerland AG 2020
S. S. Goonewardene et al., *Management of Non-Muscle Invasive Bladder Cancer*,
https://doi.org/10.1007/978-3-030-28646-0_36

   Burger presented a summary of the Second International Consultation on
Bladder Cancer recommendations on the diagnosis and treatment options for
non-muscle-invasive urothelial cancer of the bladder (NMIBC) using an evidence-based approach (Burger et al. 2012). A detailed Medline analysis was
performed for original articles addressing the treatment of NMIBC with regard
to diagnosis, surgery, intravesical chemotherapy, and follow-up. Proceedings
from the last 5 yr of major conferences were also searched (Burger et al. 2012).
Urothelial cancer of the bladder staged Ta, T1, and carcinoma in situ (CIS), also
indicated as NMIBC, poses greatly varying but uniformly demanding challenges
to urologic care. On the one hand, the high recurrence rate and low progression
rate with Ta low-grade demand risk-adapted treatment and surveillance to provide
thorough care while minimizing treatment-related burden (Burger et al. 2012). On
the other hand, the propensity of Ta high-grade, T1, and CIS to progress demands
intense care and timely consideration of radical cystectomy.

   The European Association of Urology non-muscle-invasive bladder cancer (NMIBC) guidelines recommend that all low- and intermediate-risk patients
receive a single immediate installation of chemotherapy after transurethral resection of the bladder (TURB) (Syvester et al. 2016). A systematic review and individual patient data (IPD) meta-analysis of randomized trials comparing the
efficacy of a single installation after TURB with TURB alone in NMIBC patients
was carried out to identify who would benefit from a single dose of post operative chemotherapy (Syvester et al. 2016). A total of 13 eligible studies were identified. IPD were obtained for 11 studies randomizing 2278 eligible patients, 1161
to TURB and 1117 to a single installation of epirubicin, mitomycin C, pirarubicin,
or thiotepa. A total of 1128 recurrences, 108 progressions, and 460 deaths (59
due to bladder cancer [BCa]) occurred (Syvester et al. 2016). A single installation
reduced the risk of recurrence by 35% (hazard ratio [HR]: 0.65; 95% confidence
interval [CI], 0.58-0.74; $p < 0.001$) and the 5-yr recurrence rate from 58.8% to
44.8%. The installation did not reduce recurrences in patients with a prior recurrence rate of more than one recurrence per year or in patients with an European
Organization for Research and Treatment of Cancer (EORTC) recurrence score ≥ 5
(Syvester et al. 2016). The installation did not prolong either the time to progression or death from BCa, but it resulted in an increase in the overall risk of death
(HR: 1.26; 95% CI, 1.05–1.51; $p = 0.015$; 5-yr death rates 12.0% vs. 11.2%), with
the difference appearing in patients with an EORTC recurrence score ≥ 5. A single immediate installation reduced the risk of recurrence, except in patients with
a prior recurrence rate of more than one recurrence per year or an EORTC recurrence score ≥ 5. It does not prolong either time to progression or death from BCa.
The installation may be associated with an increase in the risk of death in patients
at high risk of recurrence in whom the installation is not effective or recommended.

   Non-muscle-invasive bladder cancer (NMIBC) commonly recurs, requiring
invasive and costly transurethral resection of bladder tumor (TURBT) (Perlis
et al. 2013). A meta-analysis of seven trials published in 2004 demonstrated that
intravesical chemotherapy (IVC) following TURBT reduces recurrences. Despite
European Association of Urology endorsement, adoption of this practice has been

modest (Perlis et al. 2013) A systematic literature review of random controlled trials (RCTs) published before March 2013 was performed using the Medline, Embase, and Cochrane databases. Thirteen studies with 2548 patients were included. IVC prolonged RFI by 38% (HR: 0.62; 95% confidence interval [CI], 0.50–0.77; $p<0.001$; I(2): 69%), and ERs were 12% less likely in the intervention population (ARR: 0.12; 95% CI, -0.18 to -0.06; $p<0.001$, I(2): 0%) (Perlis et al. 2013). The number needed to treat to prevent one ER was 9 (95% CI, 6–17 patients). There was high risk of bias present in 12 of 13 publications. Quality of evidence for RFI was very low and low for ERs.

References

Babjuk M, Burger M, Zigeuner R, Shariat SF, van Rhijn BW, Compérat E, Sylvester RJ, Kaasinen E, Böhle A, Palou Redorta J, Rouprêt M. European Association of Urology. EAU guidelines on non-muscle-invasive urothelial carcinoma of the bladder: update 2013. Eur Urol. 2013;64(4):639–53.

Burger M, Oosterlinck W, Konety B, Chang S, Gudjonsson S, Pruthi R, Soloway M, Solsona E, Sved P, Babjuk M, Brausi MA, Cheng C, Comperat E, Dinney C, Otto W, Shah J, Thürof J, Witjes JA. International consultation on urologic disease-European association of urology consultation on bladder cancer 2012. ICUD-EAU international consultation on bladder cancer 2012: non-muscle-invasive urothelial carcinoma of the bladder. Eur Urol. 2013;63(1):36–44.

Gontero P, Bohle A, Malmstrom PU, O'Donnell MA, Oderda M, Sylvester R, Witjes F. The role of bacillus Calmette-Guérin in the treatment of non-muscle-invasive bladder cancer. Eur Urol. 2010;57(3):410 29.

Perlis N, Zlotta AR, Beyene J, Finelli A, Fleshner NE, Kulkarni GS. Immediate post-transurethral resection of bladder tumor intravesical chemotherapy prevents non-muscle-invasive bladder cancer recurrences: an updated meta-analysis on 2548 patients and quality-of-evidence review. Eur Urol. 2013;64(3):421–30. https://doi.org/10.1016/j.eururo.2013.06.009 Epub 2013 Jun 19.

Sylvester RJ, Oosterlinck W, Holmang S, Sydes MR, Birtle A, Gudjonsson S, De Nunzio C, Okamura K, Kaasinen E, Solsona E, Ali-El-Dein B, Tatar CA, Inman BA, N'Dow J, Oddens JR, Babjuk M. Systematic review and individual patient data meta-analysis of randomized trials comparing a single immediate instillation of chemotherapy after transurethral resection with transurethral resection alone in patients with stage pTa-pT1 urothelial carcinoma of the bladder: which patients benefit from the instillation? Eur Urol. 2016;69(2):231–44.

Chapter 37
Prognostic Factors in BCG

Ofude et al. (2015), examined prognosticators to discriminating between responders and non-responders to BCG (Ofude et al. 2015). According to univariate analysis of the prognostic significance for tumor stage, grade, loci number, sex, age and smoking, the pT1 stage and multiplicity seem to be associated in a statistically significant manner with higher risk for recurrence ($p = 0.009$, $p = 0.011$, respectively) (Ofude et al. 2015). Significant independent predictor for recurrence was multiplicity which offers important clinical information and may be a useful tool in the selection of suitable candidates for BCG-immunotherapy.

The impact of prognostic factors in T1G3 non-muscle-invasive bladder cancer (BCa) patients is critical for proper treatment decision making (Gontero et al. 2015). Gontero et al. assessed prognostic factors in patients who received bacillus Calmette-Guérin (BCG) as initial intravesical treatment of T1G3 tumors and to identify a subgroup of high-risk patients who should be considered for more aggressive treatment (Gontero et al. 2015). Most important prognostic factors for progression were age, tumor size, and concomitant carcinoma in situ (CIS); the most important prognostic factors for BCa-specific survival and OS were age and tumor size (Gontero et al. 2015). T1G3 patients ≥ 70 yr with tumors ≥ 3 cm and concomitant CIS should be treated more aggressively because of the high risk of progression.

Gontero et al. (2015). Although the majority of T1G3 patients can be safely treated with intravesical bacillus Calmette-Guérin, there is a subgroup of T1G3 patients with age ≥ 70 yr, tumor size ≥ 3 cm, and concomitant CIS who have a high risk of progression and thus require aggressive treatment.

Nguyen-Huu et al. studied the prognostic impact of muscularis mucosae (MM) invasion for pT1 bladder cancer treated by transurethral resection (TUR) and adjuvant Bacille Calmette-Guerin (BCG) intravesical immunotherapy (Nguyen-Huu et al. 2012). For pT1a patients, recurrence ($p = 0.8$) or progression rates ($p = 0.64$) were no different regarding BCG maintenance, but pT1b population had a better progression free survival with BCG maintenance than without ($p = 0.0051$)

(Nguyen-Huu et al. 2012). Only CIS had prognostic value in multivariate analysis. Tumors with muscularis mucosae muinvasion have a higher risk of progression and BCG failure (Nguyen-Huu et al. 2012). Maintenance immunotherapy should be given to improve results with these patients.

Shirakawa et al. (2012), investigated the differences in the clinical features and subsequent stage progression and disease-specific survival among patients with Bacillus Calmette-Guérin (BCG) failure, after dividing these patients into BCG-refractory, -resistant, -relapsing, and -intolerant groups.

The 10-year progression-free survival rates were 53.2, 91.1 and 93.8% in the BCG-refractory, BCG-relapsing and BCG-intolerant groups, respectively (Shirakawa et al. 2012). Stratification of BCG failure into the above-mentioned four groups can identify patients with BCG-failure in terms of their prognosis (Shirakawa et al. 2012). The potential risk for critical adverse events was higher in the BCG-refractory group than in the other BCG-failure groups, despite the fact that patients in each group all underwent induction BCG therapy, therefore, treatment decisions, protocols and recommendations should be established based on each individual BCG-failure pattern (Shirakawa et al. 2012).

References

Gontero P, Sylvester R, Pisano F, Joniau S, Vander Eeckt K, Serretta V, Larré S, Di Stasi S, Van Rhijn B, Witjes AJ, Grotenhuis AJ, Kiemeney LA, Colombo R, Briganti A, Babjuk M, Malmström PU, Oderda M, Irani J, Malats N, Baniel J, Mano R, Cai T, Cha EK, Ardelt P, Varkarakis J, Bartoletti R, Spahn M, Johansson R, Frea B, Soukup V, Xylinas E, Dalbagni G, Karnes RJ, Shariat SF, Palou J. Prognostic factors and risk groups in T1G3 non-muscle-invasive bladder cancer patients initially treated with Bacillus Calmette-Guérin: results of a retrospective multicenter study of 2451 patients. Eur Urol. 2015;67(1):74–82.
Nguyen-Huu Y, Delorme G, Lillaz J, Bedgedjian I, Le Ray-Ferrières I, Chabannes E, Bernardini S, Guichard G, Bittard H, Kleinclauss F. Muscularis mucosae invasion: prognostic factor for intravesical BCG immunotherapy failure for T1 bladder carcinoma. Prog Urol. 2012;22(5):284–90.
Ofude M, Kitagawa Y, Yaegashi H, Izumi K, Ueno S, Kadono Y, Konaka H, Mizokami A, Namiki M. Selection of adjuvant intravesical therapies using the European Organization for Research and Treatment of Cancer scoring system in patients at intermediate risk of non-muscle-invasive bladder cancer. J Cancer Res Clin Oncol. 2015;141(1):161–8.
Shirakawa H, Kikuchi E, Tanaka N, Matsumoto K, Miyajima A, Nakamura S, Oya M. Prognostic significance of Bacillus Calmette-Guérin failure classification in non-muscle-invasive bladder cancer. BJU Int. 2012;110(6 Pt B):E216–21.

Chapter 38
Intermediate and High Risk NMIBC and BCG

Witjes et al. examined the management of intermediate- and high-risk non-muscle-invasive bladder cancer (NMIBC), particularly with regard to the use of bacillus Calmette-Guérin (BCG) therapy, in North America and Europe (Witjes et al. 2013). Guideline outcomes, EAU or AUA were also compared. In all, 47% of intermediate-risk patients received EAU or AUA guideline-recommended intravesical therapy: intravesical chemotherapy, BCG induction therapy or BCG induction plus maintenance (Witjes et al. 2013). Of the high-risk patients, 50% received maintenance BCG; although not recommended for high-risk NMIBC, 12.5% received intravesical chemotherapy (Witjes et al. 2013). Of patients prescribed maintenance BCG, 93% were scheduled for at least 1 year of therapy. Notably, only 15% discontinued BCG maintenance and, of these discontinuations, 65% were due to reasons unrelated to BCG-associated adverse events (Witjes et al. 2013).

Although Bacillus Calmette-Guérin (BCG) has proven highly effective in non-muscle-invasive bladder cancer (NMIBC), but it can cause severe local and systemic side effects (Brausi et al. 2014). Brausi examined whether reducing the dose or duration of BCG was associated with fewer side effects (Brausi et al. 2014). After transurethral resection, patients with intermediate- and high-risk NMIBC without carcinoma in situ were randomised to one-third dose or full dose BCG and 1 yr or 3 yr of maintenance (Brausi et al. 2014). No significant differences in side effects were detected according to dose or duration of BCG treatment in the four arms (Brausi et al. 2014). Side effects requiring stoppage of treatment were seen more frequently in the first year, so not all patients are able to receive the 1–3 yr of treatment recommended in current guidelines (Brausi et al. 2014).

The optimal dose and duration of intravesical bacillus Calmette-Guérin (BCG) in the treatment of non-muscle-invasive bladder cancer (NMIBC) are controversial. Oddens et al. determine if a one-third dose (1/3D) is not inferior to the full dose (FD), if 1 yr of maintenance is not inferior to 3 yr of

© Springer Nature Switzerland AG 2020
S. S. Goonewardene et al., *Management of Non-Muscle Invasive Bladder Cancer*,
https://doi.org/10.1007/978-3-030-28646-0_38

maintenance, and if 1/3D and 1 yr of maintenance are associated with less toxicity (Oddens et al. 2014).

After transurethral resection, intermediate- and high-risk NMIBC patients were randomized to one of four BCG groups: 1/3rd dose for 1 year, 1/3rd dose for 3 years, full dose for 1 year, and full dose for 3 years (Oddens et al. 2014). There were no differences in toxicity between 1/3rd dose and full dose. Intermediate-risk patients should be treated with full dose for 1 year. In high-risk patients, full dose for 3 years reduces recurrences as compared with full dose for 1 year but not progressions or deaths. The benefit of the two additional years of maintenance should be weighed against its added costs and inconvenience. This demonstrates the dose of BCG can be tailored according to the situation.

Sylvester compared the long-term efficacy of BCG and epirubicin (Sylvester et al. 2010). Three hundred twenty-three patients with stage T1 or grade 3 tumors were high risk, and the remaining 497 patients were intermediate risk (Sylvester et al. 2010). The observed treatment benefit was at least as large, if not larger, in the intermediate-risk patients compared with the high-risk patients. In patients with intermediate- and high-risk stage Ta and T1 urothelial bladder cancer, intravesical BCG with or without INH is superior to intravesical epirubicin not only for time to first recurrence but also for time to distant metastases, overall survival, and disease-specific survival (Sylvester et al. 2010). The benefit of BCG is not limited to just high-risk patients; intermediate-risk patients also benefit from BCG.

References

Brausi M, Oddens J, Sylvester R, Bono A, van de Beek C, van Andel G, Gontero P, Turkeri L, Marreaud S, Collette S, Oosterlinck W. Side effects of Bacillus Calmette-Guérin (BCG) in the treatment of intermediate- and high-risk Ta, T1 papillary carcinoma of the bladder: results of the EORTC genito-urinary cancers group randomised phase 3 study comparing one-third dose with full dose and 1 year with 3 years of maintenance BCG. Eur Urol. 2014;65(1):69–76.

Oddens JR, Sylvester RJ, Brausi MA, Kirkels WJ, van de Beek C, van Andel G, de Reijke TM, et al. The effect of age on the efficacy of maintenance bacillus Calmette-Guerin relative to maintenance epirubicin in patients with stage Ta T1 urothelial bladder cancer: results from eortc genito-urinary group study 30911. Eur Urol. 2014;66(4):694–701.

Sylvester RJ, Brausi MA, Kirkels WJ, Hoeltl W, Calais Da Silva F, Powell PH, Prescott S, Kirkali Z, van de Beek C, Gorlia T, de Reijke TM. EORTC Genito-Urinary Tract Cancer Group. Long-term efficacy results of EORTC genito-urinary group randomized phase 3 study 30911 comparing intravesical instillations of epirubicin, bacillus Calmette-Guérin, and bacillus Calmette-Guérin plus isoniazid in patients with intermediate- and high-risk stage Ta T1 urothelial carcinoma of the bladder. Eur Urol. 2010;57(5):766–73.

Witjes JA, Palou J, Soloway M, Lamm D, Kamat AM, Brausi M, Persad R, Buckley R, Colombel M, Böhle A. Current clinical practice gaps in the treatment of intermediate- and high-risk non-muscle-invasive bladder cancer (NMIBC) with emphasis on the use of bacillus Calmette-Guérin (BCG): results of an international individual patient data survey (IPDS). BJU Int. 2013;112(6):742–50.

Chapter 39
NMIBC, Low Dose BCG and High-Risk Disease

Since BCG is toxic, an attempt to reduce toxicity was made by reducing the dose. CUETO group showed that 1/3 dose BCG was as effective as full dose in intermediate risk patients but not in high risk (Brausi and Olaru 2012). High risk disease still needs the full induction and maintenance courses of BCG (Merseburger et al. 2008).

Another study that evaluated the efficacy of low dose BCG is the trial 30962 from EORTC (Cambier et al. 2016). The results showed a difference of 10% in the five-years recurrence free survival only when 1/3 dose BCG for one year (54.5%) was compared to Full dose BCG for three years (64.2%) suggesting that 1/3 dose or one year full dose are suboptimal treatments (Cambier et al. 2016). For followup of endoscopic resection for those patients not fit for radical therapy, cystoscopy and cytology must be performed at three months. In the case of negative findings, following cystoscopy and cytology assessments have to be repeated every three months for three years, and every six months thereafter until five years, and then annually up to 10 years.

BCG termination was necessary in 18 patients (30%). Recurrence occurred in 16 patients (26.7%) at a median follow-up of 24.2 months while progression occurred in five patients (8.3%) at a median follow-up of 33 months (Farah et al. 2014). Recurrence-free survival and progression-free survival rates were 73% and 92% respectively. Cystectomy was performed in seven patients (12%) with a cystectomy-free survival of 88% (Farah et al. 2014). There were no cancer specific deaths. Two patients died of other causes (3.3%). The overall survival rate was 97%. This study demonstrated recurrence-free, progression-free, disease specific survival and overall survival to the reported literature and the more intense three-years South West Oncology Group (SWOG) protocol.

© Springer Nature Switzerland AG 2020
S. S. Goonewardene et al., *Management of Non-Muscle Invasive Bladder Cancer*,
https://doi.org/10.1007/978-3-030-28646-0_39

References

Brausi M, Olaru V. The management of high-risk non-muscle invasive bladder cancer. Minerva Urol Nefrol. 2012;64(4):255–60.

Cambier S, Sylvester RJ, Collette L, Gontero P, Brausi MA, van Andel G, Kirkels WJ, Silva FC, Oosterlinck W, Prescott S, Kirkali Z, Powell PH, de Reijke TM, Turkeri L, Collette S, Oddens J. EORTC nomograms and risk groups for predicting recurrence, progression, and disease-specific and overall survival in non-muscle-invasive stage Ta-T1 urothelial cell carcinoma patients treated with 1-3 Years of maintenance bacillus Calmette-Guérin. Eur Urol. 2016;69(1):60–9. https://doi.org/10.1016/j.eururo.2015.06.045 Epub 2015 Jul 23.

Farah NB, Ghanem R, Amr M. Treatment efficacy and tolerability of intravesical bacillus Calmette-Guerin (Bcg)-Rivm strain: induction and maintenance protocol in high grade and recurrent low grade non-muscle invasive bladder cancer (Nmibc). BMC Urol. 2014;14:11.

Merseburger AS, Matuschek I, Kuczyk MA. Bladder preserving strategies for muscle-invasive bladder cancer. Curr Opin Urol. 2008;18(5):513–8.

Chapter 40
Alternatives to BCG Therapy—MMC

Niehlsen et al., determined self-reported practices of use of intravesical chemo- and immunotherapy for patients with non-muscle-invasive bladder cancer (NMIBC) (Nielsen et al. 2012). An electronic survey was developed by members of the Bladder Cancer Advocacy Network (BCAN) to determine management strategies for NMIBC. In all, 63% reported routine perioperative mitomycin-c (MMC) after transurethral resection of bladder tumour (80% academic vs. 54% private practice, $p < 0.001$) (Nielsen et al. 2012). Whereas 5% of respondents reported routine induction therapy with all new low-grade (LG) diagnoses, 99% reported routinely doing so in new high-grade (HG) cases; most commonly with single-agent bacille Calmette-Guérin (BCG) (94% vs. 9% BCG/interferon and 5% MMC). Reported induction therapy was higher in the setting of high-volume (77%) or frequently recurrent (44%) LG disease (Nielsen et al. 2012). 89% reported routinely using maintenance therapy for HG versus 29% for LG disease. Routine biopsy after BCG, even with normal cystoscopy, was confirmed by 28% (39% academic vs. 22% private practice, $P < 0.001$). This demonstrates urologists report grade-specific use of IVT for NMIBC, at rates higher than suggested in some claims-based analyses (Nielsen et al. 2012).

Adjuvant therapy with different bacillus Calmette-Guérin (BCG) preparations is a well-established guideline-endorsed treatment for nonmuscle invasive bladder cancer (NMIBC) (Böhm et al. 2018). Böhm et al., demonstrated equivocal oncological outcome between BCG and mitomycin C (MMC) for NMIBC. The most outstanding feature are significant toxicity differences with higher rates in the BCG treatment group. The BCG group demonstrated minor adverse effects in 78.4% and major adverse effects in 43.3%-partially coincident. Moreover, the parallel MMC group showed in 34.7% respectively 1.4% adverse events. The adverse events for MMC were far lower.

© Springer Nature Switzerland AG 2020
S. S. Goonewardene et al., *Management of Non-Muscle Invasive Bladder Cancer*,
https://doi.org/10.1007/978-3-030-28646-0_40

References

Böhm WU, Koch R, Wenzel S, Wirth MP, Toma M. Development and treatment of localized/systemic BCGitis: retrospective studies in direct comparison to mitomycin C. Urologe A. 2018;57(5):568–576.

Nielsen ME, Smith AB, Pruthi RS, Guzzo TJ, Amiel G, Shore N, Lotan Y. Reported use of intravesical therapy for non-muscle-invasive bladder cancer (NMIBC): results from the Bladder Cancer Advocacy Network (BCAN) survey. BJU Int. 2012;110(7):967–72.

Chapter 41
BCG Versus Mitomycin C—A Systematic Review

A systematic review relating to bladder cancer epidemiology, risk factors and occupational hazards was conducted. This was to identify the oncological outcomes from BCG versus mitomycin C for NMIBC. The search strategy aimed to identify all references related to this. Search terms used were as follows: (Bladder cancer) AND (BCG) AND (Mitomycin). The following databases were screened from 1989 to June 2019:

- CINAHL
- MEDLINE (NHS Evidence)
- Cochrane
- AMed
- EMBASE
- PsychINFO
- SCOPUS
- Web of Science.

In addition, searches using Medical Subject Headings (MeSH) and keywords were conducted using Cochrane databases. Two UK-based experts in bladder cancer were consulted to identify any additional studies.

Studies were eligible for inclusion if they reported primary research focusing on bladder cancer and screening. Papers were included if published after 1984 and had to be in English. Studies that did not conform to this were excluded. Only primary research was included. The overall aim was to identify the role and components of bladder cancer screening.

Abstracts were independently screened for eligibility by two reviewers and disagreements resolved through discussion or third-party opinion. Agreement level was calculated using Cohens' Kappa to test the intercoder reliability of this screening process. Cohens' Kappa allows comparison of inter-rater reliability between papers using relative observed agreement. This also takes account of

© Springer Nature Switzerland AG 2020

S. S. Goonewardene et al., *Management of Non-Muscle Invasive Bladder Cancer*,
https://doi.org/10.1007/978-3-030-28646-0_41

the comparison occurring by chance. The first reviewer agreed all 17 papers to be included, the second, agreed on 17 (Fig. 41.1).

Data extraction was piloted by the researcher and amended in consultation with the research team (author and two academic supervisors). Data collected included authors, year and country of publication, study aims, setting, intervention aims, number of participants, study design, intervention components and delivery methods, comparison groups and outcome measures, notes and follow-up questions for the authors. Studies were quality assessed using the PRISMA criteria for randomised controlled trials, Mays et al. (Moher et al. 2009; Moher, Liberati et al. 2009; Mays et al. 2005) for the action research and qualitative studies and the Critical Skills Appraisal programme for cohort studies. This was also applied to randomised controlled trials and qualitative studies.

The search identified 17 papers (Fig. 41.1). All 17 mapped to the search terms and eligibility criteria. The current systematic reviews were examined to gain further knowledge about the subject. 14 papers were excluded due to not conforming to eligibility criteria or adding to the evidence for bladder cancer screening. Of the 17 papers left, relevant abstracts were identified and the full papers obtained (all of which were in English), to quality assure against criteria. There was considerable heterogeneity of design among the included studies therefore a narrative review of the evidence was undertaken. There was significant heterogeneity within studies, including clinical topic, numbers, outcomes, as a results a narrative review was thought to be best. The studies were randomized trials of good quality.

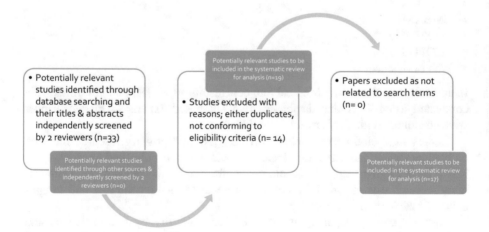

Fig. 41.1 Flow chart of studies identified through the systematic review (adapted from PRISMA)

41.1 Systematic Review Results on BCG Versus Mitomycin C for NMIBC

41.2 NMI Disease and Combination Therapy

Krege conducted a randomized multicenter trial comparing transurethral resection only to transurethral resection plus adjuvant mitomycin C and Bacillus Calmette Guerin (BCG) instillation in NMI bladder cancer (stage pTa/1 grades 1–3 except primary stage pTa grade 1) (Krege et al. 1996). At a median followup of 20.2 months, a decrease in recurrence rate was noted for both drug instillations compared to transurethral resection only. There was no significant difference between the mitomycin C and BCG instillations. Side effects occurred most frequently during or after BCG instillation, most often consisting of cystitis (Krege et al. 1996). One patient required cystectomy because of ulcerating cystitis and a prostatic abscess subsequent to unsuccessful tuberculostatic therapy (Krege et al. 1996). This study demonstrated a positive effect of adjuvant chemotherapy and immunotherapy on decreasing tumor recurrence rate. No influence was observed concerning progression rate, which was low overall.

41.3 Side Effects of Combination BCG and MMC

Intravesical Bacillus Calmette-Guérin (BCG) is a well known effective treatment for non-muscle-invasive bladder cancer (NMIBC), but it has limitations in terms of recurrence and toxicity. Solsona determine whether mitomycin C (MMC) and BCG is superior to BCG alone in increasing a disease-free interval (DFI) (Solsona et al. 2015). Solsona conducted a prospective randomized trial including 407 patients with intermediate-to high-risk NMIBC. Higher toxicity was observed with the combination, even reducing the MMC dose, especially in G3 local toxicity compared with BCG with a difference of 17.4% (95% CI, 7.6–27.2; $p<0.001$). In recurrent T1 tumors, the potential benefit of the sequential combined treatment was more evident than in the remaining subgroup (18.8% vs. 12.8%), with a number needed to treat of five versus eight to avoid an event and with similar toxicity (Solsona et al. 2015). Although combination treatment is more effective than BCG alone in reducing disease relapse, due to higher toxicity it could be offered only to patients with a high likelihood of recurrence, such as those with recurrent T1 tumors.

Witjes et al. (1998) studied toxicity and efficacy of sequential intravesical therapy with mitomycin C and Bacillus Calmette-Guerin (BCG) in intermediate or high risk NMIBC versus mitomycin C alone (Witjes et al. 1998). Patients with intermediate and high risk disease and carcinoma in situ were randomized after transurethral resection between 4 weekly instillations with 40 mg. mitomycin C followed by 6 weekly instillations with BCG (group 1, 90 patients) or 10 weekly instillations with mitomycin C (group 2, 92 patients) (Witjes et al. 1998). The frequency of bacterial and chemical cystitis, and other local side effects was similar in both groups. Allergic reactions, including skin rash, were more frequent in the mitomycin C only group and other systemic side effects were more frequent in the sequential group (Witjes et al. 1998).

The number of recurrences and progression were similar in both groups. There were no major differences in toxicity or treatment efficacy with intravesical mitomycin C and the sequential use of BCG or mitomycin C for intermediate and high risk NMI papillary bladder cancer.

41.4   Perioperative MMC Prior to BCG Induction— Intermediate Risk Patients

Badalato sought to evaluate cancer-specific outcomes among patients who received perioperative mitomycin C (MMC) prior to induction BCG versus those who received induction BCG alone (Badalato et al. 2011). A total of 212 patients were identified who received induction BCG alone, and 48 who received perioperative MMC with induction BCG. Over a median follow up of 34.5 months, there was no difference in overall survival between cohorts (Badalato et al. 2011). RFS was superior among patients who received combined therapy (5-year survival: 37.5% vs. 56.3%, $p = 0.023$) (Badalato et al. 2011). Nevertheless, the regimen of intravesical therapy did not reach significance as an independent predictor (HR 0.61, $p = 0.055$, CI 0.36–1.01). Although the combination therapy group demonstrated a significant RFS advantage, the intravesical therapy regimen did not independently modulate this benefit (Badalato et al. 2011). Further investigation is warranted to determine if immediate MMC prior to a course of induction BCG confers a benefit to RFS (Badalato et al. 2011). Nevertheless, this pilot investigation sets an important precedent on the management of NMI bladder cancer, notwithstanding the absence of contemporary large scale, randomized trials.

Mangiarotti compared intravesical BCG with intravesical mitomycin C chemotherapy in intermediate risk non-muscle invasive bladder cancer as a prospective randomised trial (Mangiarotti et al. 2008). 96 patients with low grade recurrent disease (Ta or T1) were randomly assigned to intravesical treatment with BCG or mitomycin C. Half of the patients were free of recurrence after mitomycin C (23/46) and BCG (23/46) treatment (Mangiarotti et al. 2008). Recurrences after BCG presented in the first 6-month period (>50%) or in the long term follow up

(>3 years) whereas early (<6 months) or long term (>3 years) recurrences after MMC treatment were less frequent. None progressed to muscle-invasive tumour or underwent cystectomy during the observation period. This demonstrates both MMC and BCG demonstrate efficacy in prolonging the time to recurrence and no difference in the recurrence rates was observed between MMC and BCG as primary treatment (Magariotta et al. 2008). A significant number of patients treated with MMC suffered cystitis or hypersensitivity resulting in treatment being stopped. The vast majority of patients treated with BCG had only mild or moderate side effects under BCG treatment but a serious infection was observed in one case requiring antituberculous treatment. There is a difference in side effect profile and tolerability between the two.

41.5   NMI Bladder Cancer—MMC and BCG

Malmström report the 5-year followup of a randomized comparison of mitomycin C and Bacillus Calmette-Guerin (BCG) in patients with NMI bladder carcinoma. Recurrence, progression and survival rates, crossover results, prognostic factors and long-term side effects were analysed (Malmström et al. 1999). After a median followup of 64 months 42% were disease-free (Malmström et al. 1999). A significant difference was noted in disease-free survival with BCG ($p=0.04$), which was most pronounced for stage Tis disease. No difference in tumor progression, or crude or corrected survival was found between the 2 arms. Crossover treatment was successful in 39% of patients with second line BCG and 19% with second line mitomycin C (Malmström et al. 1999). Only the completion of treatment was predictive of outcome for patients treated with BCG. Therapy with BCG was superior to mitomycin C for recurrence prophylaxis but no difference was found for progression and survival.

Based upon the results presented, the response at the first three-month evaluation has major prognostic importance (Soloway 1990). Among the 80 patients who received a treatment course of MMC, 13% of the complete responders compared to 34% of those who failed had a subsequent cystectomy, and among the 55 patients who received BCG, 6% of the complete responders compared to 25% of the failures had a subsequent cystectomy during the follow up interval (Soloway 1990).

41.6   NMI Bladder Cancer—BCG Versus MMC

Friedrich et al. (2007) conducted a randomised, parallel group, multicentre phase 4 trial comparing short- and long-term chemoprophylaxis with Mitomycin C (MMC) with short-term immunoprophylaxis with Bacillus Calmette-Guérin (BCG) after transurethral resection of the bladder for non-muscle-invasive bladder carcinoma (Freidrich et al. 2007). The 3-year recurrence-free rates were 65.5% (95% CI, 55.9–73.5%) for short-term BCG, and 68.6% (59.9–75.7%) for short-term MMC, whereas recurrence-free rates were significantly increased to 86.1% (77.9–91.4%) in patients with MMC long-term therapy (log-rank test, $p = 0.001$) (Friedrich et al. 2007). Long-term MMC significantly reduced the risk of tumour recurrence without enhanced toxicity compared with both short-term BCG and MMC in patients with intermediate- and high-risk non-muscle-invasive bladder carcinoma.

Lundholm compared the efficacy and toxicity of long-term mitomycin C versus Bacillus Calmette-Guerin (BCG) instillation in patients at high risk for recurrence and progression of NMI bladder carcinoma (Lundholm et al. 1996). After a median followup of 39 months 49% of the patients given BCG and 34% given mitomycin C were disease-free ($p<0.03$), compared to 48% and 35%, respectively, of those with stage Ta or T1 disease, and 54% and 33%, respectively, of those with dysplasia or stage Tis tumor. Tumor progressed in 13% of patients, with no statistically significant difference observed regarding progression between the mitomycin C and BCG groups. Side effects were more common after BCG instillation, with 5 cases of severe side effects compared to 1 in the mitomycin C group. Treatment was stopped due to toxicity in 10% of the patients (Lundholm et al. 1996). The majority of patients tolerated long-term intravesical therapy well. BCG instillation was hampered by more frequent side effects. BCG was superior regarding recurrence prophylaxis, since patients given BCG had fewer recurrences and a significantly longer time to treatment failure compared to those treated with mitomycin C. No statistically significant difference was observed regarding progression (Lundholm et al. 1996).

41.7 NMI Bladder Cancer—Low Dose BCG Versus MMC

Ojea examined lower doses of Bacillus Calmette-Guerin (BCG) to assess effectiveness and lower toxicity in intermediate risk disease (Ojea et al. 2007). A low dose of BCG 27 mg was compared with BCG 13.5 mg, using mitomycin C (MMC) 30 mg as the third arm. A total of 430 patients were randomised into three groups. Instillations were repeated once a week for 6 week followed by another six instillations given once every 2 week during 12 week (Ojea et al. 2007). There was a significantly longer disease-free interval for BCG 27 mg versus MMC 30 mg ($p = 0.006$) (Ojea et al. 2007). There were no statistically significant differences between BCG 27 mg and BCG 13.5 mg ($p = 0.165$) or between BCG 13.5 mg and MMC 30 mg ($p = 0.183$). There were no significant differences among the three groups with regards to time to progression and cancer-specific survival time. Local and systemic toxicity were higher in both BCG treatment groups (Ojea et al. 2007). This study demonstrates one third of the standard dose,

BCG 27 mg, seems to be the minimum effective dose as adjuvant treatment for intermediate-risk NMI bladder cancer, being more effective than MMC 30 mg. One sixth of the standard dose, BCG 13.5 mg, has the same efficacy as MMC 30 mg but it is more toxic (Ojea et al. 2007).

41.8 Intermediate Risk Non-Muscle Invasive Bladder Cancer and Outcomes

Isbarn conducted multicenter trial comparing a long-term treatment regimen with mitomycin C (MMC) with two short-term treatment approaches with MMC or bacille Calmette-Guérin (BCG) for intermediate-/high-risk bladder tumor after transurethral resection (Isbarn et al. 2008). The 3-year recurrence-free rate in the patients of the intermediate-/high-risk group was 65.5% (95% CI: 55.9–73.5%) in the BCG arm and 68.6% (95% CI: 59.9–75.7%) in the MMC short-term arm (Isbarn et al. 2008). In the MMC long-term arm, the 3-year recurrence-free rate was significantly higher at 86.1% (95% CI: 77.9–91.4%, log-rank test: $p = 0.001$). There was no increased toxicity observed with long-term administration of MMC. In the low-risk group, the 3-year recurrence-free rate after adjuvant therapy was 74% (95% CI: 60.0–83.8%) and in the patients receiving no adjuvant treatment 63% (95% CI: 46.6–75.5%, corresponding to a hazard ratio of 0.58 (95% CI: 0.28–1.18%) (Isbbarn et al. 2008). The difference between the treatment arms was not significant. This study showed no significant decrease of the recurrence rate in low-risk tumors with six adjuvant MMC instillations. This treatment approach thus does not represent an alternative to early instillation.

41.9 High Risk Non-Muscle Invasive Bladder Cancer—MMC or BCG?

Gårdmark reported the 10-year follow-up of a study randomizing between instillations of Bacillus Calmette-Guérin (BCG) and mitomycin-C (MMC) for treating high-risk none muscle invasive bladder cancer (Gårdmark et al. 2007). The patients included had frequently recurring Ta/T1G1–G2, T1G3 or primary Tis-dysplasia. The patients were randomized to treatment with either 40 mg of MMC or 120 mg of BCG (Danish strain 1331) given weekly for 6 weeks, then monthly up to a year and finally every third month for a further year (Gårdmark et al. 2007). The median follow-up for survivors was 123 months. The disease progressed in 58 (23%) of the patients, 34 in the MMC group and 24 in the BCG group ($p = 0.26$). Based on this is cannot be said MMC or BCG, differed in their effect on progression, need for subsequent treatment or survival.

41.10 Alternating BCG and MMC for CIS

Kaasinen evaluated whether, in carcinoma in situ (CIS) of the urinary bladder, alternating instillation therapy with mitomycin C (MMC) and Bacillus Calmette-Guerin (BCG) was more effective and less toxic than conventional BCG mono-therapy (Kaasinen et al. 2003). After an overall median follow-up of 56 months, the Kaplan-Meier disease-free estimate for BCG monotherapy was significantly better than alternating therapy ($p = 0.03$; log rank test) (Kaasinen et al. 2003). Risk for progression appeared lower in the BCG monotherapy group ($p = 0.07$), but no differences existed in survival. BCG monotherapy caused significantly more local side-effects than alternating therapy (Kaasinen et al. 2003). One-year BCG mon-otherapy was more effective than the alternating therapy for reducing recurrence (Kaasinen et al. 2003).

Rintala examined if alternating chemotherapeutic and immunotherapeutic instillations improved efficacy and reduced toxicity in patients with carcinoma in situ of the bladder (Rintala et al. 1995). Of 68 carcinoma in situ patients ran-domly treated with instillations 40 received mitomycin C and 28 received mito-mycin C and Pasteur Bacillus Calmette-Guerin (BCG) in alternating courses. Mean followup was 33 months (Rintala et al. 1995). The complete response rates with mitomycin C and mitomycin C/BCG were 45 and 71% at 3 months, 59 and 82% at 12 months, and 47 and 74% at 24 months, respectively ($p = 0.041$). The disease-free interval showed the superiority of alternating therapy ($p = 0.043$). Recurrence rates during the instillation period were 1.834 with mitomycin C and 0.922 with mitomycin C/BCG ($p = 0.013$) (Rintala et al. 1995). No remarka-ble side effects developed in the alternating group. Therapy of carcinoma in situ with alternating mitomycin C and BCG is more effective than mitomycin C alone. Compared to BCG monotherapy only few side effects occur.

Sekine elucidate the most efficient therapy for carcinoma in situ of the bladder, the efficacy of intravesical mitomycin C plus doxorubicin therapy was compared with Bacillus Calmette-Guerin (BCG) therapy (Sekine et al. 2001). Both thera-pies were equally effective with initial response rates of 86% (18/21) for BCG and 81% (17/21) for mitomycin C plus doxorubicin, irrespective of the tumor grade (Sekine et al. 2001). Of seven initial non-responders, five patients achieved a com-plete response by subsequent instillation, resulting in a total response rate of 95%. After a mean follow-up of 47 months, five patients (12%) developed disease pro-gression (Sekine et al. 2001). The progression rates were not different between the topical therapies but were significantly higher in grade 3 than in grade 2 cases (Sekine et al. 2001). It appears likely that mitomycin C plus doxorubicin instilla-tion has an equivalent efficacy to BCG as the initial therapy of carcinoma in situ and the combination of them would be the most efficient treatment for the disease (Sekine et al. 2001).

Witjes et al. (1993) compared intravesical instillations of mitomycin-C (MMC), Bacillus Calmette-Guerin (BCG) Tice, and BCG-RIVM in pTa-pT1 papillary carcinoma and primary carcinoma in situ (CIS) (Witjes et al. 1993).

Early recurrences were treated with additional instillations. For toxicity and efficacy 437 patients were evaluated with a median follow-up of 32 months (range
12–56). Drug-induced and bacterial cystitis were the most frequent side-effects
(Witjes et al. 1993). The number and severity of side-effects (chi 2 test) were comparable in both BCG groups, but were significantly less in the MMC group for
drug-induced cystitis ($p = 0.009$), other local side-effects ($p = 0.004$) and systemic
side-effects ($p < 0.001$) (Witjes et al. 1993). The disease-free percentage (log-rank
test) showed no significant difference for the three arms for papillary tumours
($p = 0.08$), nor the CIS ($p = 0.20$), although for CIS numbers are small. Additional
instillations did not influence toxicity or efficacy.

41.11 Alternating BCG and MMC for NMI Bladder Cancer

Rintala attempted to prove if alternating chemoprophylactic and immunoprophy-
lactic instillations improved efficacy and decreased toxicity in patients with
recurrent NMI bladder cancer (Rintala et al. 1996). A total of 188 patients with
rapidly recurring stage Ta or T1 cancer was randomly treated with mitomycin C
(group 1) or alternating mitomycin C and Pasteur strain Bacillus Calmette-Guerin
(BCG) instillations (group 2) for 2 years (Rintala et al. 1996). Mean followup
was 34 months. Median times to initial recurrence were 12 months in group 1
and 7 months in group 2 ($p = 0.976$), and treatment failed in 21.5% and 18.9%,
respectively. Recurrence rates during the instillation period were 1.01 in group 1
and 0.86 in group 2 ($p = 0.376$) (Rintala et al. 1996). There was no difference in
the disease-free interval between the 2 groups ($p = 0.976$). Instillations were discontinued because of adverse effects in 6 cases (6%) in both groups. Efficacy of
alternating mitomycin C and BCG was equal to mitomycin C monotherapy, and
both methods were effective in prophylaxis of recurrent papillary bladder cancer.
Less toxicity occurred in the alternating treatment group compared to earlier BCG
monotherapy results.

41.12 Tumour Marker Responses, Combination MMC and BCG in Non-Muscle Invasive Bladder Cancer

van der Meijden, studied intravesical mitomycin C followed by intravesical
Bacillus Calmette-Guérin (BCG) on a papillary marker tumour and examined side
effects van der Meijden et al. (1996). Thirty-five patients with multiple pTa or pT1
bladder tumours were given 4 instillations of mitomycin C at weekly intervals then
6 instillations at weekly intervals of BCG-RIVM (van der Meijden et al. 1996). All
visible tumours were resected before starting intravesical instillations except one

marker tumour. Response was determined 2 weeks after the last instillation. The incidence of adverse effects was similar to previously reported toxicity of either mitomycin C or BCG alone (van der Meijden et al. 1996). Complete response, histologically proven, was observed in 16 of 35 patients and in 3 patients without histological confirmation. One patient showed progression. The sequential combination of mitomycin C and BCG is an efficacious treatment. The measurement of response to a marker tumour is a safe and efficient method to test new drugs or combinations of drugs.

41.13   Outcomes in Recurrent Cancer Treated with BCG

The long-term prospective data on Bacillus Calmette-Guérin (BCG) and mitomycin C (MMC) instillation therapy are limited (Järvinen et al. 2009). Järvinen compared the long-term benefit of BCG and MMC maintenance therapy in patients with recurrent bladder carcinoma. Eighty-nine patients with frequently recurrent TaT1 disease without carcinoma in situ (CIS) were eligible (Järvinen et al. 2009). Originally, the patients were enrolled in the prospective FinnBladder I study between 1984 and 1987 and randomised to receive BCG or MMC. Both regimens involved five weekly instillations, followed by monthly instillations for 2 year (Järvinen et al. 2009). Thirty-six of 45 patients (80.0%) in the MMC group experienced recurrence in contrast to 26 of 44 patients (59.1%) in the BCG group (Järvinen et al. 2009). No difference existed in the overall mortality. The study population, however, was too small for conclusive evidence about progression or survival (Järvinen et al. 2009).

Results of a randomized prospective study are reported in which mitomycin C, Tice Bacillus Calmette-Guerin (BCG) and RIVM-BCG were compared in 437 patients with primary or recurrent pTa and pT1 bladder tumors, including carcinoma in situ (Vegt et al. 1995). The followup (or time in study) varied from 2 to 81 months (mean 36 months). After complete transurethral resection of all visible tumors the patients were treated with 30 mg. mitomycin C once a week for 4 consecutive weeks and thereafter every month for a total of 6 months, and $5 \times 10(8)$ colony-forming units Tice BCG or RIVM-BCG once a week for 6 consecutive weeks. For papillary tumors mitomycin C and RIVM-BCG treatments were equally effective ($p = 0.53$), and mitomycin C was more effective than Tice BCG therapy ($p = 0.01$) (Vegt et al. 1995).

References

Badalato GM, Hruby G, Razmjoo M, McKiernan JM. Maximizing intravesical therapy options: is there an advantage to the administration of perioperative mitomycin C prior to an induction course of BCG? Can J Urol. 2011;18(5):5890–5.

Friedrich MG, Pichlmeier U, Schwaibold H, Conrad S, Huland H. Long-term intravesical adjuvant chemotherapy further reduces recurrence rate compared with short-term intravesical chemotherapy and short-term therapy with Bacillus Calmette-Guérin (BCG) in patients with non-muscle-invasive bladder carcinoma. Eur Urol. 2007;52(4):1123–9.

Gårdmark T, Jahnson S, Wahlquist R, Wijkström H, Malmström PU. Analysis of progression and survival after 10 years of a randomized prospective study comparing mitomycin-C and Bacillus Calmette-Guérin in patients with high-risk bladder cancer. BJU Int. 2007;99(4):817–20. Epub 2007 Jan 22.

Isbarn H, Budäus L, Pichlmeier U, Conrad S, Huland H, Friedrich MG. Comparison of the effectiveness between long-term instillation of mitomycin C and short-term prophylaxis with MMC or Bacillus Calmette-Guérin. Study of patients with non-muscle-invasive urothelial cancer of the urinary bladder. Urologe A. 2008;47(5):608–15.

Järvinen R, Kaasinen E, Sankila A, Rintala E, FinnBladder Group. Long-term efficacy of maintenance Bacillus Calmette-Guérin versus instillation therapy in frequently recurrent TaT1 tumours without carcinoma in situ: a subgroup analysis of the prospective, randomised Finn Bladder I study with a 20-year follow-up. Eur Urol. 2009;56(2):260–5.

Kaasinen E, Wijkström H, Malmström PU, Hellsten S, Duchek M, Mestad O, Rintala E. Nordic Urothelial Cancer Group. Alternating mitomycin C and BCG instillations versus BCG alone in treatment of carcinoma in situ of the urinary bladder: a nordic study. Eur Urol. 2003;43(6):637–45.

Krege S, Giani G, Meyer R, Otto T, Rübben H. A randomized multicenter trial of adjuvant therapy in NMI bladder cancer: transurethral resection only versus transurethral resection plus mitomycin C versus transurethral resection plus Bacillus Calmette Gucrin. Participating Clinics J Urol. 1996;156(3):962–6.

Lundholm C, Norlén BJ, Ekman P, Jahnson S, Lagerkvist M, Lindeborg T, Olsson JL, Tveter K, Wijkstrom H, Westberg R, Malmström PU. A randomized prospective study comparing long-term intravesical instillations of mitomycin C and Bacillus Calmette-Guerin in patients with NMI bladder carcinoma. J Urol. 1996;156(2 Pt 1):372–6.

Malmström PU, Wijkström H, Lundholm C, Wester K, Busch C, Norlén BJ. 5-year followup of a randomized prospective study comparing mitomycin C and Bacillus Calmette-Guerin in patients with NMI bladder carcinoma. Swedish-Norwegian Bladder Cancer Study Group. J Urol. 1999;161(4):1124–7.

Mangiarotti B, Trinchieri A, Del Nero A, Montanari E. A randomized prospective study of intravesical prophylaxis in non-musle invasive bladder cancer at intermediate risk of recurrence: mitomycin chemotherapy vs. BCG immunotherapy. Arch Ital Urol Androl. 2008;80(4):167–71.

Mays N, Pope C, Popay J. Systematically reviewing qualitative and quantitative evidence to inform management and policy-making in the health field. J Health Serv Res Policy. 2005;10(Suppl. 1):6–20.

Moher D, Liberati A, Tetzlaff J, Altman DG. Preferred reporting items for systematic reviews and meta-analyses: the prisma statement. BMJ. 2009;339(7716):332–6.

Ojea A, Nogueira JL, Solsona E, Flores N, Gómez JM, Molina JR, Chantada V, Camacho JE, Piñeiro LM, Rodríguez RH, Isorna S, Blas M, Martínez-Piñeiro JA, Madero R; CUETO Group (Club Urológico Español De Tratamiento Oncológico). A multicentre, randomised prospective trial comparing three intravesical adjuvant therapies for intermediate-risk NMI bladder cancer: low-dose bacillus Calmette-Guerin (27 mg) versus very low-dose Bacillus Calmette-Guerin (13.5 mg) versus mitomycin C. Eur Urol. 2007;52(5):1398–406.

Rintala E, Jauhiainen K, Kaasinen E, Nurmi M, Alfthan O, Finnbladder Group. Alternating mito-
    mycin C and Bacillus Calmette-Guerin instillation prophylaxis for recurrent papillary (stages
    Ta to T1) NMI bladder cancer. J Urol. 1996;156(1):56–9; discussion 59–60.
Rintala E, Jauhiainen K, Rajala P, Ruutu M, Kaasinen E, Alfthan O, The Finn bladder Group.
    Alternating mitomycin C and bacillus Calmette-Guerin instillation therapy for carcinoma
    in situ of the bladder. J Urol. 1995;154(6):2050–3
Sekine H, Ohya K, Kojima SI, Igarashi K, Fukui I. Equivalent efficacy of mitomycin C plus dox-
    orubicin instillation to Bacillus Calmette-Guerin therapy for carcinoma in situ of the bladder.
    Int J Urol. 2001;8(9):483–6.
Soloway MS. Follow up of patients receiving treatment for NMI bladder cancer with mitomycin
    C and BCG. Prog Clin Biol Res. 1990;350:71–9.
Solsona E, Madero R, Chantada V, Fernandez JM, Zabala JA, Portillo JA, Alonso JM, Astobieta
    A, Unda M, Martinez-Piñeiro L, Rabadan M, Ojea A, Rodriguez-Molina J, Beardo P,
    Muntañola P, Gomez M, Montesinos M, Martinez Piñeiro JA, Members of Club Urológico
    Español de Tratamiento Oncológico. Sequential combination plus Bacillus Calmette-Guérin
    (BCG) is more effective but more toxic than BCG alone in patients with non-muscle-invasive
    bladder cancer in intermediate- and high-risk patients: final outcome of CUETO 93009, a ran-
    domized prospective trial. Eur Urol. 2015;67(3):508–16.
van der Meijden AP, Hall RR, Macaluso MP, Pawinsky A, Sylvester R, Van Glabbeke M. Marker
    tumour responses to the sequential combination of intravesical therapy with mitomycin-C
    and BCG-RIVM in multiple NMI bladder tumours. Report from the European Organisation
    for Research and Treatment on Cancer-Genitourinary Group (EORTC 30897). Eur Urol.
    1996;29(2):199–203.
Vegt PD, Witjes JA, Witjes WP, Doesburg WH, Debruyne FM, van der Meijden AP. A ran-
    domized study of intravesical mitomycin C, Bacillus Calmette-Guerin Tice and Bacillus
    Calmette-Guerin RIVM treatment in pTa-pT1 papillary carcinoma and carcinoma in situ of
    the bladder. J Urol. 1995;153(3 Pt 2):929–33.
Witjes JA, Caris CT, Mungan NA, Debruyne FM, Witjes WP. Results of a randomized phase III
    trial of sequential intravesical therapy with mitomycin C and Bacillus Calmette-Guerin versus
    mitomycin C alone in patients with NMI bladder cancer. J Urol. 1998;160(5):1668–71; dis-
    cussion 1671–2.
Witjes JA, van der Meijden AP, Witjes WP, Doesburg W, Schaafsma HE, Debruyne FM, Dutch
    South-East Cooperative Urological Group. A randomised prospective study comparing intra-
    vesical instillations of mitomycin-C, BCG-Tice, and BCG-RIVM in pTa-pT1 tumours and
    primary carcinoma in situ of the urinary bladder. Eur J Cancer. 1993;29A(12):1672–6.

Chapter 42
What the Literature Says NMIBC—BCG or MMC

Bladder cancer is the second commonest urinary tract malignancy with 70–80% being non-muscle invasive (NMIBC) at diagnosis (Veeratterapillay et al. 2016). Patients with high-risk NMIBC (T1/Tis, with high grade/G3, or CIS) are at greater risk of recurrence and progression. Intravesical Bacilli Calmette-Guerin (BCG) is first line therapy but there is a current worldwide shortage. BCG reduces recurrence in high-risk NMIBC and is more effective that other intravesical agents including mitomycin C, epirubicin, interferon-alpha and gemcitabine (Veeratterapillay et al. 2016). Primary cystectomy offers a high change of cure in this cohort (80–90%) and is a more radical treatment option which patients need to be counselled carefully about. Bladder thermotherapy and electromotive drug administration with mitomycin C are alternative therapies with promising short-term results although long-term follow-up data are lacking (Veeratterapillay et al. 2016).

Shelley assessed, in a systematic review and meta-analysis, the relative effectiveness of intravesical mitomycin C and bacillus Calmette-Guérin (BCG) for tumour recurrence, disease progression and overall survival in patients with medium- to high-risk Ta and T1 bladder cancer (Shelley et al. 2004). The major medical databases were searched comprehensively up to June 2003, and relevant journals hand-searched for randomized controlled trials, in any language, that compared intravesical mitomycin C with BCG in medium- to high-risk patients with Ta or T1 bladder cancer. Twenty-five articles were identified but only seven were considered eligible for the analysis (Shelley et al. 2004). This represented 1901 evaluable patients in all, 820 randomized to mitomycin C and 1081 to BCG. Shelley demonstrated tumour recurrence was significantly lower with intravesical BCG than with mitomycin C only in those patients at high risk of tumour recurrence (Shelley et al. 2004). However, there was no difference in disease progression or survival, and the decision to use either agent might be based on adverse events and cost.

© Springer Nature Switzerland AG 2020   221
S. S. Goonewardene et al., *Management of Non-Muscle Invasive Bladder Cancer*,
https://doi.org/10.1007/978-3-030-28646-0_42

Böhle compare the therapeutic efficacy of intravesical bacille Calmette-Guérin (BCG) with mitomycin C (MMC) on progression of Stage Ta and T1 bladder carcinoma (Böhle and Bock 2004). In nine eligible clinical trials, 1277 patients were treated with BCG and 1133 with MMC. Within the overall median follow-up of 26 months, 7.67% of the patients in the BCG group and 9.44% of the patients in the MMC group developed tumor progression. In all nine individual studies and in the combined results, no statistically significant difference in the ORs for progression between the BCG and MMC-treated groups was found (combined OR $=0.77$; 95% CI 0.57–1.03; $p=0.081$) (Böhle and Bock 2004). In the subgroup with BCG maintenance, the combined result of the five individual studies showed a statistically significant superiority of BCG over MMC (OR $=0.66$; 95% CI 0.47–0.94; $p=0.02$). In the four studies without BCG maintenance, the combined result indicated no statistically significant difference between the two treatments (OR $=1.16$; 95% CI 0.65–2.07; $p=0.612$) (Böhle and Bock 2004). Potential confounders, such as tumor risk status, duration of follow-up, BCG strain, BCG and MMC treatment regimen, and year of publication did not significantly influence these results. The results demonstrated statistically significant superiority for BCG compared with MMC for the prevention of tumor progression only if BCG maintenance therapy was provided.

References

Böhle A, Bock PR. Intravesical bacille Calmette-Guérin versus mitomycin C in NMI bladder cancer: formal meta-analysis of comparative studies on tumor progression. Urology. 2004;63(4):682–6; discussion 686–7.
Shelley MD, Wilt TJ, Court J, Coles B, Kynaston H, Mason MD. Intravesical bacillus Calmette-Guérin is superior to mitomycin C in reducing tumour recurrence in high-risk NMI bladder cancer: a meta-analysis of randomized trials. BJU Int. 2004;93(4):485–90.
Veeratterapillay R, Heer R, Johnson MI, Persad R, Bach C. High-risk non-muscle-invasive bladder cancer-therapy options during intravesical BCG shortage. Curr Urol Rep. 2016;17(9):68.

Chapter 43
NMIBC and Intravesical Chemotherapy— HIVEC I and HIVEC II

Bladder cancer (BC) is a severe health burden: and has high recurrence and progression rates. Standard treatment starts with TURB followed by intravesical chemotherapy with Mitomycin C or immunotherapy with BCG (Merseburger et al. 2008). However, successful management still remains a challenge, because approximately 30% of patients have recurrence or progression within 5 years, and treatment has considerable side effects (Crijnen and De Reijke 2018). This is compounded by BCG shortages. Due to the lack of BCG and the large cohort of patients with recurrence of NMIBC, novel therapies are key to avoid being dependant on one drug.

Disease recurrence and progression remain as significant challenges for the management of non-muscle invasive bladder cancer (NMIBC). The burden and recurrence of this disease is far greater than most realise. In recent years, novel drugs and delivery systems have been investigated as strategies to reduce recurrence, progression and mortality (Aminsharifi et al. 2018). A novel approach involving a heat-activated drug delivery system (ThermoDox®) that enables local accumulation of systemic chemotherapy. Results of this system are still pending.

BCG-RIVM strain was used in many treatment protocols for non-muscle invasive bladder cancer only as induction courses (Farah et al. 2014). Cho et al. (Anticancer Res 2012) compared BCG-RIVM induction and 'standard' maintenance (Lamm et al., J Urol. 2000) to mitomycin C. They found no statistically significant differences regarding disease recurrence and progression. Farah et al. (2014), studied the efficacy and tolerability of this specific BCG RIVM strain, using six-weekly, induction course and single monthly instillations as maintenance for one year, in high risk recurrent, multifocal low grade and multifocal high grade pTa/pT1, CIS transitional cell carcinoma of bladder.

Sixty evaluable patients–median age 63, median follow-up 3.98 years. Forty-two patients (70%) completed BCG-RIVM treatment as planned. BCG termination was necessary in 18 patients (30%). Recurrence occurred in 16 patients (26.7%) at a median follow-up of 24.2 months while progression occurred in five

© Springer Nature Switzerland AG 2020
S. S. Goonewardene et al., *Management of Non-Muscle Invasive Bladder Cancer*,
https://doi.org/10.1007/978-3-030-28646-0_43

patients (8.3%) at a median follow-up of 33 months. Recurrence-free survival and progression-free survival rates were 73% and 92% respectively. Cystectomy was performed in seven patients (12%) with a cystectomy-free survival of 88%. There were no cancer specific deaths. Two patients died of other causes (3.3%). The overall survival rate was 97%. This study demonstrated the clinical efficacy and tolerability of BCG-RIVM strain in the management of high risk NMIBC when given in a schedule of six-weekly induction with monthly maintenance for one year.

Gofrit et al. evaluated the effectiveness of combined local bladder hyperthermia and intravesical chemotherapy for the treatment of patients with high-grade (G3) NMI bladder cancer (Gofrit et al. 2004). Patients with G3 bladder tumors (Stage Ta or T1) were treated with combined intravesical chemotherapy with mitomycin-C and local radiofrequency hyperthermia of the bladder wall (Gofrit et al. 2004). Combined local bladder hyperthermia and intravesical chemotherapy has a beneficial prophylactic effect in patients with G3 NMI bladder cancer (Gofrit et al. 2004). Ablation of high-grade bladder tumors is feasible, achieving a complete response in about three quarters of the patients (Gofrit et al. 2004).

References

Aminsharifi A, Brousell SC, Chang A, León J, Inman BA, THERMODOX®. Heat-targeted drug delivery: a promising approach for organsparing treatment of bladder cancer. Arch Esp Urol. 2018;71(4):447–52.

Crijnen J, De Reijke TM. Emerging intravesical drugs for the treatment of non muscle-invasive bladder cancer. Expert Opin Emerg Drugs. 2018;23(2):135–47.

Farah NB, Ghanem R, Amr M. Treatment efficacy and tolerability of intravesical Bacillus Calmette-Guerin (BCG)-RIVM strain: induction and maintenance protocol in high grade and recurrent low grade non-muscle invasive bladder cancer (NMIBC). BMC Urol. 2014;14:11.

Gofrit ON, Shapiro A, Pode D, Sidi A, Nativ O, Leib Z, Witjes JA, van der Heijden AG, Naspro R, Colombo R. Combined local bladder hyperthermia and intravesical chemotherapy for the treatment of high-grade NMI bladder cancer. Urology. 2004;63(3):466–71.

Merseburger AS, Matuschek I, Kuczyk MA. Bladder preserving strategies for muscle-invasive bladder cancer. Curr Opin Urol. 2008;18(5):513–8.

Chapter 44
BCG Refractory Disease—Oncological Outcomes

Reasons for development of Bacillus Calmette-Guerin (BCG)-refractory NMI bladder cancers are unknown (Okamura et al. 2003). Okamura analyzed a series of cases on the influence of treatment before BCG application (Okamura et al. 2003). Thirty-three cases (34.4%) demonstrated tumor recurrence within 24 to 146 months, including 9 with progression. Pretreatments had been performed in 19 of these cases (57.6%) whereas they had been conducted for only 10 (15.9%) of the BCG-effective cases (Okamura et al. 2003). Of the total 96 patients, 29 received pretreatment with open surgery, systemic chemotherapy, intravesical instillation or oral administration of anticancer drugs, or immunotherapy (Okamura et al. 2003). Sixty-six percent of these proved BCG refractory, in contrast to only 20.9% in the no-pretreatment group. Furthermore, 7 of the 9 patients demonstrating progression had undergone pretreatment. The data suggest that intravesical instillation of BCG is more effective when no prior treatment has been attempted (Okamura et al. 2003).

Luciani assessed the risk of continued intravesical therapy and delayed cystectomy in the management of NMI bladder cancer refractory to Bacillus Calmette-Guérin (BCG) therapy. Luciani reviewed the medical records of 24 patients who underwent an experimental intravesical treatment with BCG plus interferon alpha-2b or valrubicin (Luciani et al. 2001). All patients had Stage Tis and/or T1 transitional cell carcinoma and had failed multiple prior courses of intravesical therapy, including at least one course of BCG (Luciani et al. 2001). Patients were followed up for a median of 28.5 months (range 6 to 48). One patient died of unrelated disease. All other patients were alive at last follow-up. Fourteen patients with preserved bladder were continuing cystoscopic surveillance: four had no recurrence, five had recurrence limited to the mucosa (Ta or Tis) and became free of disease after an additional course of intravesical therapy, and five had recurrent Ta or Tis or positive cytologic findings. The remaining 9 patients underwent radical cystectomy. All pathologic specimens showed no evidence of progression to muscle-invasive disease (Luciani et al. 2001). A select group of patients with

S. S. Goonewardene et al., *Management of Non-Muscle Invasive Bladder Cancer*, https://doi.org/10.1007/978-3-030-28646-0_44

BCG-refractory transitional cell carcinoma and a poor surgical risk for cystec-tomy may benefit from continued intravesical therapy without a significant risk of progression. However, a cautious approach to this treatment modality is recom-mended, and very close follow-up is necessary to detect bladder recurrences and involvement of the upper tract and prostatic urethra.

Patients with high-grade Ta, T1, or carcinoma in situ non-muscle-invasive bladder cancer (NMIBC) are at high risk for recurrence and, more importantly, progression. Thus, both the American Urological Association and European Association of Urology recommend initial intravesical treatment with Bacillus Calmette-Guerin (BCG) followed by maintenance therapy for a minimum of 1 year. The complete response rate to BCG therapy in patients with high-risk NMIBC can be as high as ~80% (Lightfoot et al. 2011) yet high-risk disease has recurrence. BCG failure can be further characterized into BCG refractory, BCG resistant, BCG relapsing, and BCG intolerant. Current recommendations include one further course of BCG or cystectomy (Lightfoot et al. 2011). In patients who continue to fail conservative treatment and who refuse surgical therapy or are not surgical candidates, treatment options become even more complicated. In this set-ting, treatment options are limited and include repeat BCG treatment, an alternate immunotherapy regimen, chemotherapy, or device-assisted therapy (Lightfoot et al. 2011).

Shirakawa examined progression and disease-specific survival among patients with Bacillus Calmette-Guérin (BCG) failure, after dividing these patients into BCG-refractory, -resistant, -relapsing, and -intolerant groups (Shirakawa et al. 2012). There were 173 patients included with initial BCG failure from 521 patients who had undergone induction BCG therapy for non-muscle-invasive blad-der cancer, excluding CIS, between 1987 and 2009. Patients were stratified into four BCG-failure groups, and each prognostic outcome was evaluated (Shirakawa et al. 2012). Median follow-up period from initial BCG failure was 4.7 years. A total of 42 patients (24.3%) were stratified into the BCG-refractory, three (1.7%) into the BCG-resistant, 106 (61.3%) into the BCG-relapsing, and 22 (12.7%) into the BCG-intolerant group. Twenty-four patients (13.9%) experienced stage pro-gression during follow-up. Multivariate analysis showed that pathological G3 at BCG failure ($p = 0.014$; risk ratio 2.84) and BCG-refractory ($p < 0.001$; risk ratio 4.68) were independent predictors for stage progression. The 10-year progres-sion-free survival rates were 53.2%, 91.1% and 93.8% in the BCG-refractory, BCG-relapsing and BCG-intolerant groups, respectively (Shirakawa et al. 2012). The stage progression rate was higher in the BCG-refractory than in the BCG-relapsing ($p < 0.001$) and BCG-intolerant ($p = 0.007$) groups. Similarly, the 10-year disease-specific survival rate in the BCG-refractory group was sig-nificantly worse than those in the other BCG failure groups ($p < 0.001$). This demonstrates stratification of BCG failure into the above-mentioned four groups can identify patients with BCG-failure in terms of their prognosis (Shirakawa et al. 2012). The potential risk for critical adverse events was higher in the BCG-refractory group than in the other BCG-failure groups, despite the fact that patients in each group all underwent induction BCG therapy, therefore, treatment decisions, protocols and recommendations should be established based on each individual BCG-failure pattern.

Patients with recurrent or persistent high-grade non-muscle-invasive bladder cancer after Bacille Calmette-Guérin (BCG) therapy are termed "BCG failures." Herr hypothesize that BCG-refractory patients who fail to respond to BCG have worse outcomes after bladder-sparing treatments compared with BCG-relapsing patients whose tumors recur after at least a 6-month disease-free interval (Herr et al. 2015). Seventeen patients were classified as BCG refractory and 15 patients defined BCG relapsing. Recurrence-free median survival time was 10 months for BCG-refractory patients receiving mycobacterial cell wall-DNA complex versus 23 months for BCG-relapsing patients who received another induction course of BCG therapy ($p = 0.002$). Progression-free survival time was 18 months for BCG-refractory versus 52 months for BCG-relapsing patients ($p = 0.001$). Of the 17 BCG-refractory patients, 8 (47%) have died versus 3 (20%) of the 15 BCG-relapsing patients (Herr et al. 2015).

References

Herr HW, Milan TN, Dalbagni G. BCG-refractory vs. BCG-relapsing non-muscle-invasive bladder cancer: a prospective cohort outcomes study. Urol Oncol. 2015;33(3):108.e1–4.
Lightfoot AJ, Rosevear HM, O'Donnell MA. Recognition and treatment of BCG failure in bladder cancer. Sci World J. 2011;11:602–13.
Luciani LG, Neulander E, Murphy WM, Wajsman Z. Risk of continued intravesical therapy and delayed cystectomy in BCG-refractory NMI bladder cancer: an investigational approach. Urology. 2001;58(3):376–9.
Okamura T, Akita H, Tozawa K, Kawai N, Nagata D, Kohri K. Bacillus Calmette-Guerin-refractory NMI bladder cancers: focus on pretreatment episodes. Int J Clin Oncol. 2003;8(3):168–73.
Shirakawa H, Kikuchi E, Tanaka N, Matsumoto K, Miyajima A, Nakamura S, Oya M. Prognostic significance of Bacillus Calmette-Guérin failure classification in non-muscle-invasive bladder cancer. BJU Int. 2012;110(6 Pt B):E216–21.

Chapter 45
NMIBC—High Grade BCG Refractory Disease

For the group of patients with initial BCG induction therapy failure that are unfit or refuse radical cystectomy or have a low or intermediate grade disease an additional course of 1 BCG is a choice (Brausi and Olaru 2012). For patients who failed before completion of maintenance BCG, radical cystectomy has to be considered in presence of a high grade T1 or CIS. BCG maintenance (full dose three years) after Re-TUR is the standard therapy in high-risk TCC of the bladder. This only applied if the patient is fit for surgery.

Dose reduction to 1/3 dose or one year full dose are suboptimal treatments in high grade disease (Brausi and Olaru 2012). Lee et al. evaluated the effectiveness of photodynamic therapy using Radachlorin in patients with high grade, nonmuscle invasive bladder cancer refractory or intolerant to bacillus Calmette-Guérin therapy who refused radical cystectomy (Lee et al. 2013). This study demonstrated Photodynamic therapy with Radachlorin is a safe, effective treatment for nonmuscle invasive bladder cancer refractory or intolerant to bacillus Calmette-Guérin therapy in select patients (Lee et al. 2013).

Patients with high-grade Ta, T1, or carcinoma in situ non-muscle-invasive bladder cancer (NMIBC) are at high risk for recurrence and, more importantly, progression (Lightfoot et al. 2011). The complete response rate to BCG therapy in patients with high-risk NMIBC can be as high as ~80%; however, most patients with high-risk disease suffer from recurrence (Lightfoot et al. 2011). BCG failure can be further characterized into BCG refractory, BCG resistant, BCG relapsing, and BCG intolerant (Lightfoot et al. 2011). In this setting, treatment options are limited and include repeat BCG treatment, an alternate immunotherapy regimen, chemotherapy, or device-assisted therapy (Lightfoot et al. 2011).

Patients with recurrent or persistent high-grade non-muscle-invasive bladder cancer after bacille Calmette-Guérin (BCG) therapy are termed "BCG failures." Herr et al. hypothesized that BCG-refractory patients who fail to respond to BCG have worse outcomes after bladder-sparing treatments compared with BCG-relapsing patients whose tumors recur after at least a 6-month disease-free interval

© Springer Nature Switzerland AG 2020
S. S. Goonewardene et al., *Management of Non-Muscle Invasive Bladder Cancer*,
https://doi.org/10.1007/978-3-030-28646-0_45

(Herr et al. 2015). This demonstrated BCG-refractory and BCG-relapsing categories differentiate BCG-failed patients into high-and lower-risk prognostic groups that may be useful in guiding treatment strategies.

Thirty to forty percent of patients with high grade nonmuscle invasive bladder cancer (NMIBC) fail to respond to intravesical therapy with bacillus Calmette-Guerin (BCG) (Correa et al. 2015). Interferon-α2B plus BCG has been shown to be effective in a subset of patients with NMIBC BCG refractory disease. Here we present a contemporary series on the effectiveness and safety of intravesical BCG plus interferon-α2B therapy in patients with BCG refractory NMIBC (Correa et al. 2015). Combination BCG plus interferon-α2B remains a reasonably safe alternative treatment for select patients with BCG refractory disease prior to proceeding to radical cystectomy.

BCG is the most efficacious intravesical treatment for NMI bladder cancer (Punnen et al. 2003). However, 30–40% of tumors are refractory. BCG failure is an indication for cystectomy but several salvage intravesical (IVe) strategies have been proposed (Punnen et al. 2003). Early results with reduced dose BCG in combination with IFN-a in patients are currently the most promising. This demonstrated 12 month data with reduced dose IVe BCG plus IFN-a salvage therapy for BCG refractory NMI TCC confirm previous reports of >50% complete response rates (Punnen et al. 2003).

Perdonà et al. investigated intravesical gemcitabine in high-risk nonmuscle-invasive bladder cancer (NMIBC) refractory to bacillus Calmette-Guérin (BCG) (Perdonà et al. 2010). This was a prospective multicentre single-arm trial. Eligible patients were those with high-risk NMIBC refractory to BCG therapy, for which radical cystectomy was indicated but not conducted because of patient refusal or ineligibility (Perdonà et al. 2010). Overall, treatment was well tolerated. Urinary symptoms represented the primary adverse events. The role of gemcitabine used as second-line treatment in high-risk BCG-refractory NMIBC patients who refused or were unsuitable for radical cystectomy remains to be defined (Perdonà et al. 2010).

Radical cystectomy is the standard of care for patients who fail intravesical bacillus Calmette-Guérin (BCG) for nonmuscle invasive bladder cancer (NMIBC) (Ahn et al. 2014). While BCG is standard treatment for intermediate and high-risk NMIBC, many patients fail therapy with recurrence or progression (Ahn et al. 2014). Early cystectomy is the standard of care for BCG failure; however, many patients are unwilling or unable to undergo cystectomy. Multiple intravesical therapies have been used in this BCG failure population with moderate success, and, recently, technologies to improve drug delivery or create novel drugs have also been applied (Ahn et al. 2014). Comparing efficacy of these therapies remain challenging as study cohorts are heterogeneous and study designs are variable (Ahn et al. 2014). However, there are an increasing number of novel treatment options that can be offered to patients faced with recurrent NMIBC after BCG who seek bladder-sparing therapy (Ahn et al. 2014).

The definitive treatment for patients with non-muscle-invasive bladder cancer (NMIBC) who fail to respond to intravesical BCG is cystectomy (Barlow et al.

2010). When a patient is deemed BCG-refractory and cannot or will not undergo cystectomy, alternative intravesical therapy may be the most effective way to minimize recurrence and progression (Barlow et al. 2010). A number of immunotherapeutic and chemotherapeutic agents have been given intravesically over the years, and several recently and currently investigated novel agents appear to be particularly promising for the management of BCG-refractory NMIBC (Barlow et al. 2010). The most effective treatments in the future will likely utilize targeted therapies based on the underlying genetic mutations associated with each individual diagnosis of NMIBC (Barlow et al. 2010).

References

Ahn JJ, Ghandour RA, McKiernan JM. New agents for bacillus Calmette-Guérin-refractory non-muscle invasive bladder cancer. Curr Opin Urol. 2014;24(5):540–5.

Barlow LJ, Seager CM, Benson MC, McKiernan JM. Novel intravesical therapies for non-muscle-invasive bladder cancer refractory to BCG. Urol Oncol. 2010;28(1):108–11.

Brausi M, Olaru V. The management of high-risk non-muscle invasive bladder cancer. Minerva Urol Nefrol. 2012;64(4):255–60.

Correa AF, Theisen K, Ferroni M, Maranchie JK, Hrebinko R, Davies BJ, Gingrich JR. The role of interferon in the management of BCG refractory nonmuscle invasive bladder cancer. Adv Urol. 2015;2015:656918.

Herr HW, Milan TN, Dalbagni G. BCG-refractory vs. BCG-relapsing non-muscle-invasive bladder cancer: a prospective cohort outcomes study. Urol Oncol. 2015;33(3):108.e1–4.

Lee JY, Diaz RR, Cho KS, Lim MS, Chung JS, Kim WT, Ham WS, Choi YD. Efficacy and safety of photodynamic therapy for recurrent, high grade nonmuscle invasive bladder cancer refractory or intolerant to bacille Calmette-Guérin immunotherapy. J Urol. 2013;190(4):1192–9.

Lightfoot AJ, Rosevear HM, O'Donnell MA. Recognition and treatment of BCG failure in bladder cancer. Sci World J. 2011;11:602–13.

Perdonà S, Di Lorenzo G, Cantiello F, Damiano R, De Sio M, Masala D, Bruni G, Gallo L, Federico P, Quattrone C, Pizzuti M, Autorino R. Is gemcitabine an option in BCG-refractory nonmuscle-invasive bladder cancer? A single-arm prospective trial. Anticancer Drugs. 2010;21(1):101–6.

Punnen SP, Chin JL, Jewett MA. Management of bacillus Calmette-Guerin (BCG) refractory NMI bladder cancer: results with intravesical BCG and Interferon combination therapy. Can J Urol. 2003;10(2):1790–5.

Chapter 46
A Systematic Review on Alternatives in BCG Refractory Disease

A systematic review relating to management in BCG refractory disease was conducted. The search strategy aimed to identify all references related to bladder cancer AND BCG refractory disease. Search terms used were as follows: (Bladder cancer) AND (BCG refractory) AND (Management). The following databases were screened from 1989 to June 2019:

- CINAHL
- MEDLINE (NHS Evidence)
- Cochrane
- AMed
- EMBASE
- PsychINFO
- SCOPUS
- Web of Science.

In addition, searches using Medical Subject Headings (MeSH) and keywords were conducted using Cochrane databases. Two UK-based experts in bladder cancer were consulted to identify any additional studies.

Studies were eligible for inclusion if they reported primary research focusing on bladder cancer and screening. Papers were included if published after 1984 and had to be in English. Studies that did not conform to this were excluded. Only primary research was included. The overall aim was to identify the role and components of bladder cancer screening.

Abstracts were independently screened for eligibility by two reviewers and disagreements resolved through discussion or third party opinion (Fig. 46.1). Agreement level was calculated using Cohen's Kappa to test the intercoder reliability of this screening process. Cohens' Kappa allows comparison of inter-rater reliability between papers using relative observed agreement. This also takes account of the comparison occurring by chance. The first reviewer agreed all 16 papers to be included, the second, agreed on 16.

© Springer Nature Switzerland AG 2020
S. S. Goonewardene et al., *Management of Non-Muscle Invasive Bladder Cancer*,
https://doi.org/10.1007/978-3-030-28646-0_46

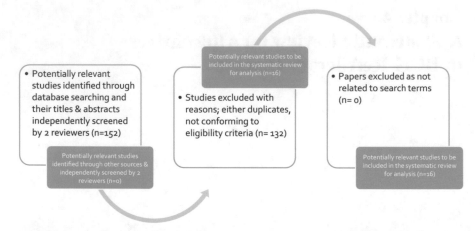

Fig. 46.1 Flow chart of studies identified through the systematic review (adapted from PRISMA)

Data extraction was piloted by the researcher and amended in consultation with the research team (author and two academic supervisors). Data collected included authors, year and country of publication, study aims, setting, intervention aims, number of participants, study design, intervention components and delivery methods, comparison groups and outcome measures, notes and follow-up questions for the authors. Studies were quality assessed using the PRISMA criteria for randomised controlled trials, Mays et al. (Moher et al. 2009; Moher, Liberati et al. 2009, 154, 153; Mays et al. 2005) for the action research and qualitative studies and the Critical Skills Appraisal programme for cohort studies. This was also applied to randomised controlled trials and qualitative studies. There were 15 cohort studies and one RCT. The RCT was of good quality, and the cohort studies were of moderate quality.

References

Mays N, Pope C, Popay J. Systematically reviewing qualitative and quantitative evidence to inform management and policy-making in the health field. J Health Serv Res Policy. 2005;10(Suppl. 1):6–20.
Moher D, Liberati A, Tetzlaff J, Altman DG. Preferred reporting items for systematic reviews and meta-analyses: the prisma statement. BMJ. 2009;339(7716):332–6.

Chapter 47
Systematic Review Results on BCG Refractory Disease Management

47.1 BCG Refractory Disease—Cystectomy or Conservative Therapy

There are no randomized controlled trials (RCTs) evaluating the clinical or benefit of mitomycin C versus radical cystectomy in high-risk non-muscle invasive bladder cancer (NMIBC) (Patel et al. 2015). Patel et al., used the Archimedes computational model to simulate an RCT to assess clinical and economic outcomes for BCG-refractory NMIBC. A total of 1300 virtual patients were evaluated (Patel et al. 2015). Progression to MIBC in the MMC arm was 30% over a lifetime. Disease specific death at 5 years was 1.6 and 8.7% for immediate cystectomy and MMC arms respectively. Overall death rate was 17.8 and 23.8% at 5 years. This demonstrated immediate radical cystectomy after BCG failure for NMIBC has improved survival as opposed to MMC (Patel et al. 2015). Simulation of clinical trials using computational models similar to the Archimedes model may prove useful in the face of current medical cost-conscious era and also help predict trial outcomes.

47.2 BCG Refractory Disease and Alternative Options—Gemcitabine

Approximately 30–40% with NMI bladder cancer treated with Bacille Calmette-Guerin (BCG) or epirubicin do not respond; of the responders 35% relapse within 5 years (Addeo et al. 2010). Addeo compared efficacy and toxicity of intravesical gemcitabine (GEM) with mitomycin (MMC) in recurrent NMI bladder cancer after treatment with BCG (Addeo et al. 2010). 120 patients were randomly assigned to either MMC or GEM treatment arm. In the GEM arm, 39 (72%) of

© Springer Nature Switzerland AG 2020
S. S. Goonewardene et al., *Management of Non-Muscle Invasive Bladder Cancer*,
https://doi.org/10.1007/978-3-030-28646-0_47

54 remained free of recurrence versus 33 (61%) of 55 in MMC arm (Addeo et al. 2010). Among patients with recurrences, 10 MMC and six GEM had progressive disease. The incidence of chemical cystitis in the MMC arm was statistically higher than in the GEM arm ($p = 0.012$) (Addeo et al. 2010). This study demonstrates GEM has better efficacy and lower toxicity than MMC; therefore, GEM appears as a logical candidate for intrabladder therapy in patients with refractory transitional cancer.

Intravesical gemcitabine (Gem) has good outcomes for transitional cell carcinomas (TCC) of the bladder, with moderate urinary toxicity and low systemic absorption. Gunelli et al. (2007) evaluated the activity of biweekly intravesical treatment with Gem using a scheme directly derived from in vitro preclinical studies (Gunelli et al. 2007). Patients with Bacille Calmette-Guérin (BCG) -refractory disease- Ta G3, T1 G1-3 TCC underwent transurethral bladder resection and then intravesical instillation (Gunelli et al. 2007). Thirty-eight (95%) of the 40 patients showed persistent negative post-treatment cystoscopy and cytology 6 months after Gem treatment, while the remaining 2 patients relapsed at 5 and 6 months. At a median follow-up of 28 months, recurrences had occurred in 14 patients. Among these, four had downstaged (T) disease, three had a lower grade (G) lesion and three had a reduction in both T and G. Urinary and systemic toxicity was very low, with no alterations in biochemical profiles (Gunelli et al. 2007). In conclusion, biweekly instillation of Gem proved active in BCG-refractory Ta G3, T1 G1-3 TCC. This highlights the importance of vitro systems that reproduce the conditions of intravesical clinical treatment.

The incidence of bladder cancer is projected to rise is 28% by 2010 for both sexes (according to the WHO). Though intravesical adjuvant therapy with bacillus Calmette-Guérin (BCG) is superior to any other agent in reducing tumor recurren and disease progression, its real efficacy remains controversial. One-third of the patients will soon develop BCG failure (Mohanty et al. 2008). Mohanty studied the efficacy, tolerability, and safety of intravesical gemcitabine in managing BCG refractory NMI bladder malignancy (Mohanty et al. 2008). Thirty-five BCG failure patients were involved. Twenty-one patients (60%) showed no recurrences, 11 patients (31.4%) had NMI recurrences, while 3 patients (8.75%) progressed to muscle invasiveness. Average time to first recurrence was 12 months and to disease progression was 16 months. Adverse events were low and mild (Mohanty et al. 2008). Therapy was well tolerated. Gemcitabine fulfills all requirements in treating BCG failure with low adverse events, is well tolerated, and highly effective in reducing tumor recurrences.

Gacci analyzed the safety and short-term efficacy of gemcitabine (GEM) as salvage intravesical therapy for bacille Calmette-Guérin (BCG)-resistant T1G3 patients (Gacci et al. 2006). Both intravesical administrations of GEM and BCG were well tolerated: no severe adverse events were reported. Of the 9 patients treated with GEM, 3 were recurrence-free after 13, 17 and 21 months. 7 kept an intact bladder, with an overall survival rate of 9 of 9. Among 10 patients treated with BCG instillation, 1 was recurrence-free after 27 months and 6 kept their bladders, with a survival rate of 8 of 10. This confirms the high risk of tumor recurrence and progression of BCG-refractory pT1G3 transitional cell carcinoma. The use of GEM in BCG-refractory pT1G3 patients has to be considered experimental until multicentric randomized studies with adequate follow-up are able to confirm the preliminary results of this pilot study (Gacci et al. 2006).

Perdonà, evaluated intravesical gemcitabine in high-risk nonmuscle-invasive bladder cancer (NMIBC) refractory to bacillus Calmette-Guérin (BCG) (Perdonà et al. 2010) as a prospective multicentre single-arm trial. Eligible patients were high-risk NMIBC refractory to BCG therapy, who did not have radical cystectomy because of patient refusal or ineligibility. Intravesical gemcitabine was administered twice weekly at a dose of 2000 mg/50 ml for 6 weeks, and then weekly for 3 weeks at 3, 6, and 12 months (Perdonà et al. 2010). Fifty-five percent (11 patients) developed disease recurrence. Mean time to the first recurrence was 3.5 months and 45% (five patients) had disease progression. Overall, treatment was well tolerated. Urinary symptoms represented the primary adverse events (Perdonà et al. 2010). The role of gemcitabine used as second-line treatment in high-risk BCG-refractory NMIBC patients who refused or were unsuitable for radical cystectomy remains to be defined. Further clinical research in this area is needed.

Gemcitabine, a chemotherapeutic agent, has been shown to be active against transitional cell cancer of the bladder. Bassi examined the pharmacokinetic profile of gemcitabine, administered intravesically in patients with carcinoma in situ(CIS) (Bassi et al. 2005). Nine patients with CIS refractory to intravesical bacillus Calmette-Guérin (BCG) therapy were enrolled. Grade 1 complications included 1 case of neutropenia, urinary frequency and hematuria were observed in 1 and 3 patients, respectively (Bassi et al. 2005). No other complications were observed. With regard to activity, after 6 instillations of this drug, 4 complete responses were observed. Intravesical gemcitabine is well tolerated and safe (Bassi et al. 2005). No systemic absorption with a clinical or pharmacological effect was detected and only slightly irritative bladder symptoms were observed. This needs further investigation in phase-II trials.

Dalbagani et al., conducted a phase II study was to determine the efficacy of intravesical gemcitabine in bacille Calmette-Guérin (BCG) -refractory transitional cell carcinoma of the bladder (Dalbagni et al. 2006). Thirty eligible patients were included. The median follow-up was 19 months (range, 0–35 months). 15 (50%; 95% CI, 32–68%) achieved a complete response (CR). Twelve patients had tumor recurrence with a median recurrence-free survival time of 3.6 months (95% CI, 2.9 to 11.0 months). Two patients had a complete response at 23 and 29 months (Dalbagni et al. 2006). The 1-year recurrence-free survival rate for complete response was 21% (95% CI, 0–43%). Two patients progressed to a higher stage while receiving gemcitabine treatment. Eleven patients (37%) underwent a cystectomy subsequent to gemcitabine therapy (Dalbagni et al. 2006). Gemcitabine has activity in a high-risk patient population and remains a viable option for some patients who refuse cystectomy.

47.3 BCG Refractory Disease—Gemcitabine and Combination Therapy

Currently, there are few options other than cystectomy for the management of BCG refractory non-muscle invasive bladder cancer (Breyer et al. 2010). Breyer examined with intravesical combination chemotherapy using gemcitabine and MMC (Breyer et al. 2010). A total of 10 patients (6 male and 4 female) had a median follow-up of 26.5 months (4–34 months). Six patients were recurrence free, with complete response at a median of 14 months (4–34 months) (Breyer et al. 2010). Four patients had biopsy proven recurrence. Median time to recurrence was 6 months (range 4–13 months). There were no major complications. Two patients experienced irritative lower urinary tract symptoms, which did not require cessation of therapy and one experienced a maculopapillary rash (Breyer et al. 2010). Intravesical combination chemotherapy with gemcitabine and MMC is well tolerated and gives good outcomes in patients.

Dalbagni et al. (2017) determined effect of everolimus and intravesical gemcitabine instead of radical cystectomy in BCG refractory disease. 14 patients were enrolled in phase I of the trial. 23 patients were enrolled in phase II of the trial and 19 were evaluable for primary and secondary endpoints (Dalbagni et al. 2017). Four patients withdrew consent prior to treatment initiation. Of the 19 patients evaluable for response, 3 (16%, 95% confidence interval [CI] 3–40%) were disease free at 1yr. The probability of RFS was 20% (95% CI 5–42%) at 12 months. However, there was significant toxicity. Ten patients out of 19 had grade 3 or greater toxicity events. Seven withdrew consent or were taken off study (Dalbagni et al. 2017). Continuous oral everolimus plus intravesical gemcitabine was not well tolerated in this patient population where the threshold for tolerability is low. This study was halted and enrolment stopped.

47.4 BCG Refractory Disease and Photodynamic Therapy

Waidelich et al. (2001) determined whether photodynamic therapy after the oral administration of 5-aminolevulinic acid in NMIBC uncontrolled by transurethral resection and intravesical bacillus Calmette-Guerin (BCG) immunotherapy would preserve the bladder and halt progression (Waidelich et al. 2001). At a median followup of 36 months (range 12–51) 3 of the 5 with carcinoma in situ and 4 of the 19 with papillary tumors were free of recurrence. Three patients were rendered disease-free by repeat photodynamic therapy and 3 underwent cystectomy (Waidelich et al. 2001). Tumor progression was stopped in 20 of 24 cases. Immediately after the oral administration of 5-aminolevulinic acid hypotension and tachycardia occurred in 19 and 10 patients, respectively, with previously known severe cardiovascular disease. These initial clinical results suggest that photodynamic therapy with orally administered 5-aminolevulinic acid is effective as an organ preserving procedure for treating NMI bladder cancer even in patients with bacillus Calmette-Guerin refractory carcinoma.

47.5 Assessment of Response Prior to Taxane Therapy

Wosnitzer et al. (2011) designed a study to identify molecular markers linked to the optimal response to such treatment modality (Wosnitzer et al. 2011). Increased total tau (cytoplasmic and nuclear) and stathmin expression before intravesical taxane therapy was significantly associated with decreased recurrence-free survival ($p < 0.0001$ and 0.007, respectively). A tau positive phenotype was an independent prognostic factor for recurrence-free survival on multivariate analysis (HR 15.66, 95% CI 2.68–91.71, $p = 0.002$). Neither the proliferation index assessed by Ki-67 expression nor p53 status was significantly associated with recurrence-free survival (Wosnitzer et al. 2011). This demonstrate assessment of tau and stathmin protein expression should be considered to select patients before intravesical taxane based chemotherapy for nonmuscle invasive, bacillus Calmette-Guérin refractory bladder cancersince those who have tumors with low tau/stathmin protein expression show a better response (Wosnitzer et al. 2011).

47.6 BCG Refractory Disease and Docetaxel

Barlow analyzed clinical effectiveness and safety of intravesical docetaxel in BCG refractory disease (Barlow et al. 2009b). A retrospective was conducted, including 18 patients treated during the Phase I trial and 15 patients treated after the trial's completion. Toxicity, efficacy and recurrence-free survival were analysed (Barlow et al. 2009b). Thirty-three patients with refractory NMIBC received salvage intravesical docetaxel therapy. Twenty of thirty-three (61%) patients had a complete response (CR) after six weekly induction treatments (Barlow et al. 2009a). Ten patients with complete responses were given maintenance docetaxel therapy, and one patient received maintenance BCG and interferon. With a median follow-up of 29 months, 1 and 2-year recurrence-free survival rates were and 45 and 32%, respectively. Twelve of thirty-three patients (36%) had Grade 1 or 2 local toxicities. No patients experienced Grade 3 or 4 toxicities. Docetaxel is a promising intravesical agent with minimal toxicity and significant efficacy and durability for the management of BCG-refractory NMIBC.

Barlow analysed the durability of response in NMIBC BCG refractory disease with intravesical docetaxel in a combined induction and maintenance regimen (Barlow et al. 2009a). Building from a phase 1 trial, a second group of patients was treated with a 6-week induction and then given monthly maintenance therapy with intravesical docetaxel. Thirteen patients with BCG-refractory Ta, T1, or

Tis transitional cell carcinoma were treated (Barlow et al. 2009a). The median follow-up was 13 months; 10 of 13 patients had a CR after induction, and six have remained disease-free during the follow-up. Of those in who the treatment failed, six had transurethral resection of the tumour and one a cystectomy. All 10 initial responders completed at least three instillations of maintenance therapy to date (median nine instillations), of whom six have remained recurrence-free (Barlow et al. 2009a). Monthly maintenance therapy with intravesical docetaxel appears to extend the durability of response to induction treatment for a selected group of patients with BCG-refractory NMIBC, and might decrease the overall risk of recurrence in high-risk NMIBC.

47.7   BCG Refractory Disease and MCNA

Patients with high risk recurrences after bacillus Calmette-Guérin failure have limited options. Morales performed an open label study to evaluate the efficacy and safety of intravesical MCNA in this setting (Morales et al. 2015). A total of 129 patients participated, 91 with carcinoma in situ with or without papillary disease and 38 with papillary only tumors. The overall disease-free survival rate was 25.0% at 1 year and 19.0% at 2 years. In patients with papillary only tumors the disease-free survival rate was 35.1% and 32.2% at 1 and 2 years, respectively (Morales et al. 2015). The median disease-free duration in the 30 responders was 32.7 months. The progression-free survival rate was 87.3%, 79.8% and 77.7% at 1, 2 and 3 years. Progression occurred in 28 patients. MCNA was well tolerated and few adverse events (Morales et al. 2015). Intravesical MCNA had good outcomes in those at high risk NMIBC with BCG refractory disease, especially those with papillary only tumors and those with bacillus Calmette-Guérin relapse.

47.8   Role of Immunotoxin in BCG Refractory Disease

Kowalski performed a Phase I study was performed to determine the maximum tolerated dose (MTD) of the immunotoxin VB4-845 in NMIBC BCG refractory disease (Kowalski et al. 2010). Sixty-four patients with Grade 2 or 3, stage Ta or T1 transitional cell carcinoma or in situ carcinoma, either refractory to or intolerant of BCG therapy, were enrolled. Treatment was administered in ascending dose cohorts ranging from 0.1 to 30.16 mg (Kowalski et al. 2010). After receiving weekly instillations of VB4-845 to the bladder via catheter for 6 consecutive weeks, patients were followed for 4–6 weeks post-therapy and assessed at week 12. By the end of the study, the majority of patients had developed antibodies to the exotoxin portion of VB4-845. A complete response was achieved in 39% of patients at the 12-week time point (Kowalski et al. 2010). VB4-845 dosed on a weekly basis for 6 weeks was very well tolerated at all dose levels. Although an MTD was not determined at the doses administered, VB4-845 showed evidence of an antitumor effect that warrants further clinical investigation for the treatment of NMIBC in this patient population.

47.9   BCG Refractory Disease and Valrubicin

BCG refractory carcinoma in situ (CIS) of the bladder can potentially receive for intravesical (IVe) valrubicin. This post hoc analysis of data from the pivotal phase 3, prospective, open-label study of valrubicin evaluated the effects of patient characteristics and past treatments on the response to valrubicin (Steinberg et al. 2011). Ninety patients enrolled; 87 patients with positive biopsy at initiation completed a valrubicin course and underwent the 3-month assessment. Five had missing data at 6 months. Of the remaining 82 patients, 18 demonstrated a complete response; 64 demonstrated partial or no response (Steinberg et al. 2011). More complete responders had evidence of inflammation before or during valrubicin treatment ($P = 0.005$ vs. nonresponders) (Steinberg et al. 2011). Complete responders to valrubicin did not differ significantly from partial or nonresponders in the number of prior courses or instillations. The results suggest that therapy with valrubicin may be considered in appropriate candidates who have not responded to prior therapies. Cystectomy should be reconsidered when valrubicin treatment fails (Steinberg et al. 2011).

Steinberg assess the efficacy of intravesical valrubicin in refractory BCG CIS who otherwise undergone cystectomy (Steinberg et al. 2000). Of 90 patients 19 (21%) had a complete response, including 7 who remained disease-free at the last evaluation, with a median followup of 30 months. Recurrence has been noted in 79 patients to date, including only 2 with clinically advanced disease (stage T2) (Steinberg et al. 2000). Of these 79 patients 44 (56%, 4 responders and 40 nonresponders) underwent radical cystectomy. Of the 41 patients with known pathological stage 6 (15%) had stage pT3 or greater at cystectomy. Four patients died of bladder cancer during the median followup of 30 months, none of whom was a complete responder or underwent cystectomy following valrubicin. The main side effects of valrubicin therapy were reversible local bladder symptoms (Steinberg et al. 2000). Valrubicin was effective and well tolerated in patients with carcinoma in situ of the bladder refractory to BCG therapy. Delaying cystectomy while attempting salvage therapy with valrubicin does not pose an undue risk to most patients.

47.10   Cystectomy Post BCG Therapy in Prior Pelvic Radiotherapy Cases

Intravesical Bacillus Calmette-Guerin (BCG) immunotherapy is indicated for high-grade nonmuscle-invasive bladder cancer (NMIBC). The efficacy of BCG in patients with a history of previous pelvic radiotherapy (RT) may be diminished (Rao et al. 2013). Rao evaluated the outcomes of radical cystectomy for

BCG-treated recurrent bladder cancer in patients with a history of RT for prostate cancer (PC). 53 patients underwent radical cystectomy for recurrent NMIBC despite BCG. Those with previous pelvic RT had a higher pathologic stage and decreased recurrence-free survival compared to the groups without prior RT exposure (Rao et al. 2013). Response rates for intravesical BCG therapy may be impaired in those with prior prostate radiotherapy. These cases were pathologically upstaged and more likely to have decreased recurrence-free survival (Rao et al. 2013). Earlier consideration of radical cystectomy may be warranted for those with NMIBC who previously received RT for PC.

47.11   Role of Inteferon or Valrubicin in BCG Refractory Disease

Luciani assessed the risk of continued intravesical therapy and delayed cystectomy in BCG refractory NMIBC. Luciani retrospectively reviewed an experimental intravesical treatment with BCG plus interferon alpha-2b or valrubicin (Luciani et al. 2001). Median follow-up was for 28.5 months (range 6–48). One patient died of unrelated disease. All other patients were alive at last follow-up. Fourteen patients with preserved bladder were continuing cystoscopic surveillance: four had no recurrence, five had recurrence limited to the mucosa (Ta or Tis) and became free of disease after an additional course of intravesical therapy, and five had recurrent Ta or Tis or positive cytologic findings (Luciani et al. 2001). The remaining 9 patients underwent radical cystectomy. All pathologic specimens showed no evidence of progression to muscle-invasive disease. Tis of the resected ureters in 6 and involvement of the prostate in 4 of the 9 patients (three in the urethral ducts and glands and one in the prostatic stroma) were noted (Luciani et al. 2001). A select group of patients with BCG-refractory transitional cell carcinoma and a poor surgical risk for cystectomy may benefit from continued intravesical therapy without a significant risk of progression (Luciani et al. 2001).

Shore et al. (2017) assessed the efficacy and safety of recombinant adenovirus interferon alfa with Syn3 (rAd-IFNα/Syn3), a replication-deficient recombinant adenovirus gene transfer vector, in high-grade (HG) BCG-refractory or relapsed NMIBC (Shore et al. 2017). Forty patients received rAd-IFNα/Syn3 (1×10^{11} vp/mL, n = 21; 3×10^{11} vp/mL, n = 19) between November 5, 2012, and April 8, 2015. Fourteen patients (35.0%; 90% CI, 22.6–49.2%) remained free of HG recurrence 12 months after initial treatment. Comparable 12-month HG RFS was noted for both doses. Of these 14 patients, two experienced recurrence at 21 and 28 months, respectively, after treatment initiation, and one died as a result of an upper tract tumor at 17 months without a recurrence (Shore et al. 2017). rAd-IFNα/Syn3 was well tolerated; no grade four or five adverse events (AEs) occurred, and no patient discontinued treatment because of an adverse event. The most frequently reported drug-related AEs were micturition urgency (n = 16;

40%), dysuria (n = 16; 40%), fatigue (n = 13; 32.5%), pollakiuria (n = 11; 28%), and hematuria and nocturia (n = 10 each; 25%) (Shore et al. 2017). rAd-IFNα/Syn3 was well tolerated. It demonstrated promising efficacy for patients with HG NMIBC after BCG therapy who were unable or unwilling to undergo radical cystectomy.

47.12 Paclitaxel for BCG Refractory CIS

Bassi evaluated the safety profile of paclitaxel-hyaluronic acid bioconjugate given by intravesical instillation to patients with carcinoma in situ refractory to bacillus Calmette-Guérin (Bassi et al. 2011). A total of 11 adverse events were reported by 7 patients and 9 (60%) showed complete treatment response (Bassi et al. 2011). Intravesical instillation of ONCOFID-P-B for carcinoma in situ refractory to bacillus Calmette-Guérin showed minimal toxicity and no systemic absorption in the first human intravesical clinical trial to our knowledge. Finally, satisfactory response rates were observed (Bassi et al. 2011).

47.13 Refractory BCG in NMI Bladder Cancer Interferon and Low Dose BCG

O'Donnell determined whether combining low dose bacillus Calmette-Guerin (BCG) interferon-alpha 2B would be effective for patients in whom previous BCG failed (O'Donnell et al. 2001). At a median followup of 30 months 63% and 53% of patients were disease-free at 12 and 24 months, respectively. Patients in whom 2 or more previous BCG courses had failed fared as well as those with 1 failure. Of the 18 failures 14 occurred at the initial cystoscopy evaluation (O'Donnell et al. 2001). Of 22 patients initially counselled to undergo cystectomy 12 (55%) are disease-free with a functioning bladder. Combination therapy was well tolerated. While longer followup and larger multicenter studies are required to validate these encouraging findings, intravesical low dose BCG plus interferon-alpha 2B appears to be effective in many cases of high risk disease previously deemed BCG refractory (O'Donnell et al. 2001). However, early failure while on this regimen should be aggressively pursued with more radical treatment options.

Gallager et al. (2008) evaluate the effect of the bacille Calmette-Guérin (BCG) failure pattern in patients with non-muscle-invasive bladder cancer on the subsequent response to intravesical immunotherapy (Gallagher et al. 2008). At a median follow-up of 24 months, the BCG-N and BCG-F patients had a cancer-free rate of 59% and 45%, respectively. The BCG-F patients with immediate recurrence (refractory disease), within 6, 6–12, 12–24, and longer than 24 months had a cancer-free rate of 34%, 41%, 43%, 53%, and 66%, respectively ($p = 0.005$ for trend) (Gallagher et al. 2008). No statistically significant difference was found in the cancer-free rates between patients with failure after 12 months and those with failure after 24 months or between BCG-N patients and those with failure after 12 and 24 months. A multivariate analysis of patients with failure after 12 months revealed that the number of previous courses of BCG did not significantly affect the treatment response (Gallagher et al. 2008). Patients with non-muscle-invasive bladder cancer with disease recurrence more than 1 year after BCG treatment and who were treated with low-dose BCG plus interferon-alpha had response rates similar to those of BCG-N patients treated with regular-dose BCG plus interferon (Gallagher et al. 2008). Although cystectomy should still be strongly considered, these patients might benefit from another trial with intravesical immunotherapy.

Belldegrum evaluated the clinical experience with recombinant interferon-alpha (Belldegrum et al. 1998). While bacillus Calmette-Guerin (BCG) is recognized as the most efficacious intravesical agent in the prophylaxis and treatment of NMI transitional cell carcinoma, it is associated with significant toxicities and a 20–40% relapse rate. Interferons, particularly recombinant interferon-alpha, have demonstrated efficacy against primary and recurrent papillary transitional cell carcinoma and carcinoma in situ with minimal toxicity, although the response and relapse rates are inferior to BCG (Belldegrum et al. 1998). Intravesical recombinant interferon-alpha therapy has also produced responses in patients who failed to respond or were refractory to BCG or chemotherapy. This highlights a role as a second line therapy following failure of BCG or chemotherapy.

Sternberg reviewed intravesical gemcitabine for bladder cancer after failed bacillus Calmette-Guérin treatment (Sternberg et al. 2013). Of 69 patients treated with intravesical gemcitabine 37 had bacillus Calmette-Guérin refractory disease. Median followup in progression-free patients was 3.3 years. Progression-free and cancer specific survival were similar in patients with refractory disease and those with other types of bacillus Calmette-Guérin failure (Sternberg et al. 2013). Overall survival was lower in patients with refractory disease (58% vs. 71%) but this was not statistically significant ($p = 0.096$). Of the patients 27 patients experienced a complete response. Progression-free, cancer specific and overall survival did not differ significantly between patients with and without a complete response. Cystectomy was subsequently performed in 20 patients (Sternberg et al. 2013). This paper suggests intravesical gemcitabine should be considered after bacillus Calmette-Guérin failure in patients with bladder cancer who refuse radical cystectomy or who are not candidates for major surgery.

Bacillus Calmette-Guerin (BCG) has shown promise in large scale studies. Karakiewiczk et al. (2006) assessed recurrence-free survival in patients treated with intravesical BCG/Interferon (IFN) (Karakiewicz et al. 2006). Thirteen patients aged from 45 to 81 years (mean: 65) were included. Recurrence was diagnosed in 5 patients (38%). Recurrence free survival (RFS) at 24 months was 66% (Karakiewiczk et al. 2006). When stratified according to T stage prior to BCG/IFN, patients with CIS fared worse than T1 patients (50% vs. 100%). Maintenance had no effect on RFS (75% vs. 69%).

The unpredictable behavior of carcinoma in situ and its high potential for recurrence and progression make identifying patient characteristics predicting a poor prognosis a priority (Rosevear et al. 2011). Roseyear assessed which factors affect the response to bacillus Calmette-Guérin plus interferon-α therapy in patients with urothelial carcinoma in situ. The complete response rate at 3 and 6 months in naïve vs previously failed bacillus Calmette-Guérin cases was 76% and 70% versus 76% and 66%, respectively (Rosevear et al. 2011). The 24-month disease-free rate was decreased in the 53 patients with a history of 2 or more failed bacillus Calmette-Guérin courses versus that in the 71 with a history of 1 failed course and bacillus Calmette-Guérin naïve patients (23% vs. 57% and 60%, respectively). The 22 patients with refractory carcinoma in situ had the worst outcome of a 23% disease-free rate at 24 months while the 59 with relapse within 1 year had an intermediate outcome of 42% versus 59% in the 33 with relapse after 1 year (Rosevear et al. 2011). Patients with a history of papillary disease did better than those without such a history ($p = 0.019$). Factors associated with a poor response to bacillus Calmette-Guérin plus interferon-α therapy in patients with carcinoma in situ are prior tumor stage, 2 or more prior bacillus Calmette-Guérin failures and a bacillus Calmette-Guérin failure pattern.

Bacillus Calmette-Guerin (BCG) has shown promise in large scale studies. Karakiewiczk et al. (2006) assessed recurrence-free survival in patients treated with intravesical BCG/Interferon (IFN) (Karakicwicz et al. 2006). Thirteen patients aged from 45 to 81 years (mean: 65) were included. Stages at TCC diagnosis were distributed as follows: 6 (46%) CIS, 3 (23%) Ta, and 4 (31%) T1. Induction BCG consisted of an average of 11 weekly instillations (range 3–24). Prior to BCG/Interferon stage distribution was as follows: 9 (69%) CIS, and 4 (31%) T1 (Karakiewiczk et al. 2006). BCG/Interferon maintenance was administered to 5 (38%) patients. Follow-up ranged from 1.5 to 32 months (mean = 15, median = 12). Recurrence was diagnosed in 5 patients (38%). Recurrence free survival (RFS) at 24 months was 66% (Karakiewiczk et al. 2006). When stratified according to T stage prior to BCG/IFN, patients with CIS fared worse than T1 patients (50% vs. 100%). Maintenance had no effect on RFS (75% vs. 69%). These results corroborate previous BCG/IFN reports. In selected patients, intravesical BCG/IFN offers a valid alternative to definitive therapy.

47.14   Nanobound Paclitaxel in BCG Refractory Disease

Up to 50% of patients treated with intravesical agents for high grade nonmuscle invasive bladder cancer will have disease recurrence. Response rates to current second line intravesical therapies are low and for these high-risk patients novel agents are necessary (McKiernan et al. 2011). 18 patients were enrolled in the study. One patient demonstrated measurable systemic absorption after 1 infusion (McKiernan et al. 2011). Grade 1 local toxicities were experienced by 10 (56%) patients with dysuria being the most common, and no grade 2, 3 or 4 drug related local toxicities were encountered. Of the 18 patients 5 (28%) had no evidence of disease at post-treatment evaluation. Intravesical nanoparticle albumin-bound paclitaxel exhibited minimal toxicity and systemic absorption in the first human intravesical phase.

Robins reported long-term follow-up results of a phase II trial of salvage intra-vesical nanoparticle albumin-bound (nab)-paclitaxel for patients with recurrent non-muscle-invasive bladder cancer after previous intravesical bacillus Calmette-Guérin (BCG) therapy (Robins et al. 2017). A total of 28 patients were enrolled with a median follow-up of 41 months (range 5–76). There were 22 men and 6 women with a median age of 79 (range 36–93), and the median number of prior intravesical therapies was 2. Twenty-one of the 28 patients (75%) were BCG refractory (Robins et al. 2017). Ten of the 28 patients (36%) achieved complete response. Six of the 28 patients remain cancer free, with a recurrence-free survival rate of 18%. Five-year overall and cancer-specific survival rates were 56% and 91%, respectively. Radical cystectomy occurred in 11 of the 28 patients (39%), of whom 2 out of 11 (18%) had pT2 or greater disease (Robins et al. 2017). With a median follow-up of 41 months, 18% of this cohort treated with nab-paclitaxel was disease free. Cystectomy-free survival was 61% and bladder cancer-specific mortality was 9%. Nab-paclitaxel is a reasonable treatment option in this high-risk population.

47.15 ADT32 in Refractory BCG Cases

Ignatoff assess the safety and effectiveness of AD32, a doxorubicin analogue who have failed prior BCG-based immunotherapy (Ignatoff et al. 2009). The study was halted due to unavailability of study drug after accrual of 48 of a planned 64 patients; 42 were included in the analysis. 28 (67%) were still alive after median follow-up of 61.1 months. Of 21 TCC patients, 18 (85.7%) experienced disease recurrence (median time to recurrence, 5.3 months) (Ignatoff et al. 2009). Of the 5 CIS patients with complete response (CR), 3 (60%) experienced disease recurrence; (median time to recurrence, 37.3 months). Recurrence-free rates at 12 and 24 months were 20% (90% CI, 7.8, 36.1%) and 15% (90 CI, 4.9, 30.2%), respectively, for patients with TCC and 80% (90% CI, 31.4, 95.8%) at both intervals for CIS patients with CR (Ignatoff et al. 2009). Infection was the most common treatment-related toxicity; no grade 4 or higher toxicity was observed. The most common GU-specific toxicity was increased frequency/urgency.

References

Addeo R, Caraglia M, Bellini S, Abbruzzese A, Vincenzi B, Montella L, Miragliuolo A, Guarrasi R, Lanna M, Cennamo G, Faiola V, Del Prete S. Randomized phase III trial on gemcitabine versus mytomicin in recurrent NMI bladder cancer: evaluation of efficacy and tolerance. J Clin Oncol. 2010;28(4):543–8.

Barlow L, McKiernan J, Sawczuk I, Benson M. A single-institution experience with induction and maintenance intravesical docetaxel in the management of non-muscle-invasive bladder cancer refractory to bacille Calmette-Guérin therapy. BJU Int. 2009a;104(8):1098–102.

Barlow LJ, McKiernan JM, Benson MC. The novel use of intravesical docetaxel for the treatment of non-muscle invasive bladder cancer refractory to BCG therapy: a single institution experience. World J Urol. 2009b;27(3):331–5.

Bassi PF, Volpe A, D'Agostino D, Palermo G, Renier D, Franchini S, Rosato A, Racioppi M. Paclitaxel-hyaluronic acid for intravesical therapy of bacillus Calmette-Guérin refractory carcinoma in situ of the bladder: results of a phase I study. J Urol. 2011;185(2):445–9.

Bassi P, De Marco V, Tavolini IM, Longo F, Pinto F, Zucchetti M, Crucitta E, Marini L, Dal Moro F. Pharmacokinetic study of intravesical gemcitabine in carcinoma in situ of the bladder refractory to bacillus Calmette-Guérin therapy. Urol Int. 2005;75(4):309–13.

Belldegrun AS, Franklin JR, O'Donnell MA, Gomella LG, Klein E, Neri R, Nseyo UO, Ratliff TL, Williams RD. NMI bladder cancer: the role of interferon-alpha. J Urol. 1998;159(6):1793–801.

Breyer BN, Whitson JM, Carroll PR, Koncty BR. Sequential intravesical gemcitabine and mitomycin C chemotherapy regimen in patients with non-muscle invasive bladder cancer. Urol Oncol. 2010;28(5):510–4.

Dalbagni G, Benfante N, Sjoberg DD, Bochner BH, Machele Donat S, Herr HW, Mc Coy AS, Fahrner AJ, Retinger C, Rosenberg JE, Bajorin DF. Single arm phase I/II study of everolimus and intravesical gemcitabine in patients with primary or secondary carcinoma in situ of the bladder who failed bacillus Calmette Guerin (NCT01259063). Bladder Cancer. 2017;3(2):113–119.

Dalbagni G, Russo P, Bochner B, Ben-Porat I., Sheinfeld J, Sogani P, Donat MS, Herr HW, Bajorin D. Phase II trial of intravesical gemcitabine in bacille Calmette-Guérin-refractory transitional cell carcinoma of the bladder. J Clin Oncol. 2006;24(18):2729–34.

Gacci M, Bartoletti R, Cai T, Nerozzi S, Pinzi N, Repetti F, Viggiani F, Ghezzi P, Nesi G, Carini M; TUR (Toscana Urologia) Group. Intravesical gemcitabine in BCG-refractory T1G3 transitional cell carcinoma of the bladder: a pilot study. Urol Int. 2006;76(2):106–11.

Gallagher BL, Joudi FN, Maymí JL, O'Donnell MA. Impact of previous bacille Calmette-Guérin failure pattern on subsequent response to bacille Calmette-Guérin plus interferon intravesical therapy. Urology. 2008;71(2):297–301.

Gunelli R, Bercovich E, Nanni O, Ballardini M, Frassineti GL, Giovannini N, Fiori M, Pasquini E, Ulivi P, Pappagallo GL, Silvestrini R, Zoli W. Activity of endovesical gemcitabine in BCG-refractory bladder cancer patients: a translational study. Br J Cancer. 2007;97(11):1499–504.

Ignatoff JM, Chen YH, Greenberg RE, Pow-Sang JM, Messing EM, Wilding G. Phase II study of intravesical therapy with AD32 in patients with papillary urothelial carcinoma or carcinoma in situ (CIS) refractory to prior therapy with bacillus Calmette-Guerin (E3897): a trial of the Eastern Cooperative Oncology Group. Urol Oncol. 2009;27(5):496–501.

Karakiewicz PI, Benayoun S, Lewinshtein DJ, Chun FK, Shahrour K, Perrotte P. Treatment of BCG failures with intravesical BCG/Interferon: the University of Montreal experience. Can J Urol. 2006;13(4):3189–94.

Kowalski M, Entwistle J, Cizeau J, Niforos D, Loewen S, Chapman W, MacDonald GC. A phase I study of an intravesically administered immunotoxin targeting EpCAM for the treatment of nonmuscle-invasive bladder cancer in BCGrefractory and BCG-intolerant patients. Drug Des Devel Ther. 2010;4:313–20.

Luciani LG, Neulander E, Murphy WM, Wajsman Z. Risk of continued intravesical therapy and delayed cystectomy in BCG-refractory NMI bladder cancer: an investigational approach. Urology. 2001;58(3):376–9.

McKiernan JM, Barlow LJ, Laudano MA, Mann MJ, Petrylak DP, Benson MC. A phase I trial of intravesical nanoparticle albumin-bound paclitaxel in the treatment of bacillus Calmette-Guérin refractory nonmuscle invasive bladder cancer. J Urol. 2011;186(2):448–51.

Mohanty NK, Nayak RL, Vasudeva P, Arora RP. Intravesicle gemcitabine in management of BCG refractory NMI TCC of urinary bladder-our experience. Urol Oncol. 2008;26(6):616–9.

Morales A, Herr H, Steinberg G, Given R, Cohen Z, Amrhein J, Kamat AM. Efficacy and safety of MCNA in patients with nonmuscle invasive bladder cancer at high risk for recurrence and progression after failed treatment with bacillus Calmette-Guérin. J Urol. 2015;193(4):1135–43.

O'Donnell MA, Krohn J, DeWolf WC. Salvage intravesical therapy with interferon-alpha 2b plus low dose bacillus Calmette-Guerin is effective in patients with NMI bladder cancer in whom bacillus Calmette-Guerin alone previously failed. J Urol. 2001;166(4):1300–4, discussion 1304–5.

Patel S, Dinh T, Noah-Vanhoucke J, Rengarajan B, Mayo K, Clark PE, Kamat AM, Lee CT, Sexton WJ, Steinberg GD. Novel simulation model of non-muscle invasive bladder cancer: a platform for a virtual randomized trial of conservative therapy vs. Cystectomy in BCG refractory patients. Bladder Cancer. 2015;1(2):143–150.

Perdonà S, Di Lorenzo G, Cantiello F, Damiano R, De Sio M, Masala D, Bruni G, Gallo L, Federico P, Quattrone C, Pizzuti M, Autorino R. Is gemcitabine an option in BCG-refractory nonmuscle-invasive bladder cancer? A single-arm prospective trial. Anticancer Drugs. 2010;21(1):101–6.

Rao MV, Quek ML, Jayram G, Ellimoottil C, Sondej T, Hugen CM, Flanigan RC, Steinberg GD. Radical cystectomy after bcg immunotherapy for high-risk nonmuscle-invasive bladder cancer in patients with previous prostate radiotherapy. ISRN Urol. 2013;2013:405064.

Robins DJ, Sui W, Matulay JT, Ghandour R, Anderson CB, DeCastro GJ, McKiernan JM. Long-term survival outcomes with intravesical nanoparticle albumin-bound paclitaxel for recurrent non-muscle-invasive bladder cancer after previous bacillus calmette-guérin therapy. Urology. 2017;103:149–153.

Rosevear HM, Lightfoot AJ, Birusingh KK, Maymí JL, Nepple KG, O'Donnell MA; National BCG/Interferon Investigator Group. Factors affecting response to bacillus Calmette-Guérin plus interferon for urothelial carcinoma in situ. J Urol. 2011;186(3):817–23.

Shore ND, Boorjian SA, Canter DJ, Ogan K, Karsh LI, Downs TM, Gomella LG, Kamat AM, Lotan Y, Svatek RS, Bivalacqua TJ, Grubb RL 3rd, Krupski TL, Lerner SP, Woods ME, Inman BA, Milowsky MI, Boyd A, Treasure FP, Gregory G, Sawutz DG, Yla-Herttuala S, Parker NR, Dinney CPN. Intravesical rAd-IFNα/Syn3 for patients with high-grade, bacillus Calmette-Guerin-refractory or relapsed non-muscle-invasive bladder cancer: a phase II randomized study. J Clin Oncol. 2017;35(30):3410–3416.

Steinberg G, Bahnson R, Brosman S, Middleton R, Wajsman Z, Wehle M. Efficacy and safety of valrubicin for the treatment of Bacillus Calmette-Guerin refractory carcinoma in situ of the bladder. The Valrubicin Study Group. J Urol. 2000;163(3):761–7.

Steinberg GD, Smith ND, Ryder K, Strangman NM, Slater SJ. Factors affecting valrubicin response in patients with bacillus Calmette-Guérin-refractory bladder carcinoma in situ. Postgrad Med. 2011;123(3):28–34.

Sternberg IA, Dalbagni G, Chen LY, Donat SM, Bochner BH, Herr HW. Intravesical gemcitabine for high risk, nonmuscle invasive bladder cancer after bacillus Calmette-Guérin treatment failure. J Urol. 2013;190(5):1686–91.

Waidelich R, Stepp H, Baumgartner R, Weninger E, Hofstetter A, Kriegmair M. Clinical experience with 5-aminolevulinic acid and photodynamic therapy for refractory NMI bladder cancer. J Urol. 2001;165(6 Pt 1):1904–7.

Wosnitzer MS, Domingo-Domenech J, Castillo-Martin M, Ritch C, Mansukhani M, Petrylack DP, Benson MC, McKiernan JM, Cordon-Cardo C. Predictive value of microtubule associated proteins tau and stathmin in patients with nonmuscle invasive bladder cancer receiving adjuvant intravesical taxane therapy. J Urol. 2011;186(5):2094–100.

Chapter 48
What the Literature Says on BCG Refractory Disease and Alternatives

High-risk non-muscle-invasive bladder cancer (NMIBC) should receive an adjuvant course of intravesical Bacille Calmette-Guerin (BCG) as first-line treatment (Yates and Rouprêt 2011). However, a large amount will have refractory or relapsing disease. Guideline recommendation in the 'refractory' setting is radical cystectomy, however, morbidity, a patient's desire for bladder preservation or reluctance to undergo surgery can mean this does not happen (Yates and Rouprêt 2011). The other options are immunotherapy, chemotherapy, device-assisted therapy and combination therapy (Yates and Rouprêt 2011). However, the current data are still inadequate to formulate definitive recommendations, and data from ongoing trials and maturing studies will give us an insight into whether there is a realistic efficacious second-line treatment for patients who fail intravesical BCG but are not candidates for definitive surgery.

Patients with high-grade muscle invasive bladder cancer (NMIBC) receive intravesical therapy with bacillus Calmette-Guérin (BCG) as the well-established standard-of-care (Velaer et al. 2016). However, 40% will recur within 2 years. For patients who fail BCG, options include radical cystectomy, repeat BCG therapy, or alternative intravesical salvage therapy. Salvage intravesical therapy can involve sequential gemcitabine and docetaxel intravesical therapy. Based on the results of phase I studies, gemcitabine has unremarkable systemic and local side effects (Gontero and Frea 2006). The currently available phase II studies have assessed the activity of intravesical gemcitabine on a marker lesion in intermediate risk NMIBC with complete responses in up to 56%. Unexpected complete responses in BCG refractory CIS were noted with intravesical gemcitabine (Gontero and Frea 2006). Gemcitabine seems to have fulfilled the requirements to be a promising new candidate for standard intravesical therapy in SBC so far.

© Springer Nature Switzerland AG 2020
S. S. Goonewardene et al., *Management of Non-Muscle Invasive Bladder Cancer*,
https://doi.org/10.1007/978-3-030-28646-0_48

References

Gontero P, Frea B. Actual experience and future development of gemcitabine in NMI bladder cancer. Ann Oncol. 2006;17(Suppl. 5):v123–8.

Velaer KN, Steinberg RL, Thomas LJ, O'Donnell MA, Nepple KG. Experience with sequential intravesical gemcitabine and docetaxel as salvage therapy for non-muscle invasive bladder cancer. Curr Urol Rep. 2016;17(5):38.

Yates DR, Rouprêt M. Contemporary management of patients with high-risk non-muscle-invasive bladder cancer who fail intravesical BCG therapy. World J Urol. 2011;29(4):415–22.

Chapter 49
NMIBC—BCG Refractory Disease and Use of Interferon

Thirty to forty percent of patients with high grade nonmuscle invasive bladder cancer (NMIBC) fail to respond to intravesical therapy with bacillus Calmette-Guerin (BCG). Interferon-α2B plus BCG has been shown to be effective in a subset of patients with NMIBC BCG refractory disease (Correa et al. 2015). Correa et al. (2015) reviewed a contemporary series on the effectiveness and safety of intravesical BCG plus interferon-α2B therapy in patients with BCG refractory NMIBC. High risk disease was found in 88.6% of patients at induction. The 12-month and 24-month recurrence-free survival were 38.6% and 18.2%, respectively. 25 (56.8%) ultimately had disease recurrence. Radical cystectomy was performed in 16 (36.4%) patients.

It is advocated that patients with high-risk non-muscle-invasive bladder cancer (NMIBC) receive an adjuvant course of intravesical Bacille Calmette-Guerin (BCG) as first-line treatment (Yates and Rouprêt 2011). However, a substantial proportion of patients will 'fail' BCG, either early with persistent (refractory) disease or recur late after a long disease-free interval (relapsing) (Yates and Rouprêt 2011). Guideline recommendation in the 'refractory' setting is radical cystectomy, but there are situations when extirpative surgery is not feasible due to competing co-morbidity, a patient's desire for bladder preservation or reluctance to undergo surgery. These options can be categorised as immunotherapy, chemotherapy, device-assisted therapy and combination therapy (Yates and Rouprêt 2011). However, data is lacking from trials.

References

Correa AF, Theisen K, Ferroni M, Maranchie JK, Hrebinko R, Davies BJ, Gingrich JR. The role of interferon in the management of BCG refractory nonmuscle invasive bladder cancer. Adv Urol. 2015;2015:656918.
Yates DR, Rouprêt M. Contemporary management of patients with high-risk non-muscle-invasive bladder cancer who fail intravesical BCG therapy. World J Urol. 2011;29(4):415–22.

Chapter 50
Novel Agents in BCG Refractory Disease

50.1 BCG Refractory Disease and Use of Inteferon

BCG refractory disease has noted oncological outcomes (Rosevear et al. 2011) assessed response factors to bacillus Calmette-Guérin plus interferon-α therapy for CIS. The complete response rate at 3 and 6 months in naïve versus previously failed bacillus Calmette-Guérin cases was 76% and 70% versus 76% and 66% (Rosevear et al. 2011). The 24-month disease-free rate was decreased in the 53 patients with a history of 2 or more failed bacillus Calmette-Guérin courses versus that in the 71 with a history of 1 failed course and bacillus Calmette-Guérin naïve patients (23% vs. 57% and 60%, respectively) (Rosevear et al. 2011). The 22 patients with refractory CIS had the worst outcome of a 23% disease-free rate at 24 months. The 59 with relapse at less than 1 year had an intermediate outcome of 42% versus 59% in 33 with relapse after 1 year. Papillary disease did better than those without such a history ($p = 0.019$). Factors associated with a poor response are prior tumor stage, 2 or more prior bacillus Calmette-Guérin failures and a bacillus Calmette-Guérin failure pattern.

50.2 BCG Refractory Disease and Use of MCNA

Due to an aging population, and a cohort which may not be fit for radical cystectomy novel agents are required (Morales and Cohen 2016). A cell wall-nucleic acid complex (MCNA) from M. phlei has been investigated for possible application in patients with BCG refractory NMIBC. MCNA has shown activity against high risk BCG refractory bladder cancer and offers an alternative to current treatments. The clinical experience remains limited and the optimal therapeutic regimen (dose, frequency) have not been firmly established (Morales and Cohen 2016).

© Springer Nature Switzerland AG 2020
S. S. Goonewardene et al., *Management of Non-Muscle Invasive Bladder Cancer*,
https://doi.org/10.1007/978-3-030-28646-0_50

Patients and clinicians would welcome the introduction of a compound that may delay or prevent the risks and negative impact in quality of life of cystectomy and urinary diversion.

50.3   BCG Refractory Disease and Immunotoxin

Kowalski examined a Phase I study on immunotoxin VB4-845 in nonmuscle-invasive bladder cancer (NMIBC) refractory to or intolerant of bacillus Calmette-Guerin (BCG) (Kolwalski et al. 2010). Sixty-four patients were enrolled. VB4-845 therapy was safe and well tolerated with most adverse events reported as mild; as a result, no patients were removed from the study in response to toxicity (Morales and Cohen 2016). By the end of the study, the majority had developed antibodies to the exotoxin portion of VB4-845. A complete response was achieved in 39% of patients at the 12-week time point (Morales and Cohen 2016). VB4-845 dosed on a weekly basis for 6 weeks was very well tolerated at all dose levels (Morales and Cohen 2016). Although an MTD was not determined at the doses administered, VB4-845 showed evidence of an antitumor effect that warrants further clinical investigation for the treatment of NMIBC in this patient population.

BCG is a good treatment for NMIBC. However, 30–40% of tumors are refractory (Punnen et al. 2003). BCG failure is an indication for cystectomy yet there are salvage intravesical (IVe) strategies. At 12 months after induction salvage BCG/IFN-a, 6 of the 12 (50%) were tumor free. Of the six recurrences, 3(50%) did not respond to the IVe therapy and had residual/recurrent tumor at the first follow-up visit. The combinative therapy was well tolerated with minimal toxicity compared to previous full dose BCG.

50.4   BCG Refractory Disease and Immunotherapy

CIS refractory to BCG can is usually treated with BCG (Autenrieth et al. 2018). Autenrieth et al. (2018) examined a novel targeted alpha-emitter immunotherapy for CIS after BCG (Autenrieth et al. 2018). This demonstrated intravesical instillation of the ^{213}Bi-immunoconjugate targeting EGFR is feasible. No adverse effects were observed and all blood and urine parameters determined remained in their normal ranges. Therapeutic efficacy was considered satisfactory, in that three of the 12 patients showed no signs of CIS 44, 30 and 3 months after treatment (Autenrieth et al. 2018). This demonstrates intravesical instillation of ^{213}Bi-anti-EGFR monoclonal antibody was well tolerated and showed therapeutic efficacy (Autenrieth et al. 2018). Repeated instillation and/or instillation of higher activities of the ^{213}Bi-immunoconjugate might lead to better therapeutic outcomes, however further studies are needed.

50.5 Immunotherapy for BCG Refractory Disease

Until recently, there were very limited options for patients who are refractory to chemotherapy, or do not tolerate chemotherapy due to toxicities and overall outcomes have remained very poor (Gupta et al. 2017). While the role of immunotherapy was first established in non-muscle invasive bladder cancer, no systemic immunotherapy was approved for advanced disease until the recent approval of a programmed death ligand-1 (PD-L1) inhibitor, atezolizumab, in patients with advanced/metastatic UC who have progressed on platinum-containing regimens (Gupta et al. 2017).

The introduction of novel immunotherapy agents has led to rapid changes in the field of urothelial carcinoma. Numerous checkpoint inhibitors are being tested alone or in combination in the first and subsequent-line therapies of metastatic disease, as well as neoadjuvant and adjuvant settings. They are also being studied in combination with radiation therapy and for non-muscle invasive bladder cancer refractory to BCG. Furthermore, immunotherapy is being utilized for those ineligible for firstline platinum-based chemotherapy. This review outlines the novel immunotherapy agents which have either been approved or are currently being investigated in clinical trials in UC.

50.6 BCG Refractory Disease and Nanoparticle Albumin Bound Paclitaxel

Up to 50% of patients treated with intravesical agents for high grade nonmuscle invasive bladder cancer will have disease recurrence (McKiernan et al. 2011). Nanoparticle albumin-bound paclitaxel (Abraxane®, ABI-007) has been shown to have increased solubility and lower toxicity compared to docetaxel in systemic therapy (McKiernan et al. 2011). A total of 18 patients were enrolled (McKiernan et al. 2011). One patient demonstrated measurable systemic absorption after 1 infusion. Grade 1 local toxicities were experienced by 10 (56%) patients with dysuria being the most common, and no grade 2, 3 or 4 drug related local toxicities were encountered. Of the 18 patients 5 (28%) had no evidence of disease at posttreatment evaluation (McKiernan et al. 2011). Intravesical nanoparticle albumin-bound paclitaxel exhibited minimal toxicity and systemic absorption in the first human intravesical phase I trial to our knowledge. A larger phase II study has begun to formally evaluate the activity of this regimen.

50.7 Strategies to Enhance Intravesical Chemotherapy in BCG Refractory Disease

BCG Refractory recurrence occurs. When it does, the cancer is a lot more aggressive. Clinical trial evidence demonstrating the efficacy of BCG plus interferon 2B, gemcitabine and anthracyclines (doxorubicin, epirubicin, valrubicin) in refractory or BCG is accumulating (Smaldone et al. 2009). Phase I trials investigating alternative agents such as apaziquone, taxanes (docetaxel, paclitaxel), and suramin are reporting promising data (Smaldone et al. 2009). Current efforts are also being directed towards optimizing the administration of existing chemotherapeutic regimens, including the use of novel modalities including hyperthermia, photodynamic therapy, magnetically targeted carriers, and liposomes (Smaldone et al. 2009). Despite recent enthusiasm for new intravesical agents, radical cystectomy remains the treatment of choice for patients with NMIBC who have failed intravesical therapy and select patients with naive T1 tumors and aggressive features.

50.8 Use of Dócetaxe; in BCG Refractory Disease

Barlow examined the safety and efficacy of intravesical docetaxel in a larger patient population with extended follow-up in BCG refractory disease (Barlow et al. 2009).

Thirty-three patients with refractory NMIBC received salvage intravesical docetaxel therapy (Barlow et al. 2009). Twenty of thirty-three (61%) patients had a complete response (CR) after six weekly induction treatments. Ten patients with a complete response were given maintenance docetaxel therapy, and one patient received maintenance BCG and interferon. With a median follow-up of 29 months, 1 and 2-year recurrence-free survival rates were and 45 and 32%, respectively. Twelve of thirty-three patients (36%) had Grade 1 or 2 local toxicities. No patients experienced Grade 3 or 4 toxicities (Barlow et al. 2009). Docetaxel is a promising intravesical agent with minimal toxicity and significant efficacy and durability for the management of BCG-refractory NMIBC.

References

Autenrieth ME, Seidl C, Bruchertseifer F, Horn T, Kurtz F, Feuerecker B, D'Alessandria C, Pfob C, Nekolla S, Apostolidis C, Mirzadeh S, Gschwend JE, Schwaiger M, Scheidhauer K, Morgenstern A. Treatment of carcinoma in situ of the urinary bladder with an alpha-emitter immunoconjugate targeting the epidermal growth factor receptor: a pilot study. Eur J Nucl Med Mol Imaging. 2018;45(8):1364–71.
Barlow LJ, McKiernan JM, Benson MC. The novel use of intravesical docetaxel for the treatment of non-muscle invasive bladder cancer refractory to BCG therapy: a single institution experience. World J Urol. 2009;27(3):331–5.

Gupta S, Gill D, Poole A, Agarwal N. Systemic immunotherapy for urothelial cancer: current trends and future directions. Cancers (Basel). 2017;9(2).

Kowalski M, Entwistle J, Cizeau J, Niforos D, Loewen S, Chapman W, MacDonald GC. A Phase I study of an intravesically administered immunotoxin targeting EpCAM for the treatment of nonmuscle-invasive bladder cancer in BCGrefractory and BCG-intolerant patients. Drug Des Devel Ther. 2010;15(4):313–20.

McKiernan JM, Barlow LJ, Laudano MA, Mann MJ, Petrylak DP, Benson MC. A phase I trial of intravesical nanoparticle albumin-bound paclitaxel in the treatment of bacillus Calmette-Guérin refractory nonmuscle invasive bladder cancer. J Urol. 2011;186(2):448–51.

Morales A, Cohen Z. Mycobacterium phlei cell wall-nucleic acid complex in the treatment of nonmuscle invasive bladder cancer unresponsive to bacillus Calmette-Guerin. Expert Opin Biol Ther. 2016;16(2):273–83.

Punnen SP, Chin JL, Jewett MA. Management of bacillus Calmette-Guerin (BCG) refractory NMI bladder cancer: results with intravesical BCG and Interferon combination therapy. Can J Urol. 2003;10(2):1790–5.

Rosevear HM, Lightfoot AJ, Birusingh KK, Maymí JL, Nepple KG, O'Donnell MA; National BCG/Interferon Investigator Group. Factors affecting response to bacillus Calmette-Guérin plus interferon for urothelial carcinoma in situ. J Urol. 2011;186(3):817–23.

Smaldone MC, Gayed BA, Tomaszewski JJ, Gingrich JR. Strategies to enhance the efficacy of intravescical therapy for non-muscle invasive bladder cancer. Minerva Urol Nefrol. 2009;61(2):71–89.

Chapter 51
A Scoring System for Intravesical Therapy and NMIBC

An accurate prediction of progression is critically important in the management of non-muscle-invasive bladder cancer ~(Fujii 2018). At present, three risk models are widely known for prediction of the risk of tumor recurrence and progression of non-muscle-invasive bladder cancer: the European Organization for Research and Treatment of Cancer, Club Urológico Español de Tratamiento Oncológico, and new European Organization for Research and Treatment of Cancer models (2018).

Ofude et al. (2015) investigated whether the European Organization for Research and Treatment of Cancer (EORTC) scoring system is appropriate for selection of adjuvant intravesical therapies for non-muscle-invasive bladder cancer (NMIBC) (Ofude et al. 2015). Tumor number, size, and grade were significant predictors of time to recurrence. In groups with intermediate recurrence the recurrence prevention effects in those with an EORTC score of ≥5 were significantly greater with intravesical Bacillus Calmette-Guérin therapy than with weekly intravesical chemotherapy (Ofude et al. 2015).

References

Fujii Y. Prediction models for progression of non-muscle-invasive bladder cancer: a review. Int J Urol. 2018;25(3):212–8.
Ofude M, Kitagawa Y, Yaegashi H, Izumi K, Ueno S, Kadono Y, Konaka H, Mizokami A, Namiki M. Selection of adjuvant intravesical therapies using the European organization for research and treatment of cancer scoring system in patients at intermediate risk of non-muscle-invasive bladder cancer. J Cancer Res Clin Oncol. 2015;141(1):161–8.

© Springer Nature Switzerland AG 2020
S. S. Goonewardene et al., *Management of Non-Muscle Invasive Bladder Cancer*,
https://doi.org/10.1007/978-3-030-28646-0_51

Chapter 52
High Risk NMIBC and TURBT

Risk stratification is important for management of transitional cell carcinoma (TCC) of the bladder (Amin et al. 2013). When stratified as high risk bladder cancer, transurethral resection (TUR) is the gold standard for initial diagnosis and treatment of non muscle invasive bladder cancer (NMIBC) (Kamat et al. 2013). Inorder to correctly stage the tumour, detrusor muscle must be present in the pathological specimen. When muscle is not present, the tumor has to be staged as Tx.

A second TUR done after two six weeks of the first resection reduces the rate of tumor left behind and improves staging. This is key to EAU guidelines on muscle invasive bladder cancer. It also allows the bladder to be cleared prior to definitive therapy such as BCG or if fit radical cystectomy or radical radiotherapy.

Non-muscle invasive urothelial carcinoma is a heterogeneous disease that requires the practicing urologist to implement a variety of surgical and non-surgical treatment strategies (Pagano et al. 2014). The disease course can range from recurrent low-grade papillary disease to aggressive disease concerning for progression from initial presentation (Pagano et al. 2014). As per tailor made patient care, treatments similarly span the range from minimally invasive resection to immediate radical cystectomy (Pagano et al. 2014).

For most patients some form of intravesical therapy will bridge the gap between transurethral resections (TUR) and radical surgery (Pagano et al. 2014). Recent advances in the field continue to emphasize the importance of quality TUR and its strong impact on outcomes (Pagano et al. 2014). In addition, continued research to optimize intravesical therapies has provided more information about how, when, and in whom these agents should be utilized to enhance their efficacy.

If a patient is fit for surgery, with high risk disease immediate radical cystectomy should be considered for high grade, multiple T1 tumors, T1 tumors located at a site difficult to resect, residual T1 tumors after resection or high grade tumors with CIS and lymphovascular invasion.

© Springer Nature Switzerland AG 2020
S. S. Goonewardene et al., *Management of Non-Muscle Invasive Bladder Cancer*,
https://doi.org/10.1007/978-3-030-28646-0_52

The treatment of high-risk non muscle-invasive bladder cancer (NMIBC) is difficult given its unpredictable natural history and patient comorbidities. Because current case series are mostly limited in size, the Thomas et al. (2012) report the outcomes from a large, single-center series. Progression to muscle invasion occurred in 110 patients (15.8%; 95% confidence interval [CI], 13–18.3%) at a median of 17.2 months (interquartile range, 8.9–35.8 months), including 26.5% (95% CI, 22.2–31.3%) of the 366 patients who had >5 years follow-up. This paper demonstrated, within a program of conservative treatment, progression of high-risk NMIBC was associated with a poor prognosis. Surveillance and bacillus Calmette-Guerin were ineffective in altering the natural history of this disease.

References

Amin MB, McKenney JK, Paner GP, Hansel DE, Grignon DJ, Montironi R, Lin O, et al. Icud-Eau international consultation on bladder cancer 2012: pathology. Eur Urol. 2013;63(1):16–35.

Kamat AM, Hegarty PK, Gee JR, Clark PE, Svatek RS, Hegarty N, Shariat SF, et al. Icud-Eau international consultation on bladder cancer 2012: screening, diagnosis, and molecular markers. Eur Urol. 2013;63(1):4–15.

Pagano MJ, Badalato G, McKiernan JM. Optimal treatment of non-muscle invasive urothelial carcinoma including perioperative management revisited. Curr Urol Rep. 2014;15(11):450.

Thomas F, Rosario DJ, Rubin N, Goepel JR, Abbod MF, Catto JW. The long-term outcome of treated high-risk nonmuscle-invasive bladder cancer: time to change treatment paradigm? Cancer. 2012;118(22):5525–34.

Chapter 53
G3T1 Bladder Cancer: Cystectomy Versus BCG

Although both radical cystectomy and intravesical immunotherapy are initial treatment options for high-risk, T1, grade 3 (T1G3) bladder cancer, controversy regarding the optimal strategy persists (Kulkarni et al. 2009). Immediate cystectomy was the dominant (more effective and less expensive) therapy for patients aged <60 years, whereas BCG therapy was dominant for patients aged >75 years (Kulkarni et al. 2009). With increasing comorbidity, BCG therapy was dominant at lower age thresholds. Compared with BCG therapy, immediate radical cystectomy for average patients with high-risk, T1G3 bladder cancer yielded better health outcomes and lower costs (Kulkarni et al. 2009). Tailoring therapy based on patient age and comorbidity may increase survival while yielding significant cost-savings for the healthcare system (Kulkarni et al. 2009).

Lida et al. reported on the long-term clinical outcome of high-grade (G3) non-muscle-invasive bladder cancer (NMIBC) patients treated at a single institution. RC provides excellent survival rates in patients with high-grade NMIBC (Lida et al. 2009). Adjuvant therapy with BCG after a complete TUR of the bladder may be an effective treatment for high-grade NMIBC (Lida et al. 2009). If a conservative treatment is preferred to RC, co-existence of a concomitant CIS should be considered with caution.

Clarke et al. (2006) assessed the use of mitomycin C, by urologists within the UK, as a single-dose intravesical agent (Clarke et al. 2006). Maintenance treatment with mitomycin C was advocated by 44 (15%) of respondents, mainly for recurrent multifocal Ta/T1 tumours (Clarke et al. 2006). The perception of the side-effects of mitomycin C was favourable, with 69% of respondents judging mitomycin C to be well tolerated with mild side-effects (Clarke et al. 2006). Urologists adopt new ideas rapidly, as shown by the wide acceptance of the UK Medical Research Council study. The prompt use of mitomycin C needs to be reinforced, as efficacy is optimum within 6 h of resection (Clarke et al. 2006).

Immunotherapy with Bacillus Calmette Guerin (BCG) has been widely used recently as primary option for treatment of high grade NMI (G3T1) carcinoma of

© Springer Nature Switzerland AG 2020

S. S. Goonewardene et al., *Management of Non-Muscle Invasive Bladder Cancer*,
https://doi.org/10.1007/978-3-030-28646-0_53

the bladder. Pansodoro examined long term experience of therapy of G3T1 bladder cancer (Pansadoro et al. 2003). Of these patients, 12 (14%) had progression at a median follow-up of 16 months (range 8–58 months). Cystectomy was needed in 8 (9%) patients. Death due to disease occurred in 5/86 (6%) patients (Pansadoro et al. 2003). One patient died due to adenocarcinoma at the ureterosigmoidostomy site. Sixty-four (74%) patients are alive at a median follow-up of 71 months (range 28-197 months). Sixty patients (70%) are alive with an intact bladder (Pansadoro et al. 2003). Treatment with BCG is a feasible conservative therapy for patients with primary G3T1 transitional bladder cancer. Long term results of BCG treatment are excellent (Pansadoro et al. 2003). Cystectomy shouldn't be considered first line treatment for high grade NMI carcinoma of the bladder.

Immunotherapy with bacille Calmette-Guérin (BCG) has been proposed in the past decade as first-line treatment for high-grade NMI bladder cancer (G3T1). Pansadoro et al. (2002) reported an 18-year experience in the treatment of patients with G3T1 bladder cancer. Cystectomy was required in 7 patients (8%) (Pansodoro et al. 2002). Death from disease occurred in 5 (6%) of 81 patients. One patient died of adenocarcinoma at the ureterosigmoidostomy site. Sixty patients (74%) were alive at a median follow-up of 79+months (range 15–182) (Pansodoro et al. 2002). Of these, 56 (69%) were alive with a functioning bladder. Conservative treatment with BCG is a reasonable approach for patients with primary G3T1 transitional cell carcinoma of the bladder (Pansodoro et al. 2002). The long-term results of BCG therapy are good. Cystectomy may not be justified as the therapy of choice in first-line treatment of high-grade NMI carcinoma of the bladder (Pansodoro et al. 2002).

Pieras Ayala et al. evaluated outcomes after TUR in patients with G3T1 transitional carcinoma treated with BCG (Pieras Ayala et al. 2001). Cystoscopy performed at 3 months is very useful since it detected 61% of the NMI recurrences and 66% of the cases with progression to muscle invasion during the first 6 months (Pieras Ayala et al. 2001). Routine biopsy of erythematous areas detected during cystoscopy is of little value since a large number of these biopsies are unnecessary in view of its diagnostic yield (5%) (Pieras Ayala et al. 2001). Since 90% of the Cis detected during the first 6 months of follow-up were patients with Cis in the initial tumor, it would be appropriate to perform standard multiple biopsy for control only in this subgroup of patients if the sensitivity of cytology is low in high grade tumors or Cis (Pieras Ayala et al. 2001).

Cookson et al., reported the results of 15 years of followup of high risk patients treated initially with aggressive local therapy, including transurethral resection alone or combined with intravesical bacillus Calmette-Guerin (Cookson et al. 1997). Disease stage progressed in 46 patients (53%) and 31 (36%) eventually underwent cystectomy for progression (28) or refractory carcinoma in situ (3), while 18 (21%) had upper tract tumors at a median of 7.3 years (Cookson et al. 1997). The 10 and 15-year disease specific survival rates were 70 and 63%, respectively. At 15 years 34% of patients overall were dead of bladder cancer, 27% were dead of other causes and 37% were alive, including 27% with an intact functioning bladder (Cookson et al. 1997). Despite aggressive local therapy patients with high risk NMI bladder cancer are at lifelong risk for development of stage progression and upper tract tumors (Cookson et al. 1997). A third of patients are at risk for death from bladder cancer, justifying careful and vigilant long-term followup. These results support the use of initial aggressive local therapy in patients with high risk NMI bladder cancer.

References

Clarke NS, Basu S, Prescott S, Puri R. Chemo-prevention in NMI bladder cancer using mitomy-cin C: a survey of the practice patterns of British urologists. BJU Int. 2006;97(4):716–9.

Cookson MS, Herr HW, Zhang ZF, Soloway S, Sogani PC, Fair WR. The treated natural history of high risk NMI bladder cancer: 15-year outcome. J Urol. 1997;158(1):62–7.

Kulkarni GS, Alibhai SM, Finelli A, Fleshner NE, Jewett MA, Lopushinsky SR, Bayoumi AM. Cost-effectiveness analysis of immediate radical cystectomy versus intravesical Bacillus Calmette-Guerin therapy for high-risk, high-grade (T1G3) bladder cancer. Cancer. 2009;115(23):5450–9.

Lida S, Kondo T, Kobayashi H, Hashimoto Y, Goya N, Tanabe K. Clinical outcome of high-grade non-muscle-invasive bladder cancer: a long-term single center experience. Int J Urol. 2009;16(3):287–92.

Pansadoro V, Emiliozzi P, depaula F, Scarpone P, Pizzo M, Federico G, Martini M, Pansadoro A, Sternberg CN. High grade NMI (G3t1) transitional cell carcinoma of the bladder treated with intravesical Bacillus Calmette-Guerin (BCG). J Exp Clin Cancer Res. 2003;22(4 Suppl):223–7.

Pansadoro V, Emiliozzi P, de Paula F, Scarpone P, Pansadoro A, Sternberg CN. Long-term follow up of G3T1 transitional cell carcinoma of the bladder treated with intravesical bacille Calmette-Guérin: 18 year experience. Urology. 2002;59(2):227–31.

Pieras Ayala E, Palou J, Rodríguez-Villamil L, Millán Rodríguez F, Salvador Bayarri J, Vicente Rodríguez J. Cytoscopic follow-up of initial G3T1 bladder tumors treated with BCG. Arch Esp Urol. 2001;54(3):211–7.

Chapter 54
A Systematic Review of High-Grade Bladder Cancer—Methods

A systematic review relating to management of high-grade bladder cancer was conducted. The search strategy aimed to identify all references related to bladder cancer AND high-grade disease management. Search terms used were as follows: (Bladder cancer) AND (high grade) AND (Management) The following databases were screened from 1989 to June 2019:

- CINAHL
- MEDLINE (NHS Evidence)
- Cochrane
- AMed
- EMBASE
- PsychINFO
- SCOPUS
- Web of Science

In addition, searches using Medical Subject Headings (MeSH) and keywords were conducted using Cochrane databases. Two UK-based experts in bladder cancer were consulted to identify any additional studies.

Studies were eligible for inclusion if they reported primary research focusing on bladder cancer and screening. Papers were included if published after 1984 and had to be in English. Studies that did not conform to this were excluded. Only primary research was included. The overall aim was to identify the role and components of bladder cancer screening.

Abstracts were independently screened for eligibility by two reviewers and disagreements resolved through discussion or third-party opinion (Fig. 54.1). Agreement level was calculated using Cohen's Kappa to test the intercoder reliability of this screening process. Cohen's Kappa allows comparison of inter-rater reliability between papers using relative observed agreement. This also takes account of the comparison occurring by chance. The first reviewer agreed all 18 papers to be included, the second, agreed on 18.

© Springer Nature Switzerland AG 2020   269
S. S. Goonewardene et al., *Management of Non-Muscle Invasive Bladder Cancer*,
https://doi.org/10.1007/978-3-030-28646-0_54

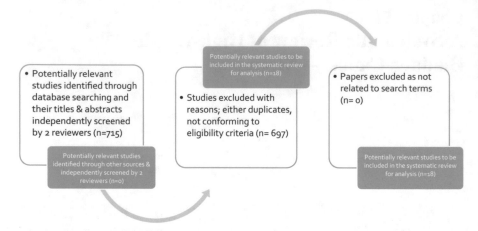

Fig. 54.1 Flow chart of studies identified through the systematic review (adapted from PRISMA)

Data extraction was piloted by the researcher and amended in consultation with the research team (author and two academic supervisors). Data collected included authors, year and country of publication, study aims, setting, intervention aims, number of participants, study design, intervention components and delivery methods, comparison groups and outcome measures, notes and follow-up questions for the authors. Studies were quality assessed using the PRISMA criteria for randomised controlled trials, Mays et al. (Moher et al. 2009; Moher, Liberati et al. 2009, 154, 153; Mays et al. 2005) for the action research and qualitative studies and the Critical Skills Appraisal programme for cohort studies. This was also applied to randomised controlled trials and qualitative studies. There was one RCT and the rest were cohort studies.

References

Mays N, Pope C, Popay J. Systematically reviewing qualitative and quantitative evidence to inform management and policy-making in the health field. J Health Serv Res Policy. 2005;10(Suppl. 1):6–20.

Moher D, Liberati A, Tetzlaff J, Altman DG. Preferred reporting items for systematic reviews and meta-analyses: the prisma statement. BMJ (Online). 2009;339(7716):332–36.

Chapter 55
Systematic Review of G3T1 Bladder Cancer

55.1 Conservative Management in High Grade Bladder Cancer

The treatment of high-risk NMIBC is difficult given its variable pathology (Thomas et al. 2012). Thomas reported outcomes from a large, single-center series. 712 patients (median age, 73.7 years) were included. Progression to muscle invasion occurred in 110 patients (15.8%) with a median follow-up of 17.2 months including 26.5% of the 366 patients who had >5 years follow-up (Thomas et al. 2012). Progression was associated with age, dysplastic urothelium, urothelial cell carcinoma variants and recurrence ($p < 0.001$). Disease-specific mortality occurred in 134 (18.8%). Neither progression nor disease-specific mortality were associated with BCG ($p > 0.6$). Within a program of conservative treatment, progression of high-risk NMIBC was associated with a poor prognosis (Thomas et al. 2012). Surveillance and bacillus Calmette-Guerin were ineffective in altering the natural history of this disease.

55.2 Intravenous Chemotherapy Versus Intravesical Chemotherapy

The management of T1G3 bladder cancer is controversial (Zhang et al. 2016). Zhang compared intravenous chemotherapy and intravesical chemotherapy versus intravesical chemotherapy alone for T1G3 bladder cancer after TURBT (Zhang et al. 2016). The recurrence rate was 36.7% for intravesical chemotherapy alone, compared with 19.9% for combination therapy ($p < 0.001$) (Zhang et al. 2016). The progression rate was 10.6% for intravesical chemotherapy alone and 2.3% for combined chemotherapy ($p = 0.003$). Kaplan-Meier curves showed significant differences in

© Springer Nature Switzerland AG 2020
S. S. Goonewardene et al., *Management of Non-Muscle Invasive Bladder Cancer*,
https://doi.org/10.1007/978-3-030-28646-0_55

recurrence-free survival and progression-free survival between the two treatment strategies, with a log-rank p-value of <0.001 and 0.003, respectively (Zhang et al. 2016). Multivariable analyses revealed that intravenous chemotherapy was the independent prognostic factor for tumor recurrence and progression in the cohort.

55.3   Chemotherapy in Elderly Patients

Although maintenance bacillus Calmette-Guérin (BCG) is the gold standard in high-risk non-muscle-invasive bladder cancer (NMIBC), its efficacy in older patients is controversial. Oddens studied the impact of age on prognosis and treatment in Ta T1 NMIBC (Oddens et al. 2014). 546 had BCG with or without INH arms and 276 in the epirubicin arm. In BCG with or without INH, 34.1% were >70 yr of age and 3.7% were >80 (Oddens et al. 2014). With a median follow-up of 9.2 yr, patients >70 yr had a shorter time to progression ($p = 0.028$), overall survival ($p < 0.001$), and NMIBC-specific survival ($p = 0.049$). The time to recurrence was similar compared with the younger patients. BCG was more effective than epirubicin for all four end points, and there was no evidence that BCG was any less effective compared with epirubicin in patients >70 yr (Oddens et al. 2014). In intermediate- and high-risk Ta T1 Urothelial cell carcinomapatients treated with BCG, patients >70 yr of age have a worse long-term prognosis; however, BCG is more effective than epirubicin independent of patient age.

55.4   Novel Chemotherapy for High Grade T1 Disease

Management of high-grade G3T1 bladder cancer continues to be controversial (Yang et al. 2017). Gemcitabine and cisplatin (GC) adjuvant chemotherapy may offer a third path between intravesical therapy and early cystectomy. Yang et al. (2017) assessed outcomes of GC adjuvant chemotherapy in T1G3 bladder cancer after transurethral resection of bladder tumor (TURBT) (Yang et al. 2017). Complete response was achieved in 44 (91.7%). Of these, 5 patients experienced recurrence and 5 patients showed progression. The progression rate and disease-specific survival rate were 10.4 and 91.7% at 3 years, respectively. More than 80% of survivors preserved their bladder (Yang et al. 2017). Kaplan-Meier curves showed that concomitant carcinoma in situ (CIS) was the only factor that had an influence on progression-free survival ($p = 0.022$) and disease-specific survival ($p = 0.017$). Concomitant CIS was the prognostic factor for progression rate and disease-specific survival rate at 3 years ($p = 0.008$ and $p = 0.035$) (Yang et al. 2017). GC adjuvant chemotherapy is a safe conservative treatment for T1G3 bladder cancer, but effective is really a phase II study. Patients with T1G3 bladder cancer with concomitant CIS should be treated more aggressively because of the high risk of progression.

55.5 Surveillance for T1G3 Disease

Páez Borda et al. (2001), examined outcomes in surveillance for primary T1G3 bladder cancer (Páez Borda et al. 2001). Thirty-two patients were allocated into a surveillance program. Risk factors for progression to muscle-invasive disease were determined. Five patients (15.6%) were lost in follow-up (Páez Borda et al. 2001). Twenty-three (85%) had NMI recurrences. Four patients (14.8%) progressed to muscle-invasive or metastatic disease. Median disease-free survival was 8 months. Projection of the risk of recurrence at 79 months was 84.9%. Projection of progression at 79 months was 46.3% (Páez Borda et al. 2001). This treatment has very high recurrence rates. In addition, recurrences are very frequent. However, projections of progression suggest that surveillance can be an alternative to other treatments in the management of T1G3 TCC of the bladder.

55.6 Complications of Cystectomy for High Grade Bladder Cancer

Cystectomy has a high morbidity and mortality rate (Jerlström et al. 2014). Jerlström conducted a population-based study with prospective collation of data until 90 days after cystectomy (Jerlström et al. 2014). During 2011, 285 (65%) of 435 cystectomies performed in Sweden were registered in the database, the majority reported by the seven academic centres. Median blood loss was 1000 ml, operating time 318 min, and length of hospital stay 15 days. Any complications were registered for 103 patients (36%) (Jerlström et al. 2014). Clavien grades 1–2 and 3–5 were noted in 19% and 15%, respectively. Thirty-seven patients (13%) were reoperated on at least once. There are a risk of complications in patients with longer operating time and higher age (Jerlström et al. 2014). The results agree with some previously published series but should be interpreted with caution considering the relatively low coverage, which is expected to be higher in the future.

55.7 Management of G3T1-TURBT Versus BCG Versus Cystectomy

Lida et al. (2009) reported on epirubicine versus BCG versus cystectomy (Lida et al. 2009). Forty-seven patients received adjuvant intravesical epirubicine after TUR of the bladder (Group 1) (Lida et al. 2009). Twenty-four patients received intravesical bacillus Calmette-Guérin (BCG) (Group 2). A radical cystectomy (RC) was performed on twenty-two patients (Group 3). Median follow up was 68.7 months. Overall, thirty patients (33%) experienced tumor recurrence. The survival rates of Group 3 were significantly higher than the 71 patients undergoing conservative therapy (Group 1 and 2). Treatment failure with epirubicine was significantly higher than with BCG. Cases without concomitant carcinoma in situ (CIS) showed statistically significantly higher survival rates than with concomitant CIS. RC provides excellent survival rates in patients with high-grade NMIBC. Adjuvant therapy with BCG after a complete TUR of the bladder may be an effective treatment for high-grade NMIBC. If a conservative treat.

55.8   Immediate Cystectomy and Age-Related Outcomes in G3T1 Disease

Controversy exists about treatment for high-risk NMI (stage T1; grade G3) bladder cancer (Kulkarni et al. 2007). Immediate cystectomy offers a good chance of survival but can affect quality of life compared with conservative therapy. Kulkarni estimated life expectancy and quality-adjusted life expectancy for both (Kulkarni et al. 2007). This highlights younger patients with high-risk T1G3 bladder have a higher life expectancy and quality adjusted life expectancy with immediate cystectomy (Kulkarni et al. 2007). The decision to pursue immediate cystectomy should review patient age, comorbid status, and patient preference (Kulkarni et al. 2007). Patients over the age of 70y or patients with a strong emphasis on sexual function, gastrointestinal, or bladder function may benefit from a more conservative initial therapeutic approach.

Badalato determined whether a survival difference exists in highgrade T1 having immediate radical cystectomy (IRC) or bladder-sparing therapy (Badalato et al. 2012). 113 underwent IRC and 236 had CM. From 1990 to 1999, only 90 patients were diagnosed with HG cT1 disease, and a majority of patients ($n = 54$) underwent IRC. From 2000 to 2010, only 23% (59/259) of the patients with HG cT1 underwent IRC (Badalato et al. 2012). Despite 42.3% more patients successfully maintaining their bladder in the long-term, no difference in 5-year bladder CSS was noted between decades (77% vs. 80% consecutively, $p = 0.566$). A subset analysis of risk factors for bladder cancer progression/recurrence demonstrated more patients with lymphovascular invasion (LVI) on TUR underwent IRC in the current era (13/59 (22.0%) vs. 13/200 (6.5%), $p < 0.001$) (Badalato et al. 2012). These findings remain to be validated in prospective work at other institutions. Conservative management strategies are a viable treatment option within a well selected subset of patients with HG cT1 UCC.

T1 high-grade (formerly T1G3) bladder cancer is a difficult problem (Boström et al. 2010). The option of radical cystectomy should be discussed with patients with restaging TUR stage T1 or higher and it is highly recommended to all patients with recurrent T1 of carcinoma in situ during bacillus Calmette-Guérin maintenance (Boström et al. 2010). In addition to restaging TUR stage, several other clinicopathological factors, such T1 substaging, associated carcinoma in situ, tumor size and appearance, lymphovascular invasion, and hydronephrosis, aid in the decision making between radical and conservative treatment (Boström et al. 2010).

55.9   Prognostic Risk Factors for BCG in G3T1 Disease

Identification of prognostic factors in T1G3 NMIBC are significant for achieving good outcomes (Gontero et al. 2015). Gontero assess prognostic factors in intravesical BCG therapy for T1G3 tumors to identify high-risk patients who need more invasive therapy (Gontero et al. 2015). With a median follow-up of 5.2 yr, 465 patients (19%) progressed, 509 (21%) underwent cystectomy, and 221 (9%) died due to their disease. The most important prognostic factors for progression were age, tumor size, and concomitant carcinoma in situ (CIS); the most important prognostic factors for bladder cancer specific survival and overall survival were age and tumor size (Gontero et al. 2015). Risk groups for progression were identified by number of adverse factors among age ≥70 yr, size ≥3 cm, and presence of CIS. Progression rates at 10 yr ranged from 17 to 52%. Bladder cancer specific death rates at 10 yr were 32% in patients ≥70 yr with tumor size ≥3 cm and 13% otherwise (Gontero et al. 2015). T1G3 patients ≥70 yr with tumors ≥3 cm and concomitant CIS should be treated more aggressively because of the high risk of progression.

55.10   BCG for G3T1 Disease

The treatment of T1G3 bladder cancer is still a controversial issue (Bogdanović et al. 2002). Intravesical bacillus Calmette-Guérin (BCG) instillation is the gold standard in high-grade NMIBC after transurethral resection (Bogdanović et al. 2002). Bogdanović et al. (2002) determined recurrence and progression rates in T1G3 NMI bladder tumours (Bogdanović et al. 2002). After one or more initial courses of therapy, 33 patients were disease-free. Twelve patients (27.90%) had recurrent tumour after a median of 7 (range 3–46) months. After a second course of BCG treatment, 6 patients had no evidence of disease, 3 patients had progression and 3 had recurrence (Bogdanović et al. 2002). Progression occurred in 7 (16.27%) patients after a median of 19 (range 3–43) months. Five patients underwent radical cystectomy and the remaining 2 underwent bladder-preserving therapies. Two patients died of TCC and 3 due to disease-unrelated conditions (Bogdanović et al. 2002). Intravesical BCG instillation can be recommended as treatment modality for responders with T1G3 TCC bladder tumour. The benefit of the second course of intravesical BCG therapy has to be confirmed in further investigations (Bogdanović et al. 2002).

55.11   Cystectomy for G3T1 Disease

Malkowicz, examined outcomes of cystectomy in G3T1 disease. 411 consecutive patients were considered candidates for bilateral pelvic iliac lymph node dissection and radical cystectomy for the management of bladder cancer

(Malkowicz et al. 1990). From this group 160 were identified as having pathological stage T2 or less disease, including 11 who also had positive nodes. The 5-year actuarial survival rate for the respective stages at 95% confidence limits was 100% for stage T0/A, 80% for stage T1, 78% for stage T1 with stage TIS, 85% for pure stage TIS, 76% for stage T2 and 87% for stage T2 with stage TIS (Malkowicz et al. 1990). Additionally, Malkowicz identified a group of patients with stage T2 transitional cell carcinoma who were at significant risk for development of metastatic disease. Of 46 patients with stage T2 transitional cell carcinoma 18 had vascular space invasion resulting in 6 of 18 cancer-related deaths (33%). Malkowicz demonstrates that radical cystectomy has been highly effective in curing patients with high grade NMI disease, including those with NMIly invasive disease associated with nodal metastases (Malkowicz et al. 1990).

Canter et al. (2013) analyzed the Surveillance Epidemiology and End Results (SEER) database to examine cystectomy in clinical HGT1 bladder cancer (Canter et al. 2013). 8,467 patients were diagnosed with HGT1 bladder cancer, and 397 (4.7%) patients underwent RC. Patients who underwent RC for clinical HGT1 disease were significantly younger ($p < 0.0001$) and married ($p < 0.0001$) (Canter et al. 2013). Surgical patients also had a significantly improved overall ($p = 0.004$) and other cause of death ($p = 0.0053$) survival probabilities yet CSM at 1, 2, and 3 years was not statistically different between the surgical and nonsurgical groups ($p = 0.134$) (Canter et al. 2013). This demonstrated definitive surgical therapy is uncommonly employed for HGT1 bladder cancer (Canter et al. 2013).

55.12   Pathological Implications on Clinical Management for G3T1 Bladder Cancer

Management of high-grade T1 (HGT1) bladder cancer represents a major challenge. Orsola et al. (2015) studied a treatment strategy by depth of lamina propria invasion (Orsola et al. 2015). In a prospective observational cohort study, primary transurethral resection (TUR), mitomycin-C, and BCG instillation were conducted. Cases with shallower lamina propria invasion (HGT1a) were followed without further surgery, whereas subjects with HGT1b received a second TUR (Orsola et al. 2015). Median age was 71 years; 89.5% were males, with 89 (44.5%) cases T1a and 111 (55.5%) T1b. At median follow-up of 71 months, disease progression was observed in 31 (15.5%) and in univariate analysis, substaging, carcinoma in situ, tumour size, and tumour pattern predicted progression (Orsola et al. 2015). In HGT1 bladder cancer, the strategy of performing a second TUR only in T1b cases results in a low progression rate of 15.5% (Orsola et al. 2015). Tumours deeply invading the lamina propria (HGT1b) showed a three-fold increase in risk of progression. Substaging should be routinely evaluated, with HGT1b cases being thoroughly evaluated for cystectomy. Inclusion in the TNM system should also be carefully considered (Orsola et al. 2015).

55.13   Redo-TURBT in High Grade Bladder Cancer

Sanseverino et al. (2016) evaluated pathological outcomes of a redo turbt prognosis in on recurrence and progression of T1HG bladder cancer (Sanseverino et al. 2016). Primary T1HG TCC of bladder underwent restaging TURB (ReTURB). Patients with muscle invasive disease at ReTURB underwent radical cystectomy; those with non-muscle invasive residual (NMI-RT) and those with no residual tumour (NRT) received an intravesical BCG therapy (Sanseverino et al. 2016). At redo TURBT, recurrence occurred in 92 of 196 (46.9%): 14.3% of these were upstaged to T2 (Sanseverino et al. 2016). At follow up of 26.3 ± 22.8 months, there were differences in recurrence and progression rates between NRT and NMIRT: 26.9% and 45.3% ($p < 0.001$), 10.6% and 23.4% (p 0.03), respectively. Recurrence-free and progression-free survivals were significantly higher in NRT compared to NMIRT patients: 73.1% and 54.7% ($p < 0.001$), 89.4% and 76.6 (p 0.03), respectively (Sanseverino et al. 2016). Redo TURBT allows to identify a considerable number of residual and understaged cancer. Patients with NMIRT on redo TURBT have worse prognosis than those with NRT in terms of recurrence and progression free survival. These outcomes seem to suggest a prognostic impact of findings on ReTURB that could be a valid tool in management of high grade T1 TCC.

Lipsker also looked at recurrence after redo TURBT of pTa high-grade versus pT1 high-grade patients (Lipsker et al. 2014). 53 cases of NMIBC with a high-risk of recurrence and progression underwent a second systematic resection (Lipsker et al. 2014) 17 were pTa high grade (32.1%) and 36 pT1 high-grade (67.9%). There was a significant difference between the 2 groups of patients (Ta high-grade vs. T1 high-grade) concerning the rate of residual tumor on second look resection (11.8% vs. 66.7%, $p=0.0002$) (Lipsker et al. 2014). The predictive factors of residual tumor after second resection were the pT1 stage ($p=0.0002$), tumor multifocality ($p=0.02$) and presence of associated Cis ($p=0.0005$). The high rate of residual tumor in our series confirmed the importance of a systematic second look resection for high-risk non-muscle-invasive bladder cancers (Lipsker et al. 2014). However, for the pTa tumors without associated Cis, the interest of this second look seemed of less concern.

55.14   Rate of Recurrence and Risk of Progression in High Grade Bladder Cancer

Multiple recurrences can occur in high-risk non-muscle-invasive bladder cancer. Chamie examined whether the increasing number of recurrences is associated with higher treatment and mortality rates (Chamie et al. 2015). Of 4,521 subjects, 2,694 (59.6%) had multiple recurrences within 2 years of diagnosis. Compared with 1 recurrence, ≥ 4 recurrences were less likely to undergo radical cystectomy (hazard ratio [HR] = 0.73, 95% CI: 0.58–0.92), yet more likely to have radiotherapy (HR = 1.51, 95% CI: 1.23–1.85) and systemic chemotherapy (HR = 1.58, 95% CI: 1.15–2.18) (Chamie et al. 2015). For patients with ≥ 4 recurrences, only 25% were treated with curative intent. The 10-year cancer-specific mortality rates were 6.9%, 9.7%, 13.7%, and 15.7% for those with 1, 2, 3, and ≥ 4 recurrences, respectively (Chamie et al. 2015). Only 25% of patients with high-risk non-muscle-invasive bladder cancer who experienced recurrences at least 4 times underwent radical cystectomy or radiotherapy. Despite portending worse outcomes, increasing recurrences do not necessarily translate into higher treatment rates.

55.15   Recurrent High-Grade Bladder Cancer

The treatment of high-risk non-muscle-invasive bladder cancer (BCa) is problematic given the variable natural history of the disease. Few reports have compared outcomes for primary high-risk tumours with those that develop following previous BCas (relapses) (Thomas et al. 2013). The latter represent a self-selected cohort, having failed previous treatments. Thomas, compared outcomes in patients with primary, progressive, and recurrent high-risk non-muscle-invasive BCa (Thomas et al. 2013). Muscle invasion occurred most commonly in recurrent (23%) tumours, when compared to progressive (20%) and primary (14.6%) cohorts (log rank $p < 0.001$). Disease-specific mortality (DSM) occurred more frequently in patients with recurrent (25.5%) and progressive (24.6%) tumours compared to primary disease (19.2%; log rank $p = 0.006$) (Thomas et al. 2013). overall mortality was highest in the progressive cohort (62%) compared with the recurrent (58%) and primary groups (54%; log rank $p < 0.001$). Patients with relapsing, high-risk, BCa tumors have higher progression, DSM, and overall mortality rates than those with primary cancers. The use of bladder-sparing strategies in these patients should approached cautiously (Thomas et al. 2013). Carcinoma in situ has little predicative role in relapsing, high-risk, BCa tumors.

55.16   Systematic Reviews on High Grade Disease Management

Kulkarni et al. (2010) reviewed the current literature on the management of T1G3 BCa and to provide recommendations for its treatment (Kulkarni et al. 2010). This demonstrated the diagnosis of T1G3 disease is difficult because pathologic staging is often unreliable and because of the risk of significant understaging at initial transurethral resection (TUR) of bladder tumour. A secondary restaging TUR is recommended for all cases of T1G3 (Kulkarni et al. 2010). A single dose of immediate post-TUR chemotherapy is recommended. For a bladder-sparing approach, intravesical BCG should be given as induction with maintenance dosing (Kulkarni et al. 2010). Immediate or early radical cystectomy (RC) should be offered to all patients with recurrent or multifocal T1G3 disease, those who are at high risk of progression, and those failing BCG treatment (Kulkarni et al. 2010). Both bladder preservation and RC are appropriate options for T1G3 BCa. Risk stratification of patients based on pathologic features at initial TUR or at recurrence can select those most appropriate for bladder preservation compared to those for whom cystectomy should be strongly considered.

High-grade T1 (formerly T1G3) bladder cancer (BCa) has a high propensity to recur and progress. As a result, decisions pertaining to its treatment are difficult (Kulkarni et al. 2010). Treatment with bacillus Calmette-Guérin (BCG) risks progression and metastases but may preserve the bladder. Cystectomy may offer the best opportunity for cure but is associated with morbidity and a risk of mortality, and it may constitute potential overtreatment for many cases of T1G3 tumours. T Kulkarni reviewed the current literature on the management of T1G3 BCa and to provide recommendations for its treatment (Kulkarni et al. 2010). The diagnosis of T1G3 disease is difficult because pathologic staging is often unreliable and because of the risk of significant understaging at initial transurethral resection (TUR) of bladder tumour. A secondary restaging TUR is recommended for all cases of T1G3. A single dose of immediate post-TUR chemotherapy is recommended (Kulkarni et al. 2010). For a bladder-sparing approach, intravesical BCG should be given as induction with maintenance dosing. Immediate or early radical cystectomy (RC) should be offered to all patients with recurrent or multifocal T1G3 disease, those who are at high risk of progression, and those failing BCG treatment (Kulkarni et al. 2010). Both bladder preservation and RC are appropriate options for T1G3 BCa. Risk stratification of patients based on pathologic features at initial TUR or at recurrence can select those most appropriate for bladder preservation compared to those for whom cystectomy should be strongly considered.

Some studies report that tumour progression in patients with non-muscle-invasive bladder cancer (NMIBC) is associated with a poor prognosis (van den Bosch and Alfred Witjes 2011). van den Bosch determined the long-term cancer-specific survival in patients with high-risk NMIBC (T1G3, multifocal, highly recurrent, or carcinoma in situ) having tumour progression (van den Bosch and Alfred Witjes 2011). Literature was systematically reviewed, and 19 trials were included, producing a total of 3088 patients, of which 659 (21%) showed progression to MIBC and 428 (14%) died as a result of BCa after a median follow-up of 48-123 mo (van den Bosch and Alfred Witjes 2011). Survival after progression from high-risk NMIBC to MIBC was 35%. Progression to MIBC and BCa-related death in high-risk NMIBC were found to be relatively early events, occurring mainly within 48 mo. Finally, even in cases of early cystectomy in patients with high-risk NMIBC, a relevant proportion of these patients appear not be cured of their disease (van den Bosch and Alfred Witjes 2011).

References

Badalato GM, Gaya JM, Hruby G, Patel T, Kates M, Sadeghi N, Benson MC, McKiernan JM. Immediate radical cystectomy vs conservative management for high grade cT1 bladder cancer: is there a survival difference? BJU Int. 2012;110(10):1471–7.
Bogdanović J, Marusić G, Djozić J, Sekulić V, Budakov P, Dejanović N, Stojkov J. The management of T1G3 bladder cancer. Urol Int. 2002;69(4):263–5.

Boström PJ, Alkhateeb S, van Rhijn BW, Kuk C, Zlotta AR. Optimal timing of radical cystectomy in T1 high-grade bladder cancer. Expert Rev Anticancer Ther. 2010;10(12):1891–902.

Canter D, Egleston B, Wong YN, Smaldone MC, Simhan J, Greenberg RE, Uzzo RG, Kutikov A. Use of radical cystectomy as initial therapy for the treatment of high-grade T1 urothelial carcinoma of the bladder: a SEER database analysis. Urol Oncol. 2013;31(6):866–70.

Chamie K, Ballon-Landa E, Daskivich TJ, Bassett JC, Lai J, Hanley JM, Konety BR, Litwin MS. Saigal CS Treatment and survival in patients with recurrent high-risk non-muscle-invasive bladder cancer. Urol Oncol. 2015;33(1):20.e9–17.

Gontero P, Sylvester R, Pisano F, Joniau S, Vander Eeckt K, Serretta V, Larré S, Di Stasi S, Van Rhijn B, Witjes AJ, Grotenhuis AJ, Kiemeney LA, Colombo R, Briganti A, Babjuk M, Malmström PU, Oderda M, Irani J, Malats N, Baniel J, Mano R, Cai T, Cha EK, Ardelt P, Varkarakis J, Bartoletti R, Spahn M, Johansson R, Frea B, Soukup V, Xylinas E, Dalbagni G, Karnes RJ, Shariat SF, Palou J. Prognostic factors and risk groups in T1G3 non-muscle-invasive bladder cancer patients initially treated with Bacillus Calmette-Guérin: results of a retrospective multicenter study of 2451 patients. Eur Urol. 2015;67(1):74–82.

Jerlström T, Gårdmark T, Carringer M, Holmäng S, Liedberg F, Hosseini A, Malmström PU, Ljungberg B, Hagberg O, Jahnson S. Urinary bladder cancer treated with radical cystectomy: perioperative parameters and early complications prospectively registered in a national population-based database. Scand J Urol. 2014;48(4):334–40.

Kulkarni GS, Finelli A, Fleshner NE, Jewett MA, Lopushinsky SR, Alibhai SM. Optimal management of high-risk T1G3 bladder cancer: a decision analysis. PLoS Med. 2007;4(9):e284.

Kulkarni GS, Hakenberg OW, Gschwend JE, Thalmann G, Kassouf W, Kamat A, Zlotta A. An updated critical analysis of the treatment strategy for newly diagnosed high-grade T1 (previously T1G3) bladder cancer. Eur Urol. 2010;57(1):60–70.

Lida S, Kondo T, Kobayashi H, Hashimoto Y, Goya N, Tanabe K. Clinical outcome of high-grade non-muscle-invasive bladder cancer: a long-term single center experience. Int J Urol. 2009;16(3):287–92.

Lipsker A, Hammoudi Y, Parier B, Drai J, Bahi R, Bessede T, Patard JJ, Pignot G. Should we propose a systematic second transurethral resection of the bladder for all high-risk non-muscle invasive bladder cancers? Prog Urol. 2014;24(10):640–5.

Malkowicz SB, Nichols P, Lieskovsky G, Boyd SD, Huffman J, Skinner DG. The role of radical cystectomy in the management of high grade NMI bladder cancer (PA, P1, PIS and P2). Urol. 1990;144(3):641–5.

Oddens JR, Sylvester RJ, Brausi MA, Kirkels WJ, van de Beek C, van Andel G, de Reijke TM, Prescott S, Witjes JA, Oosterlinck W. The effect of age on the efficacy of maintenance bacillus Calmette-Guérin relative to maintenance epirubicin in patients with stage Ta T1 urothelial bladder cancer: results from EORTC genito-urinary group study 30911. Eur Urol. 2014;66(4):694–701.

Orsola A, Werner L, de Torres I, Martin-Doyle W, Raventos CX, Lozano F, Mullane SA, Leow JJ, Barletta JA, Bellmunt J, Morote J. Re-examining treatment of high-grade T1 bladder cancer according to depth of lamina propria invasion: a prospective trial of 200 patients. Br J Cancer. 2015;112(3):468–74.

Páez Borda A, Luján Galán M, Gómez de Vicente JM, Moreno Santurino A, Abate F, Berenguer Sánchez A. Preliminary results of the treatment of high grade (T1G3) NMI tumors of the bladder with transurethral resection. Actas Urol Esp. 2001;25(3):187–92.

Sanseverino R, Napodano G, Campitelli A, Addesso M. Prognostic impact of ReTURB in high grade T1 primary bladder cancer. Arch Ital Urol Androl. 2016;88(2):81–5.

Thomas F, Rosario DJ, Rubin N, Goepel JR, Abbod MF, Catto JW. The long-term outcome of treated high-risk nonmuscle-invasive bladder cancer: time to change treatment paradigm? Cancer. 2012;118(22):5525–34.

Thomas F, Noon AP, Rubin N, Goepel JR, Catto JW. Comparative outcomes of primary, recurrent, and progressive high-risk non-muscle-invasive bladder cancer. Eur Urol. 2013;63(1):145–54.

van den Bosch S, Alfred Witjes J. Long-term cancer-specific survival in patients with high-risk, non-muscle-invasive bladder cancer and tumour progression: a systematic review. Eur Urol. 2011;60(3):493–500.

Yang GL, Zhang LH, Liu Q, Wang ZL, Duan XH, Huang YR, Bo JJ. A novel treatment strategy for newly diagnosed high-grade T1 bladder cancer: Gemcitabine and cisplatin adjuvant chemotherapy-A single-institution experience. Urol Oncol. 2017;35(2):38.e9–15.

Zhang Y, Xie L, Chen T, Xie W, Wu Z, Xu H, Xing C, Sha N, Shen Z, Qie Y, Liu X, Hu H, Wu C. Intravenous chemotherapy combined with intravesical chemotherapy to treat T1G3 bladder urothelial carcinoma after transurethral resection of bladder tumor: results of a retrospective study. Onco Targets Ther. 2016;28(9):605–11.

Chapter 56
Radical Cystectomy in High Grade NMI Bladder Cancer

Solsana et al., establish the best time of radical cystectomy (RC) for recurrent high-risk NMI bladder tumours after BCG failure (Solsana et al. 2004). In recurrent high-risk NMI bladder cancer the survival rate similar to muscle-invasive disease (Solsana et al. 2004). Radical cystectomy might have been used too late-highlighted by extravesical urothelial recurrence after RC (Solsana et al. 2004). Predictive factors for progression are needed to indicate early RC in patients with recurrent high-risk NMI tumours (Solsana et al. 2004).

Radical cystectomy is usually curative for NMI tumors, although an aggressive measure. Orthotopic urinary reconstruction may increase patient acceptance of cystectomy as therapy for high risk NMIBC, although this is not the gold standard. Pathologic upstaging to muscle-invasive or metastatic tumors occurs in one third of highly selected patients post-radical cystectomy, half of whom have extravesical pathological disease (Freeman et al. 1995). Survival is significantly decreased in this group of upstaged patients. With the alternative of orthotopic urinary diversion, radical cystectomy is a viable alternative to continued conservative measures for selected patients with aggressive NMIBC bladder tumors (Freeman et al. 1995).

Puppo et al., report the oncological and functional results of potency sparing cystectomy with intrafascial prostatectomy for high risk NMIBC (Puppo et al. 2008). A significant decrease in the median International Index of Erectile Function score from baseline was recorded for 2 years of follow-up (25 vs. 21) (Puppo et al. 2008). 32 patients (86%) had an IIEF score of greater than 17 at 2 years after cystectomy (Puppo et al. 2008). Median scores from the International Continence Society male short form questionnaire were not significantly difference prior to and after surgery. Prostate specific antigen was lower than 0.2 ng/ml in all cases. The main criticism has been the presence of consistent prostatic remnants (Puppo et al. 2008). Performing this procedure however, gives good functional results with while better preserving oncological safety (Puppo et al. 2008).

© Springer Nature Switzerland AG 2020   283
S. S. Goonewardene et al., *Management of Non-Muscle Invasive Bladder Cancer*,
https://doi.org/10.1007/978-3-030-28646-0_56

Huguet et al., reviewed understaging and outcome of radical cystectomy (RC) for high risk NMIBC in BCG refractory disease (Huguet et al. 2005). This demonstrated RC should be performed prior to progression in high risk NMIBC in BCG refractory disease (Huguet et al. 2005). In NMIBC, RC provides very good disease-free survival. One third who underwent RC after BCG failure were understaged and had a shorter survival (Huguet et al. 2005). Tumor in the prostatic urethra at endoscopic staging was the only factor associated to understaging and shorter survival (Huguet et al. 2005).

Brauers et al., evaluated the prognostic significance of a second TURBT in moderately and poorly differentiated T1 bladder cancer (Brauers et al. 2001). The second transurethral resection offers the possibility to preserve the bladder (Brauers et al. 2001). In case of up staging to muscle infiltrating tumor, cystectomy is the next therapeutic step.

Herr and Sogani, compared survival after early versus delayed cystectomy in high risk NMIBC (Herr and Sogani 2001). Of the 90 patients who underwent cystectomy 44 (49%) survived a median of 96 months. Of 35 patients with recurrent NMIBC 92% and 56% survived who underwent cystectomy less than 2 years after initial BCG therapy and after 2 years of followup, respectively (Herr and Sogani 2001). Of 55 patients with recurrent NMIBC 41% and 18% survived when cystectomy was performed within and after 2 years, respectively (Herr and Sogani 2001). Multivariate analysis showed that survival was improved in patients who underwent earlier rather than delayed cystectomy for nonmuscle invasive tumor relapse. Earlier cystectomy improves the long-term survival of patients with high risk NMIBC that is BCG refractory.

References

Brauers A, Buettner R, Jakse G. Second resection and prognosis of primary high risk NMI bladder cancer: is cystectomy often too early? J Urol. 2001;165(3):808–10.

Freeman JA, Esrig D, Stein JP, Simoneau AR, Skinner EC, Chen SC, Groshen S, Lieskovsky G, Boyd SD, Skinner DG. Radical cystectomy for high risk patients with NMI bladder cancer in the era of orthotopic urinary reconstruction. Cancer. 1995;76(5):833–9.

Herr HW, Sogani PC. Does early cystectomy improve the survival of patients with high risk NMI bladder tumors? J Urol. 2001;166(4):1296–9.

Huguet J, Crego M, Sabaté S, Salvador J, Palou J, Villavicencio H. Cystectomy in patients with high risk NMI bladder tumors who fail intravesical BCG therapy: pre-cystectomy prostate involvement as a prognostic factor. Eur Urol. 2005;48(1):53–9.

Puppo P, Introini C, Bertolotto F, Naselli A. Potency preserving cystectomy with intrafascial prostatectomy for high risk NMI bladder cancer. J Urol. 2008;179(5):1727–32; discussion 1732.

Solsona E, Iborra I, Rubio J, Casanova J, Almenar S. The optimum timing of radical cystectomy for patients with recurrent high-risk NMI bladder tumour. BJU Int. 2004;94(9):1258–62.

Part VIII
Bladder Cancer in the Elderly and Females

Chapter 57
Bladder Cancer in the Elderly

Bladder cancer is inherently a disease of the elderly with the highest incidence occurring in the eighth decade of life (Weizer et al. 2010). Approximately a third of the 70,000 patients diagnosed with bladder cancer in the USA in 2009 will have presented with muscle-invasive bladder cancer (MIBC) requiring aggressive management (Weizer et al. 2010). Left untreated, most patients with MIBC suffer significant morbidity and die of the disease within 2 years of the diagnosis. While radical cystectomy, the best treatment option for local control of bladder cancer, has been shown to be safe in the elderly, outcomes depend more heavily on the functional status of the patient than on chronologic age (Weizer et al. 2010).

Although maintenance bacillus Calmette-Guérin (BCG) is the recommended treatment in high-risk non-muscle-invasive bladder cancer (NMIBC), its efficacy in older patients is controversial (Oddens et al. 2014) Oddens et al. determined the effect of age on prognosis and treatment outcome in patients with stage Ta T1 NMIBC treated with maintenance BCG. With a median follow-up of 9.2 yr, patients >70 yr had a shorter time to progression ($p = 0.028$), overall survival ($p < 0.001$), and NMIBC-specific survival ($p = 0.049$) after adjustment for EORTC risk scores in the multivariate analysis (Oddens et al. 2014). The time to recurrence was similar compared with the younger patients. BCG was more effective than epirubicin for all four end points considered, and there was no evidence that BCG was any less effective compared with epirubicin in patients >70 yr. In intermediate- and high-risk Ta T1 Urothelial cell carcinoma patients treated with BCG, patients >70 yr of age have a worse long-term prognosis; however, BCG is more effective than epirubicin independent of patient age.

National guidelines recommend adjuvant intravesical Bacillus Calmette-Guérin (BCG) therapy for higher-risk non-muscle-invasive bladder cancer (NMIBC). Although a survival benefit has not been demonstrated, randomized trials have shown reduced recurrence and delayed progression after its use. Spencer et al., investigated predictors of BCG receipt and its association with survival for older

S. S. Goonewardene et al., *Management of Non-Muscle Invasive Bladder Cancer*,
https://doi.org/10.1007/978-3-030-28646-0_57

patients with NMIBC (Spencer et al. 2013). Of 23,932 patients with NMIBC identified, 22% received adjuvant intravesical BCG. Predictors of receipt were stages Tis and T1, higher grade, and urban residence (Spencer et al. 2013). Age >80 years, fewer than two comorbidities, and not being married were associated with decreased use. In the survival analysis, BCG use was associated with better OS (hazard ratio [HR], 0.87; 95% CI, 0.83–0.92) in the entire cohort and BCSS among higher-grade cancers (poorly differentiated: HR, 0.78; 95% CI, 0.72–0.85; undifferentiated: HR, 0.66; 95% CI, 0.56–0.77) (Spencer et al. 2013). Despite guidelines recommending its use, BCG is administered to less than one quarter of eligible patients. This large population-based study found improved OS and BCSS were associated with use of adjuvant intravesical BCG among older patients with NMIBC (Spencer et al. 2013). Better-designed clinical trials focusing on higher-grade cancers are needed to confirm these findings.

Age is now widely accepted as the greatest single risk factor for developing bladder cancer, and bladder cancer is considered as primarily a disease of the elderly. Because of the close link between age and incidence of bladder cancer, it can be expected that this disease will become an enormous challenge with the growth of an aging population in the years ahead (Shariat et al. 2009). The decision to undergo treatment for cancer is a tradeoff between loss of function and/ or independence and extension of life, which is complicated by a host of concomitant issues such as comorbid medical conditions, functional declines and "frailty", family dynamics, and social and psychologic issues (Shariat et al. 2009). Chronological age should not preclude definitive surgical therapy. It is imperative that healthcare practitioners and researchers from disparate disciplines collectively focus efforts towards gaining a better understanding of what the consequences of bladder cancer and its treatments are for older adults and how to appropriately meet the multifaceted medical and psychosocial needs of this growing population (Shariat et al. 2009).

Bladder carcinoma often occurs in older patients who also may have other comorbid conditions that could influence the administration of surgical therapy. Prout et al. (2005) distribution of comorbid conditions in patients with bladder carcinoma and ascertain whether these conditions, as grouped by the American Society of Anesthesiologists physical status classification, affected the choice of surgical therapy (Prout et al. 2005). Hypertension, chronic pulmonary disease, arthritis, and heart disease were found to affect at least 15% of the study population (Prout et al. 2005). Approximately 38% of patients were current or former smokers. Greater than 90% of patients with NMI disease were treated with transurethral resection alone (Prout et al. 2005). Among those patients with muscle invasion, only 55% of those ages 55–59 years underwent cystectomy; this percentage dropped to 4% in patients age 85 years and older (Prout et al. 2005). Among patients with an American Society of Anesthesiologists physical status classification of 0–2, the cystectomy rate ranged from 53% in those ages 55–59 years to 9% in those age 85 years and older (Prout et al. 2005). There were no significant treatment differences noted with regard to age among patients with NMI disease. Among those patients with muscle invasion, those age 75 years and older were less likely to undergo radical cystectomy (14%) compared with patients ages 55–64 years (48%) and those ages 65–74 years (43%). Patient age may contribute to treatment decisions in patients with muscle-invasive disease, even when comorbidity is taken into account.

Saika et al. (2007) compare the health-related quality of life of elderly patients after radical cystectomy for bladder cancer in urinary diversion groups: ileal conduit, ureterocutaneostomy, or orthotopic urinary reservoir (Saika et al. 2007). The 109 participating elderly patients aged 75 or older completed self-reporting questionnaires: the QLQ-C30, and on satisfaction with urinary diversion methods. Regardless of the type of urinary diversion, the majority of patients reported having good overall quality of life, although with some problem of pain (Saika et al. 2007). No significant differences among urinary diversion subgroups were found in any quality of life area in the QLQ-C30 questionnaire. More patients in the OUR sub-group felt disappointment than those in the ileal conduit or cutaneostomy sub-groups (Saika et al. 2007). However, a questionnaire which asked which diversion method would be preferable showed a trend that more patients in the OUR subgroup would have chosen the same one. Health-related quality of life appeared relatively good in these 3 groups. Patient demands and expectations may be so different from the results that the details of each urinary diversion method should be explained thoroughly (Saika et al. 2007). OUR construction could be a candidate even for elderly patients.

Harano et al. (2007), assessed the functional results, health-related quality of life (QOL) outcomes, and complications in patients with an ileal neobladder in comparison to those with cutaneous diversion (ileal conduit and cutaneostomy) (Harano et al. 2007). The data from 41 patients (21 ileal neobladder procedures and 20 cutaneous diversions) were available for the analysis (Harano et al. 2007). No differences in the overall QOL were observed between the two groups. The findings regarding the health-related QOL and the frequency of complications in the neobladder group and those in the cutaneous diversion group were similar (Harano et al. 2007). However, the functional results and the status of urinary continence in the neobladder patients were satisfactory.

The objectives of the study were to evaluate morbidity, survival, and quality of life (QoL) (Sogni et al. 2008) in elderly patients with invasive bladder cancer who received an orthotopic neobladder or an ileal conduit (Sogni et al. 2008). The scores of all the QLQ multi-item scales and single-item measures were comparable in the 2 groups (Sogni et al. 2008). Overall, 56% and 25% daytime and nighttime complete continence rates were observed in patients with an orthotopic neobladder. The results suggest that an orthotopic neobladder can be suitable for elderly patients with no additional morbidity compared with an ileal conduit. Both types of diversion seem to result in acceptable scores for most aspects of QoL, including urinary symptoms and continence rate. These figures may be helpful in the preoperative counselling of elderly patients with bladder cancer (Sogni et al. 2008).

Assessing the unmet needs of cancer patients can help providers tailor health care services to patients' specific needs (Mohamed et al. 2016). This study examines whether the unmet informational and supportive care needs of the patients with muscle-invasive bladder cancer vary by the patients' age, sex, or individual treatment choices (Mohamed et al. 2016). Younger patients (<60y) were less satisfied with the treatment information received presurgery and more likely to report posttreatment complications, choose a neobladder, and seek and receive professional support regarding sexual function, than were older patients ($p < 0.05$) (Mohamed et al. 2016). Patients with neobladder were more likely to report difficulties with urinary incontinence and deterioration in sexual function, whereas patients with ileal conduit were more likely to require spousal help with self-care. Patients who received chemotherapy were significantly more likely to report changes in everyday life ($p < 0.05$). Lastly, regardless of age, sex, or treatment choice, up to 50% of patients reported feeling depressed before or after treatment (Mohamed et al. 2016). Unmet informational and supportive needs of patients with muscle-invasive bladder cancer during survivorship, and vary by age, sex, and treatment choices. Educational and psychological assessments as well as clinical interventions should be tailored to a patient's specific unmet needs, and to specific clinical and demographic characteristics (Mohamed et al. 2016).

References

Harano M, Eto M, Nakamura M, et al. A pilot study of the assessment of the quality of life, functional results, and complications in patients with an ileal neobladder for invasive bladder cancer. Int J Urol. 2007;14(2):112–7.

Mohamed NE, Pisipati S, Lee CT, Goltz HH, Latini DM, Gilbert FS, Wittmann D, Knauer CJ, Mehrazin R, Sfakianos JP, McWilliams GW, Quale DZ, Hall SJ. Unmet informational and supportive care needs of patients following cystectomy for bladder cancer based on age, sex, and treatment choices. Urol Oncol. 2016;34(12):531.e7–14.

Oddens JR, Sylvester RJ, Brausi MA, Kirkels WJ, van de Beek C, van Andel G, de Reijke TM, Prescott S, Witjes JA, Oosterlinck W. The effect of age on the efficacy of maintenance bacillus Calmette-Guérin relative to maintenance epirubicin in patients with stage Ta T1 urothelial bladder cancer: results from EORTC genito-urinary group study 30911. Eur Urol. 2014;66(4):694–701.

Prout GR Jr, Wesley MN, Yancik R, Ries LAG, Havlik RJ, Edwards BK. Age and comorbidity impact surgical therapy in older bladder carcinoma patients: as population-based study. Cancer. 2005;104(8):1638–47.

Saika T, Arata R, Tsushima T, et al. Health-related quality of life after radical cystectomy for bladder cancer in elderly patients with an ileal conduit, ureterocutaneostomy, or orthotopic urinary reservoir: a comparative questionnaire survey. Acta Med Okayama. 2007;61(4):199–203.

Shariat SF, Milowsky M, Droller MJ. Bladder cancer in the elderly. Urol Oncol. 2009;27(6):653–67.

Sogni F, Brausi M, Frea B, et al. Morbidity and quality of life in elderly patients receiving ileal conduit or orthotopic neobladder after radical cystectomy for invasive bladder cancer. Urology. 2008;71(5):919–23.

Spencer BA, McBride RB, Hershman DL, Buono D, Herr HW, Benson MC, Gupta-Mohile S, Neugut AI. Adjuvant intravesical bacillus calmette-guérin therapy and survival among elderly patients with non-muscle-invasive bladder cancer. J Oncol Pract. 2013;9(2):92–8.

Weizer AZ, Palella GV, Montgomery JS. Managing muscle-invasive bladder cancer in the elderly. Expert Rev Anticancer Ther. 2010;10(6):903–15.

Chapter 58
Systematic Review on Bladder Cancer Management in Elderly Patients

The number of cases of muscle-invasive bladder cancer is increasing along with the age of the population (Rose and Milowsky 2015). Management of muscle-invasive bladder cancer in the elderly is complex. A geriatric assessment should be used to guide treatment (Rose and Milowsky 2015). There is increasing evidence to support aggressive therapy in appropriate elderly patients, including radical cystectomy and neoadjuvant chemotherapy. Adjuvant chemotherapy also has a role with high-risk disease after cystectomy (Rose and Milowsky 2015). A bladder preservation approach with trimodality therapy is a well tolerated and effective alternative to cystectomy in appropriately selected patients (Rose and Milowsky 2015). Treatment decisions should not be based on chronologic age alone and advanced age should not preclude aggressive or curative therapy. The recent molecular characterization of bladder cancer and several recent immunotherapy trials provide hope of a more targeted approach to treatment of bladder, potentially improving both effectiveness and tolerability of treatment regimens in the elderly.

A systematic review relating to bladder cancer management in the elderly was conducted. The search strategy aimed to identify all references related to bladder cancer AND elderly AND management. Search terms used were as follows: (Bladder cancer) AND (trimodal therapy). The following databases were screened from 1989 to June 2019:

- CINAHL
- MEDLINE (NHS Evidence)
- Cochrane
- AMed
- EMBASE
- PsychINFO
- SCOPUS
- Web of Science.

© Springer Nature Switzerland AG 2020   291
S. S. Goonewardene et al., *Management of Non-Muscle Invasive Bladder Cancer*,
https://doi.org/10.1007/978-3-030-28646-0_58

In addition, searches using Medical Subject Headings (MeSH) and keywords were conducted using Cochrane databases. Two UK-based experts in bladder cancer were consulted to identify any additional studies.

Studies were eligible for inclusion if they reported primary research focusing on bladder cancer and screening. Papers were included if published after 1984 and had to be in English. Studies that did not conform to this were excluded. Only primary research was included. The overall aim was to identify the role and components of bladder cancer screening.

Abstracts were independently screened for eligibility by two reviewers and disagreements resolved through discussion or third-party opinion (Fig. 58.1). Agreement level was calculated using Cohens' Kappa to test the intercoder reliability of this screening process. Cohens' Kappa allows comparison of inter-rater reliability between papers using relative observed agreement. This also takes account of the comparison occurring by chance. The first reviewer agreed all 19 papers to be included, the second, agreed on 19 (Fig. 58.1).

Data extraction was piloted by the researcher and amended in consultation with the research team (author and two academic supervisors). Data collected included authors, year and country of publication, study aims, setting, intervention aims, number of participants, study design, intervention components and delivery methods, comparison groups and outcome measures, notes and follow-up questions for the authors. Studies were quality assessed using the PRISMA criteria for randomised controlled trials, Mays et al. (Moher et al. 2009; Moher, Liberati et al. 2009, 154, 153; Mays et al. 2005) for the action research and qualitative studies and the Critical Skills Appraisal programme for cohort studies. This was also applied to randomised controlled trials and qualitative studies. All the studies were cohort studies.

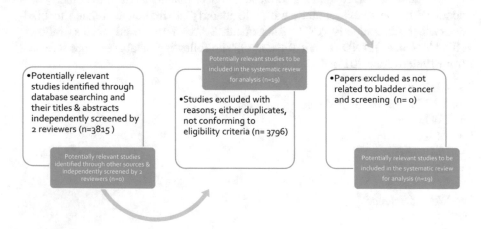

Fig. 58.1 Flow chart of studies identified through the systematic review (adapted from PRISMA)

References

Mays N, Pope C, Popay J. Systematically reviewing qualitative and quantitative evidence to inform management and policy-making in the health field. J Health Serv Res Policy. 2005;10(Suppl. 1):6–20.

Moher D, Liberati A, Tetzlaff J, Altman DG. Preferred reporting items for systematic reviews and meta-analyses: the prisma statement. BMJ (Online). 2009;339(7716):332–36.

Rose TL, Milowsky MI. Management of muscle-invasive bladder cancer in the elderly. Curr Opin Urol. 2015;25(5):459–67.

Chapter 59
Systematic Review—Results on Bladder Cancer Management in the Elderly

59.1 Radical Cystectomy and Adjuvant Chemotherapy in the Elderly

Leveridge assessed radical cystectomy (RC) outcomes and adjuvant chemotherapy (ACT) use in the elderly in routine practice (Leveridge et al. 2015). Bladder cancer occurs most commonly in the elderly. RC, standard treatment for muscle-invasive bladder cancer, presents challenges in older patients. Suboptimal evidence guides ACT use (Leveridge et al. 2015). Leveridge identified 3320 patients: 1362 (41%) aged <70 years; 674 (20%) aged 70–74 years; 674 (19%) aged 75–79 years, and 657 (20%) aged ≥80 years (Leveridge et al. 2015). Among ACT patients, 87% aged <70 years received cisplatin versus 73% aged ≥70 years ($p = 0.003$). ACT was associated with improved cancer-specific survival (hazard ratio [HR] = 0.73 and 95% confidence interval [CI] = 0.59–0.89 for age <70 years and HR = 0.73 [95% CI = 0.59–0.89] for ≥70 years) and overall survival (HR = 0.70 [95% CI = 0.58–0.85] for age <70 years and HR = 0.70 [95% CI = 0.59–0.84] for ≥70 years) across all age groups (Leveridge et al. 2015). Cystectomy carries a higher risk of postoperative mortality in elderly patients in routine clinical practice. ACT is used infrequently in older patients despite a substantial survival benefit observed across all age groups.

59.2 Adverse Effects from Cystectomy

Radical cystectomy and urinary diversion for muscle invasive bladder cancer is a demanding surgical procedure usually followed by a variable period of inability (Maffezzini et al. 2004). It might be even more delicate in the elderly (Maffezzini et al. 2004). Maffezzini described a protocol of pre, intra, and post

© Springer Nature Switzerland AG 2020
S. S. Goonewardene et al., *Management of Non-Muscle Invasive Bladder Cancer*,
https://doi.org/10.1007/978-3-030-28646-0_59

operative management aimed at minimising the impact of bladder cancer surgery (Maffezzini et al. 2004).

The patients were submitted to reduced pre-operative fasting (6–8 hours), no mechanical bowel preparation, and insertion of an epidural cannula (Maffezzini et al. 2004). Intra-operative Intra-operatively the protocol included: combined anesthesia (general + epidural), controlled hypotension, correction of blood losses in excess of 10% of the estimated total blood volume, O_2 supplementation and insertion of a jejunal cannula for nutrition (Maffezzini et al. 2004). Post-operatively: early removal of naso-gastric tubing (2–6 hours), parenteral and enteral nutrition started ion POD1 (Maffezzini et al. 2004). The feasibility study was conducted on 18 patients, 14 males and 4 women, median age 70 years (range 55–82). Six patients belonged to category ASA II, and 12 to ASA III-IV (Maffezzini et al. 2004). The protocol was completed by 10 patients and no completed by 8. The only step of the protocol that was not completed was the enteral nutrition that caused symptoms of bowel distension (Maffezzini et al. 2004). Among the patients who completed the protocol the return of peristalsis and of normal bowel function were observed on POD 1, and POD 2, respectively, whereas, the recovery required one day more in the remaining patients (Maffezzini et al. 2004). The protocol was feasible, and contributed to an accelerated recovery of intestinal function. Compliance to the protocol was independent from age. The study is ongoing for a more precise evaluation of the outcomes of the protocol.

59.3   Mortality and Survival from Radical Cystectomy in Elderly Patients

Madersbacher analyzed demographics, perioperative mortality and overall survival of radical cystectomy (RC) in patients aged 70+ years in Austria in a nationwide registry cohort (Madersbacher et al. 2010). A total of 845 patients aged 70–89 years (mean 74) entered the analysis. The annual number of cystectomies in this age group increased from 27 in 1992 to 79 (+292%) in 2004. The mean length of hospital stay declined from 37.1 days (in 1992) to 27.1 days (in 2004) (Madersbacher et al. 2010). The 60-day mortality of the entire cohort was 1.5% and increased to 5.2% in patients aged 80+ years. Almost 50% of patients had to be rehospitalized within 30 days. The 5-year overall survival declined from 62% in those aged 70–74 years to 61% in those aged 75–79 years to 46% in the oldest age group (80+ years) (Madersbacher et al. 2010). The annual number of cystectomies in patients aged 70+ years increased substantially during the study period. These nation-wide registry data provide insights into the current status of RC in the elderly in Austria and demonstrate that cystectomy in this age cohort can be done with an acceptable perioperative mortality and overall survival.

Soulié evaluated the morbidity of radical cystectomy for invasive bladder cancer in select patients older than 75 years using recent data from 2 academic hospitals (Soulié et al. 2002). 73 radical cystectomies were performed from January 1995 to June 2000 in patients 75–89 years old (median age 79.3). 2. External urinary diversion was performed in 51 cases and an ileal neobladder was constructed in 22. The perioperative mortality rate was 2.7% (Soulié et al. 2002). The intraoperative, early and late postoperative complication rates were 38.4%, 46.5% and 16.4%, respectively. Three reoperations (4.1%) were necessary. The most common early complications were pyelonephritis in 12.3% of cases, disorientation in 10.9%, pneumonia in 8.2% and prolonged ileus in 12.3% (Soulié et al. 2002). The most common late complications were ureteroileal anastomotic stenosis in 5 cases and hernia in 3. Median postoperative care unit and hospital stays were 12 and 34 days, respectively. At a median followup of 14.4 months (range 6–74) the overall mortality rate was 31.5% (Soulié et al. 2002). Hospital stay was significantly higher in patients with complications. The incidence of complications was similar in the 2 groups. These data support the aggressive surgical management of bladder cancer in select elderly patients (Soulié et al. 2002).

Bladder carcinoma often occurs in older patients who also may have other comorbid conditions that could influence the administration of surgical therapy (Prout et al. 2005). Prout conducted a study to describe the distribution of comorbid conditions in patients with bladder carcinoma and ascertain whether these conditions, as grouped by the American Society of Anesthesiologists physical status classification, affected the choice of surgical therapy (Prout et al. 2005). A total of 820 individuals age 55 years and older was found. A random sample of newly diagnosed bladder carcinoma patients were stratified according to registry, age group (ages 55–64 years, ages 65–74 years, and age 75 years and older), and gender (Prout et al. 2005). Greater than 90% of patients with NMI disease were treated with transurethral resection alone. Among those patients with muscle invasion, only 55% of those ages 55–59 years underwent cystectomy; this percentage dropped to 4% in patients age 85 years and older (Prout et al. 2005). Among patients with an American Society of Anesthesiologists physical status classification of 0–2, the cystectomy rate ranged from 53% in those ages 55–59 years to 9% in those age 85 years and older (Prout et al. 2005). There were no significant treatment differences noted with regard to age among patients with NMI disease. Among those patients with muscle invasion, those age 75 years and older were less likely to undergo radical cystectomy (14%) compared with patients ages 55–64 years (48%) and those ages 65–74 years (43%) (Prout et al. 2005). Patient age may contribute to treatment decisions in patients with muscle-invasive disease, even when comorbidity is taken into account.

Radical cystectomy (RC) is an effective but underused treatment for bladder cancer in elderly patients. Lin performed analysis of propensity scores (PSs) to determine the outcomes of RC for elderly patients, with results generalizable at the population-based level (Lin et al. 2018). 430 patients with bladder cancer who underwent RC between 2000 and 2010 (Lin et al. 2018). Older age was not significantly associated with 30-day readmission (odds ratio [OR] = 0.80, 95% confidence interval [CI] = 0.38–1.70), 90-day readmission (OR = 1.10, 95% CI = 0.60–2.00), 30-day mortality (OR = 3.07, 95% CI = 0.31–30.0), or 90-day mortality

(OR = 2.98, 95% CI = 0.91–9.70) in the PS-matched group (Lin et al. 2018). Similar trends were also observed for both groups regarding the mean length of ICU stay, LOS, and overall medical expenditure within the same admission (Lin et al. 2018). No significant differences existed between the older and younger groups for 30- and 90-day mortality and readmission rates, length of ICU stay, LOS, and medical expenditure in patients undergoing RC for bladder cancer. Some healthy elderly patients may be good candidates for this extensive curative treatment.

59.4 Cystectomy Versus Other Treatments in Elderly Patients

Chen assessed the impacts of age, performance status, and clinical stage on advanced urothelial carcinoma of the bladder (UCB) in patients treated with different treatment modalities (Chen et al. 2015). This retrospective study included 160 patients who underwent radical cystectomy (RC) with/without neoadjuvant or adjuvant chemoradiotherapy, palliative chemotherapy/radiotherapy/chemoradiotherapy (CRT) , and transurethral resection of bladder tumor (TURBT) monotherapy for advanced UCB in one institution (Chen et al. 2015). The median age of the patients was 74.0 years, and the mean survival interval was 31.5 months. The 2-year OS was significantly different among the three modalities [RC > TURBT monotherapy, odds ratio (OR): 1.86, 95% CI: 1.17–2.96, $p = 0.009$; CRT > TURBT monotherapy, OR: 1.65, 95% CI: 1.06–2.57, $p = 0.026$] (Chen et al. 2015). There were no significant differences in the 5- and 10-year OS rates between the three treatment modalities. Those younger than 76 years receiving RC had a significantly better 2-year OS than those undergoing CRT and TURBT monotherapy (RC > TURBT monotherapy, OR: 2.38; 95% CI: 1.30–4.33, $p = 0.005$) (Chen et al. 2015). The number and duration of re-hospitalizations were highest in the CRT group and lowest in the TURBT group. The short- and long-term OS rates of the three modalities were similar in those older than 76 years. Therefore, patients younger than age 76 years are likely to have a better outcome undergoing radical cystectomy for advanced UCB.

59.5 Undertreatment of Bladder Cancer in the Elderly

Bladder cancer (BC) predominantly affects the elderly and is often the cause of death among patients with muscle-invasive disease (Noon et al. 2013). Clinicians lack quantitative estimates of competing mortality risks when considering treatments for BC. Noon determined the bladder cancer-specific mortality (CSM) rate and other-cause mortality (OCM) rate for patients with newly diagnosed BC

(Noon et al. 2013). At 5 years after diagnosis, 1246 (40%) patients were dead: 617 (19%) from BC and 629 (19%) from other causes. The 5-year BC mortality rate varied between 1 and 59%, and OCM rate between 6 and 90%, depending primarily on the tumour type and patient age (Noon et al. 2013). Cancer-specific mortality was highest in the oldest patient groups. Few elderly patients received radical treatment for invasive cancer (52% vs. 12% for patients <60 vs. >80 years, respectively) (Noon et al. 2013). Female patients with high-risk non-muscle-invasive BC had worse CSM than equivalent males (Gray's $p < 0.01$). Bladder CSM is highest among the elderly. Female patients with high-risk tumours are more likely to die of their disease compared with male patients. Clinicians should consider offering more aggressive treatment interventions among older patients (Noon et al. 2013).

59.6   NMIBC, BCG Therapy and Elderly Patients

Oddens determined the relationship of age to side-effects leading to discontinuation of treatment in patients with stage Ta-T1 non-muscle-invasive bladder cancer (NMIBC) treated with maintenance bacille Calmette-Guérin (BCG) (Oddens et al. 2016). 487 eligible patients with intermediate- or high-risk Ta-T1 (without carcinoma in situ) NMIBC randomised to receive 3 years of maintenance BCG therapy (247 BCG alone and 240 BCG + isoniazid) in European Organisation for Research and Treatment of Cancer Genito-Urinary Group trial 30911 (Oddens et al. 2016). The percentage of patients who stopped for toxicity and the number of treatment cycles that they received were compared in four age groups, $\leq$60, 61–70, 71–75 and >75 years, using the Mantel-Haenszel chi-square test for trend (Oddens et al. 2016). The percentage of patients stopping BCG for toxicity was 17.9% in patients aged $\leq$60 years, 21.9% in patients aged 61–70 years, 22.9% in patients aged 71–75 years, and 16.4% in patients aged >75 years ($p = 0.90$). For both systemic and local side-effects, there was likewise no significant difference. In patients with intermediate- and high-risk Ta-T1 NMIBC treated with BCG, no differences in toxicity as a reason for stopping treatment were detected based on patient age.

Although maintenance bacillus Calmette-Guérin (BCG) is the recommended treatment in high-risk non-muscle-invasive bladder cancer (NMIBC), its efficacy in older patients is controversial.

Oddens determine the effect of age on prognosis and treatment outcome in patients with stage Ta T1 NMIBC treated with maintenance BCG (Oddens et al. 2014). A total of 957 patients with intermediate- or high-risk Ta T1 (without carcinoma in situ) NMIBC were randomized in European Organization for Research and Treatment of Cancer (EORTC) trial 30911 comparing six weekly instillations of epirubicin, BCG, and BCG plus isoniazid followed by three weekly maintenance instillations over 3 year (Oddens et al. 2014). Overall, 822 eligible patients were included: 546 patients in the BCG with or without INH arms and 276 in the epirubicin arm. In patients treated with BCG with or without INH, 34.1% were >70 year of age and 3.7% were >80 year (Oddens et al. 2014). With a median follow-up of 9.2 year, patients >70 year had a shorter time to progression ($p = 0.028$), overall survival ($p < 0.001$), and NMIBC-specific survival ($p = 0.049$) after adjustment for EORTC risk scores in the multivariate analysis. The time to recurrence was similar compared with the younger patients (Oddens et al. 2014). BCG was more effective than epirubicin for all four end points considered, and there was no evidence that BCG was any less effective compared with epirubicin in patients >70 year (Oddens et al. 2014). In intermediate- and high-risk Ta T1 Urothelial cell carcinomapatients treated with BCG, patients >70 year of age have a worse long-term prognosis; however, BCG is more effective than epirubicin independent of patient age.

National guidelines recommend adjuvant intravesical Bacillus Calmette-Guérin (BCG) therapy for higher-risk non-muscle-invasive bladder cancer (NMIBC) (Spencer et al. 2013). Although a survival benefit has not been demonstrated, randomized trials have shown reduced recurrence and delayed progression after its use. Spencer investigated predictors of BCG receipt and its association with survival for older patients with NMIBC (Spencer et al. 2013). Of 23,932 patients with NMIBC identified, 22% received adjuvant intravesical BCG. Predictors of receipt were stages Tis and T1, higher grade, and urban residence. Age >80 years, fewer than two comorbidities, and not being married were associated with decreased use (Spencer et al. 2013). In the survival analysis, BCG use was associated with better OS (hazard ratio [HR], 0.87; 95% CI, 0.83–0.92) in the entire cohort and BCSS among higher-grade cancers (poorly differentiated: HR, 0.78; 95% CI, 0.72–0.85; undifferentiated: HR, 0.66; 95% CI, 0.56–0.77) (Spencer et al. 2013). This large population-based study found improved OS and BCSS were associated with use of adjuvant intravesical BCG among older patients with NMIBC (Spencer et al. 2013).

59.7   MIBC and Radiation Therapy for Elderly Patients

Santacaterina evaluated clinical results in elderly and frail patients with bladder cancer treated with curative radiation alone (Santacaterina et al. 2015). A total of 27 ambulatory patients were treated. Median age was 84.5 years and a median CCI of 6.5 was recorded. Median delivered radiation dose was 64 Gy (Santacaterina et al. 2015). Grade 1–2 gastrointestinal (GI) and genitourinary (GU) toxicities were observed in 55.5% of patients (15/27) (Santacaterina et al. 2015). At the last follow-up, no late G3+ toxicities have been observed, with G1–2 toxicities reported in 11.1% of patients (3/27). Higher values of CCI were associated with higher acute GU/GI toxicities; there was a correlation between CCI and acute GU toxicity ($r = 0.43$, $p = 0.027$) (Santacaterina et al. 2015). The mean survival time was 23.5 months (95% confidence interval 20.9–26.1) and no median was reached. Locoregional disease-free events and metastasis-free survival showed a 2-year actuarial rate of 90% and 87%, respectively, with an actuarial 2-year overall survival of 84.5% (Santacaterina et al. 2015). Santacaterina, results demonstrate safety and feasibility of curative radiation therapy in very elderly and frail patients with bladder cancer using 3D conformal radiation therapy (Santacaterina et al. 2015).

There are only scarce data on the optimal management of patients who preset with a bladder carcinoma and who are aged 90 years and older (Méry et al. 2015). Méry et al, examined 14 patients aged 90 years or older receiving RT for bladder malignant tumors were identified (Méry et al. 2015). Mean age was 92.7 years. Ten patients (71%) had a general health status altered (PS 2–3) at the beginning of RT. A total of 14 RT courses were delivered, including six treatments (43%) with curative intent and eight treatments (57%) with palliative intent (Méry et al. 2015). Palliative intent mainly encompassed hemostatic RT (36%). At last follow-up, two patients (14%) experienced complete response, one patient (7%) experienced partial response, three patients (21%) had their disease stable, and three patients (21%) experienced tumor progression, of whom two patients with the progression of symptoms. There was no reported high-grade acute local toxicity in 14 patients (100%) (Méry et al. 2015). One patient experienced delayed grade 2 toxicity with pain and lower urinary tract symptoms. At last follow-up, seven patients (50%) were deceased. Cancer was the cause of death for five patients (Méry et al. 2015).

The current study was conducted to compare the overall survival (OS) of concurrent chemoradiotherapy (CCRT) versus radiotherapy (RT) alone in elderly patients (those aged $\geq$80 years) with muscle-invasive bladder cancer (MIBC) (Korpics et al. 2017). Patients aged $\geq$80 years with cT2–4, N0–3, M0 transitional cell MIBC who were treated with curative RT (60–70 Gray) or CCRT were identified in the National Cancer Data Base (Korpics et al. 2017). A total of 1369 patients who were treated with RT from 2004 through 2013 met eligibility criteria: 739 patients (54%) received RT alone and 630 patients (46%) received CCRT. The median age of the patients was 84 years (range, 80–90 years). The median follow-up was 21 months (Korpics et al. 2017). The 2-year OS rate was 48%. When comparing CCRT with RT alone, the 2-year OS rate was 56% versus 42% ($p < 0.0001$), respectively. Multivariable analysis demonstrated that CCRT (hazard ratio [IIR], 0.74; 95% confidence interval [95% CI] , 0.65–0.84 [$p < 0.0001$]) and a higher RT dose (HR, 0.78; 95% CI, 0.67–0.90 [$p < 0.001$]) were associated with improved OS. T4 disease was associated with worse OS (HR, 1.42; 95% CI, 1.15–1.76 [$p = 0.001$]) (Korpics et al. 2017). After using 1-to-1 propensity score matching, there remained an OS benefit for the use of CCRT (HR, 0.77; 95% CI, 0.67–0.90 [$p < 0.001$]) (Korpics et al. 2017). CCRT is associated with improved OS compared with the use of RT alone in elderly patients with MIBC, independent of Charlson-Deyo comorbidity score, suggesting that CCRT should be used in this population. Cancer 2017;123:3524–31.

Aizawa evaluate the clinical results of external-beam radiotherapy (EBRT) for muscle-invasive bladder cancer (MIBC) in elderly or medically-fragile patients (Aizawa et al. 2017). Twenty-five consecutive patients with MIBC (cT2-4N0-1M0) receiving EBRT were retrospectively analysed (Aizawa et al. 2017). Their median age was 82 years. Radiotherapy median dose was 60 Gy administered in 30 fractions.

Median follow-up period was 14.7 months. Median overall survival (OS) and progression-free survival (PFS) were 14.7 months and 7.8 months, respectively (Aizawa et al. 2017). The OS, cause-specific survival (CSS), and PFS rates at 1-year were 56.0%, 68.5%, and 40.0%, respectively. The local progression-free rates (LPFR) at 6 months and 1 year were 89.3% and 59.5%, respectively (Aizawa et al. 2017). Performance status 3 was a significantly unfavorable factor for OS, CSS, and progression-free survival; clinical N stage was a significantly unfavorable factor for progression-free survival; and lower irradiation dose ($\leq$50.4 Gy) was a significantly unfavorable factor for LPFR (Aizawa et al. 2017). EBRT for elderly or medically-fragile patients is feasible, and achieves acceptable local progression-free status.

59.8 Chemoraditherapy Versus Radiation Therapy in the Elderly

The current study was conducted to compare the overall survival (OS) of concurrent chemoradiotherapy (CCRT) versus radiotherapy (RT) alone in elderly patients (those aged $\geq$80 years) with muscle-invasive bladder cancer (MIBC) (Korpics et al. 2017). Patients aged $\geq$80 years with cT2–4, N0–3, M0 transitional cell MIBC who were treated with curative RT (60–70 Gray) or CCRT were identified in the National Cancer Data Base (Korpics et al. 2017). A total of 1369 patients who were treated with RT from 2004 through 2013 met eligibility criteria: 739 patients (54%) received RT alone and 630 patients (46%) received CCRT. The median age of the patients was 84 years (range, 80–90 years). The median follow-up was 21 months (Korpics et al. 2017). The 2-year OS rate was 48%. When comparing CCRT with RT alone, the 2-year OS rate was 56% versus 42% ($p < 0.0001$), respectively. Multivariable analysis demonstrated that CCRT (hazard ratio [HR], 0.74; 95% confidence interval [95% CI] , 0.65–0.84 [$p < 0.0001$]) and a higher RT dose (HR, 0.78; 95% CI, 0.67–0.90 [$p < 0.001$]) were associated with improved OS. T4 disease was associated with worse OS (HR, 1.42; 95% CI, 1.15–1.76 [$p = 0.001$]) (Korpics et al. 2017). After using 1-to-1 propensity score matching, there remained an OS benefit for the use of CCRT (HR, 0.77; 95% CI, 0.67–0.90 [$p < 0.001$]) (Korpics et al. 2017). CCRT is associated with improved OS compared with the use of RT alone in elderly patients with MIBC, independent of Charlson-Deyo comorbidity score, suggesting that CCRT should be used in this population. Cancer 2017;123:3524–31.

59.9 MIBC and Conservative Management in the Elderly

Tran reported the long-term results of bladder conservation strategies in elderly patients with muscle-invasive bladder cancer and evaluate the different factors affecting locoregional control and patient survival (Tran et al. 2009). Tran reviewed the records of 39 elderly patients aged 70 or older, treated with curative intent with radiotherapy, with or without chemotherapy after transurethral resection of bladder for T2–T4aN0 carcinoma of the bladder (Tran et al. 2009). Twenty-seven men and 12 women were identified with a median age of 78 (range 70–87). Sixteen of the patients had a previous history of NMI bladder cancer. Twenty-five patients had T2 lesions, 13 patients had T3 lesions, and 1 patient had T4a lesion. The majority of patients were unsuitable for surgery because of medical reasons (67%), whereas the others refused radical cystectomy (33%) (Tran et al. 2009). Patients were treated with radical radiation therapy with or without chemotherapy. At a median follow-up time of 35.5 months for patients at risk, the 5-year overall survival is 28.9% for all stages, 31.9% for T2 lesions, and 26.8% for T3–T4a lesions (Tran et al. 2009). Significant prognostic factors for overall survival on univariate analysis were performance status and age. Five-year cause-specific survival is 37.5% for all stages, 41.5% for T2 lesions, and 34.7% for T3–T4a lesions. No significant prognostic factors for cause-specific survival were indentified on univariate analysis. Toxicity was acceptable (Tran et al. 2009).

Younger age and good performance status were favorable prognostic factors for overall survival. Bladder conservation strategies achieved satisfactory results and were well-tolerated in this elderly population with invasive bladder cancer.

Bolenz studied guideline recommendation (GR)-concordance rates of treatment in elderly patients with urothelial carcinoma of the bladder (UCB) and to identify predictors of survival (Bolenz et al. 2010).The records of 206 consecutive patients aged $\geq$ 75 years (median age 79 years; range 75–95) were reviewed. All patients underwent transurethral resection (TUR) or biopsy of UCB. The overall GR-concordance rate of treatment was 88.8% (183 of 206 patients). Patients who were older ($p = 0.017$), who underwent prior treatment for UCB ($p = 0.010$), and had greater comorbidities ($p = 0.001$) were less likely to undergo treatment following GRs (Bolenz et al. 2010). With a median (mean; range) follow-up of 14.7 (22.6; 0.3–111.5) months, 79 patients died (38.3%). More comorbidities (unadjusted Charlson comorbidity index; $p = 0.007$), a Karnofsky performance status (KPS) score of $\leq$80 ($p = 0.001$) and more advanced initial pathological tumour stage ($p = 0.019$) independently predicted reduced overall survival (OS) (Bolenz et al. 2010). In the subgroup of patients with indication for cystectomy ($n = 99$), there was a trend for longer OS in patients treated with curative intent (cystectomy or radio-chemotherapy) compared with conservative treatment with TUR $\pm$ intravesical therapy only ($p = 0.095$) (Bolenz et al. 2010). The vast majority of elderly patients with UCB received adequate treatment at our tertiary institution. The KPS score, more comorbidities and more advanced pathological tumour stage are predictors for reduced OS and should be considered to optimize patient care.

59.10   Trimodal Therapy in the Elderly

Radical cystectomy is the guidelines-recommended treatment of muscle-invasive bladder cancer, but a resurgence of trimodal therapy has occurred. Limited comparative data are available on outcomes and costs attributable to these 2 treatments.

Williams compared the survival outcomes and costs between trimodal therapy and radical cystectomy in older adults with muscle-invasive bladder cancer (Williams et al. 2018). This population-based cohort study used data from the Surveillance, Epidemiology, and End Results-Medicare linked database. Patients who received radical cystectomy underwent either only surgery or surgery in combination with radiotherapy or chemotherapy. Patients who received trimodal therapy underwent transurethral resection of the bladder followed by radiotherapy and chemotherapy (Williams et al. 2018). Patients who underwent trimodal therapy had significantly decreased overall survival (hazard ratio [HR], 1.49; 95% CI, 1.31–1.69) and cancer-specific survival (HR, 1.55; 95% CI, 1.32–1.83) (Williams et al. 2018). These findings have important health policy implications regarding the appropriate use of high value-based care among older adults with invasive bladder cancer who are candidates for either radical cystectomy or trimodal therapy.

59.11 MIBC—The Orthotopic Neobladder and Elderly Patients

Saika compared the clinical results of orthotopic neobladder reconstruction in elderly patients and those in younger patients retrospectively in order to verify whether age is a critical factor in selecting a method of urinary diversion (Saika et al. 2001). Following radical cystectomy for bladder cancer, 12 patients aged 75 or older and 17 patients under 75 who underwent orthotopic neobladder reconstruction between January 1992 and May 1999 were investigated in this study (Saika et al. 2001).

The follow-up periods for elderly and younger groups ranged from 21.3 to 82.7 months and from 8.8 to 94.2 months, respectively (Saika et al. 2001). No difference in operation time, amount of bleeding or postoperative length of hospitalization was observed between elderly and younger patients. The rates of early complications in elderly and younger patients were 41.7% and 35.3%, respectively. Late complication rates were 33.3% and 47.1%, respectively (Saika et al. 2001). The difference in these complication rates was not statistically significant. One of the elderly and two of the younger patients had local recurrence and metastasis postoperatively (Saika et al. 2001). Those three patients had died of their bladder cancer. No statistically significant difference between groups was recognized in either cause-specific survival or overall survival, nor was there such a difference in relation to micturition/continence (Saika et al. 2001).

References

Aizawa R, Sakamoto M, Orito N, Kono M, Ogura M, Negoro Y, Sagoh T, Tsukahara K, Komatsu K, Noguchi M. The use of external-beam radiotherapy for muscle-invasive bladder cancer in elderly or medically-fragile patients. Anticancer Res. 2017;37(10):5761–6.

Bolenz C, Ho R, Nuss GR, Ortiz N, Raj GV, Sagalowsky AI, Lotan Y. Management of elderly patients with urothelial carcinoma of the bladder: guideline concordance and predictors of overall survival. BJU Int. 2010;106(9):1324–9.

Chen CL, Liu CY, Cha TL, Hsu CY, Chou YC, Wu ST, Meng E, Sun GH, Yu DS, Tsao CW. Does radical cystectomy outperform other bladder preservative treatments in elderly patients with advanced bladder cancer? J Chin Med Assoc. 2015;78(8):469–74.

Korpics MC, Block AM, Martin B, Hentz C, Gaynor ER, Henry E, Harkenrider MM, Solanki AA. Concurrent chemotherapy is associated with improved survival in elderly patients with bladder cancer undergoing radiotherapy. Cancer. 2017;123(18):3524–31.

Leveridge MJ, Siemens DR, Mackillop WJ, Peng Y, Tannock IF, Berman DM, Booth CM. Radical cystectomy and adjuvant chemotherapy for bladder cancer in the elderly: a population-based study. Urology. 2015;85(4):791–8.

Lin WY, Wu CT, Chen MF, Chang YH, Lin CL, Kao CH. Cystectomy for bladder cancer in elderly patients is not associated with increased 30- and 90-day mortality or readmission, length of stay, and cost: propensity score matching using a population database. Cancer Manag Res. 2018;31(10):1413–8.

Madersbacher S, Bauer W, Willinger M, Wehrberger C, Berger I, Brössner C. Radical cystectomy for bladder cancer in the 70+ population: a nation-wide registry analysis of 845 patients. Urol Int. 2010;85(3):287–90.

Maffezzini M, Gerbi G, Campodonico F, Parodi D, Capponi G, Spina A, Guerrieri AM. Perioperative management of ablative and reconstructive surgery for invasive bladder cancer in the elderly. Surg Oncol. 2004;13(4):197–200.

Méry B, Falk AT, Assouline A, Trone JC, Guy JB, Rivoirard R, Auberdiac P, Escure JL, Moncharmont C, Moriceau G, Almokhles H, de Laroche G, Pacaut C, Guillot A, Chargari C, Magné N. Hypofractionated radiation therapy for treatment of bladder carcinoma in patients aged 90 years and more: a new paradigm to be explored? Int Urol Nephrol. 2015;47(7):1129–34.

Noon AP, Albertsen PC, Thomas F, Rosario DJ, Catto JW. Competing mortality in patients diagnosed with bladder cancer: evidence of undertreatment in the elderly and female patients. Br J Cancer. 2013;108(7):1534–40.

Oddens JR, Sylvester RJ, Brausi MA, Kirkels WJ, van de Beek C, van Andel G, de Reijke TM, Prescott S, Witjes JA, Oosterlinck W. The effect of age on the efficacy of maintenance bacillus Calmette-Guérin relative to maintenance epirubicin in patients with stage Ta T1 urothelial bladder cancer: results from EORTC genito-urinary group study 30911. Eur Urol. 2014;66(4):694–701.

Oddens JR, Sylvester RJ, Brausi MA, Kirkels WJ, van de Beek C, van Andel G, de Reijke TM, Prescott S, Alfred Witjes J, Oosterlinck W. Increasing age is not associated with toxicity leading to discontinuation of treatment in patients with urothelial non-muscle-invasive bladder cancer randomised to receive 3 years of maintenance bacille Calmette-Guérin: results from European Organisation for Research and Treatment of Cancer Genito-Urinary Group study 30911. BJU Int. 2016;118(3):423–8.

Prout GR Jr, Wesley MN, Yancik R, Ries LA, Havlik RJ, Edwards BK. Age and comorbidity impact surgical therapy in older bladder carcinoma patients: a population-based study. Cancer. 2005;104(8):1638–47.

Rose TL, Milowsky MI. Management of muscle-invasive bladder cancer in the elderly. Curr Opin Urol. 2015;25(5):459–67.

Saika T, Suyama B, Murata T, Manabe D, Kurashige T, Nasu Y, Tsushima T, Kumon H. Orthotopic neobladder reconstruction in elderly bladder cancer patients. Int J Urol. 2001;8(10):533–8.

Santacaterina A, Platania A, Palazzolo C, Spatola C, Acquaviva G, Crispi M, Privitera G, Settineri N, Pergolizzi S. Very elderly (>80 years), frail patients with muscle-invasive bladder cancer and comorbidities: is curative irradiation feasible? Tumori. 2015;101(6):609–13.

Soulié M, Straub M, Gamé X, Seguin P, De Petriconi R, Plante P, Hautmann RE. A multicenter study of the morbidity of radical cystectomy in select elderly patients with bladder cancer. J Urol. 2002;167(3):1325–8.

Spencer BA, McBride RB, Hershman DL, Buono D, Herr HW, Benson MC, Gupta-Mohile S, Neugut AI. Adjuvant intravesical bacillus calmette-guérin therapy and survival among elderly patients with non-muscle-invasive bladder cancer. J Oncol Pract. 2013;9(2):92–8.

Tran E, Souhami L, Tanguay S, Rajan R. Bladder conservation treatment in the elderly population: results and prognostic factors of muscle-invasive bladder cancer. Am J Clin Oncol. 2009;32(4):333–7.

Williams SB, Shan Y, Jazzar U, Mehta HB, Baillargeon JG, Huo J, Senagore AJ, Orihuela E, Tyler DS, Swanson TA, Kamat AM. Comparing survival outcomes and costs associated with radical cystectomy and trimodal therapy for older adults with muscle-invasive bladder cancer. JAMA Surg. 2018.

Chapter 60
Reviews Relating to Management of Bladder Cancer in the Elderly

60.1 Perioperative Assessment

Extrapolating the available evidence to the population of older patients with bladder cancer requires careful assessment of an individual patient's functional status and comorbidities to estimate the likelihood of treatment-related harms (Stensland and Galsky 2014). This should be coupled with an understanding of an individual patient's goals of therapy, independence, estimated longevity, and social support to facilitate a shared medical decision regarding treatment (Stensland and Galsky 2014). The use of validated approaches to geriatric assessment may refine risk stratification in older adults, although practical challenges have prevented uniform adoption in routine clinical practice (Stensland and Galsky 2014).

60.2 Radical Cystectomy

Total cystectomy is the reference treatment for infiltrating nonmetastatic bladder cancers. With the progress in anesthesia and postoperative intensive care, this treatment can be applied to a population of elderly subjects provided there is a strict oncological and geriatric evaluation of the patient (Quintens et al. 2009). Recent series reporting total cystectomies in subjects over 75 years of age report comparable morbidity and mortality rates to the general population. Strategies to preserve the vesical reservoir can be indicated in selected cases (Quintens et al. 2009). Thus, with multidisciplinary consensus and adapted management, elderly patients with significant comorbidities should not be automatically excluded from access to effective treatment of these cancers (Quintens et al. 2009).

© Springer Nature Switzerland AG 2020
S. S. Goonewardene et al., *Management of Non-Muscle Invasive Bladder Cancer*,
https://doi.org/10.1007/978-3-030-28646-0_60

60.3   Radical Cystectomy and Orthotopic Neobladders

The incidence of bladder cancer increases with advancing age (Froehner et al. 2009). Considering the increasing life expectancy and the increasing proportion of elderly people in the general population, radical cystectomy will be considered for a growing number of elderly patients who suffer from muscle-invasive or recurrent bladder cancer (Froehner et al. 2009). Perioperative morbidity and mortality are increased and continence rates after orthotopic urinary diversion are impaired in elderly patients undergoing radical cystectomy (Froehner et al. 2009). Complications are frequent in this population, particularly when an extended postoperative period (90 d instead of 30 d) is considered (Froehner et al. 2009). Although age alone does not preclude radical cystectomy for muscle-invasive or recurrent bladder cancer or for certain types of urinary diversion, careful surveillance is required, even after the first 30 d after surgery (Froehner et al. 2009). Excellent perioperative management may contribute to the prevention of morbidity and mortality of radical cystectomy, supplementary to the skills of the surgeon, and is probably a reason for the better perioperative results obtained in high-volume centers (Froehner et al. 2009).

60.4   Radiotherapy in the Elderly

Radiotherapy is a commonly employed modality in the treatment of older men with urologic malignancies. The treatment recommendations should not be solely based on age even though optimal therapy for older patients continues to evolve (Sandhu and Mundt 2009). Radiotherapy is well tolerated by elderly prostate cancer patients and comparisons with other modalities should incorporate validated health-related quality of life measures, which is an important consideration in this age group. Due to lack of quality data, there is a need to optimize decision making process for older prostate cancer patients with more robust evidence-based measures (Sandhu and Mundt 2009). The new and emerging radiotherapeutic technologies are likely to benefit older patients with improvement in therapeutic ratio resulting from reduced dose delivery to normal tissues. The use of novel techniques, such as intensity modulated radiation therapy, image guidance and proton beam therapy, and their potential benefits for older population are discussed (Sandhu and Mundt 2009). This article also reviews the role of radiotherapy in older patients with other urologic malignancies, such as testicular tumor, bladder cancer, renal carcinoma, and penile cancer.

60.5 Conclusions

Patients over the age of 70 years will become an increasingly important component of uro-oncologic practice. Although few published studies have specifically addressed this population, it is clear that the elderly can expect outcomes similar to younger patients in the management of advanced bladder cancer provided care is taken in planning. Of particular importance is an understanding of the pathophysiology of aging, of the possible implications of the causative factors for bladder cancer, and of the potential impact of advanced age on the biology of urothelial malignancy. Future studies should specifically address the problems of older patients with this malignancy to ensure the optimal possible outcome and definition of the most appropriate balance of toxicity and efficacy. Cystectomy appears to be reasonable in elderly people who have a life expectancy of more than 2 years, provided that a rigorous pre-operative assessment and anaesthetic management are performed. Transurethral resection alone should be proposed only to patients with poor health status and/or very advanced age. Although radical cystectomy remains the treatment of choice for muscle invasive bladder cancer, it has a well-recognized risk of perioperative complications and mortality.

References

Froehner M, Brausi MA, Herr HW, Muto G, Studer UE. Complications following radical cystectomy for bladder cancer in the elderly. Eur Urol. 2009;56(3):443–54.

Quintens H, Guy L, Mazerolles C, Théodore C, Amsellem D, Roupret M, Wallerand H, Roy C, Saint F, Bernardini S, Lebret T, Soulié M, Pfister C. Treatment of infiltrating nonmetastatic bladder cancers in elderly patients. Prog Urol. 2009;19(Suppl. 3):S135–41.

Rose TL, Milowsky MI. Management of muscle-invasive bladder cancer in the elderly. Curr Opin Urol. 2015;25(5):459–67.

Sandhu A, Mundt AJ. Radiation therapy for urologic malignancies in the elderly. Urol Oncol. 2009;27(6):643–52.

Stensland KD, Galsky MD. Current approaches to the management of bladder cancer in older patients. Am Soc Clin Oncol Educ Book. 2014:e250–6.

Chapter 61
Female Outcomes in Bladder Cancer

Stein et al. compared oncological outcomes in women undergoing radical cystectomy and orthotopic diversion for bladder transitional cell carcinoma (Stein et al. 2009). Overall 3 of 120 women (2.5%) who received a neobladder died perioperatively. In this group the tumor was pathologically organ confined in 73 patients (61%), extravesical in 18 (15%) and lymph node positive in 29 (24%). Overall 5 and 10-year recurrence-free survival was 62% and 55%, respectively (Stein et al. 2009). Five and 10-year recurrence-free survival in patients with organ confined and extravesical disease was similar at 75% and 67%, and 71% and 71%, respectively (Stein et al. 2009). Patients with lymph node positive disease had significantly worse 5 and 10-year recurrence free survival (24% and 19%, respectively). One woman had recurrence in the urethra and 2 (1.7%) had local recurrence. As stratified by pathological subgroups, similar outcomes were observed when comparing women with an orthotopic neobladder to the 81 who underwent cutaneous diversion (Stein et al. 2009). Orthotopic diversion does not compromise the oncological outcome in women after radical cystectomy for bladder transitional cell carcinoma (Stein et al. 2009). This demonstrates excellent local and urethral control may be expected. Women with node positive disease are at highest risk for recurrence. Similar outcomes were observed in women undergoing cutaneous diversion.

On study examined radical cystectomy (RC) series, female sexual dysfunction and whether the type of diversion affected the occurrence of sexual dysfunction (Zippe et al. 2004). Outcome data after RC with and without orthotopic diversion has focused primarily on cure, urethral recurrence, and continence.

With a mean follow-up of 24.2 months (range 15–65.1), the total mean baseline Index of Female Sexual Function score decreased from 17.4 ± 7.23 to 10.6 ± 6.62 after RC ($p <$ or $= 0.05$) (Zippe et al. 2004). The most common symptoms reported by the patients included diminished ability or inability to achieve orgasm in 12 (45%), decreased lubrication in 11 (41%), decreased sexual desire in 10 (37%), and dyspareunia in 6 patients (22%). Only 13 (48%) of the 27 patients were able

© Springer Nature Switzerland AG 2020
S. S. Goonewardene et al., *Management of Non-Muscle Invasive Bladder Cancer*,
https://doi.org/10.1007/978-3-030-28646-0_61

to have successful vaginal intercourse, with 14 (52%) reporting decreased satisfaction in overall sexual life after RC (Zippe et al. 2004). Eight partners (30%) had a decrease in desire for sexual activity owing to apprehension after cancer diagnosis and treatment. Although the numbers were small, the preliminary data suggested no differences in sexual function between patients undergoing Studor orthotopic diversions and those undergoing Indiana cutaneous diversions. Sexual dysfunction is a prevalent problem after female RC (Zippe et al. 2004). The nature of the dysfunction involves multiple domains, including decreased orgasm, decreased lubrication, lack of sexual desire, and dyspareunia. Our early results suggest that the type of continent diversion does not affect sexual function (Zippe et al. 2004). Surgical modifications such as urethral and vaginal sparing, neurovascular preservation, and tubular vaginal reconstruction sparing may improve female sexual function after RC.

Orthotopic urinary diversion is a feasible and optimal technique for many women undergoing cystectomy (Lee et al. 2004). Although successful outcomes have been achieved, groups at most centers have strict selection criteria. Lee et al. evaluated experience with female orthotopic diversion in traditional and nontraditional candidates. Complications were detected in 20 patients, including 9 who were traditional (23%) and 11 who were nontraditional (50%) (Lee et al. 2004). Daytime and nighttime continence was reported by 46 (87%) and 45 (85%) patients, respectively, of whom 11 (21%) required intermittent catheterization. Of the patients with cancer 42 were disease-free, 2 were alive with disease and 6 died of disease (Lee et al. 2004). The nontraditional subset was older ($p < 0.0003$) and had shorter followup ($p = 0.05$), a higher American Society of Anesthesiologists score ($p = 0.01$) and a shorter overall survival ($p = 0.001$) than the traditional group. Continence was seen in 19 of 22 nontraditional patients (86%) and 4 (18%) required intermittent catheterization. This demonstrates orthotopic neobladder diversion offers excellent clinical and functional results, and should be the diversion of choice in most women following cystectomy. A subset of less favorable candidates can also successfully undergo orthotopic substitution with a tolerable toxicity profile.

References

Lee CT, Hafez KS, Sheffield JH, Joshi DP, Montie JE. Orthotopic bladder substitution in women: nontraditional applications. J Urol. 2004;171(4):1585–158.

Stein JP, Penson DF, Lee C, Cai J, Miranda G, Skinner DG. Long-term oncological outcomes in women undergoing radical cystectomy and orthotopic diversion for bladder cancer. J Urol. 2009;181(5):2052–9.

Zippe CD, Raina R, Shah AD, Massanyi EZ, Agarwal A, Ulchaker J, Jones S, Klein E. Female sexual dysfunction after radical cystectomy: a new outcome measure. Urology. 2004;63:1153–7.

Chapter 62
A Systematic Review on Bladder Cancer and Female Gender

A systematic review relating to bladder cancer and female gender was conducted. The search strategy aimed to identify all references related to bladder cancer AND female gender. Search terms used were as follows: (Bladder cancer) AND (female gender). The following databases were screened from 1989 to June 2019:

- CINAHL
- MEDLINE (NHS Evidence)
- Cochrane
- AMed
- EMBASE
- PsychINFO
- SCOPUS
- Web of Science.

In addition, searches using Medical Subject Headings (MeSH) and keywords were conducted using Cochrane databases. Two UK-based experts in bladder cancer were consulted to identify any additional studies.

Studies were eligible for inclusion if they reported primary research focusing on bladder cancer and female gender. Papers were included if published after 1984 and had to be in English. Studies that did not conform to this were excluded. Only primary research was included. The overall aim was to identify the role and components of bladder cancer screening.

Abstracts were independently screened for eligibility by two reviewers and disagreements resolved through discussion or third party opinion (Fig. 62.1). Agreement level was calculated using Cohen's Kappa to test the intercoder reliability of this screening process. Cohens' Kappa allows comparison of inter-rater reliability between papers using relative observed agreement. This also takes account of the comparison occurring by chance. The first reviewer agreed all 11 papers to be included, the second, agreed on 11.

© Springer Nature Switzerland AG 2020
S. S. Goonewardene et al., *Management of Non-Muscle Invasive Bladder Cancer*,
https://doi.org/10.1007/978-3-030-28646-0_62

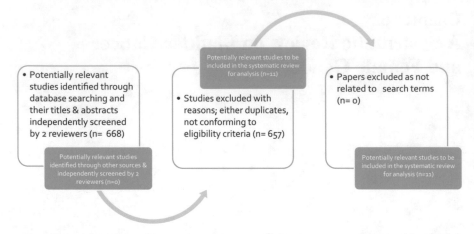

Fig. 62.1 Flow chart of studies identified through the systematic review (adapted from PRISMA)

Data extraction was piloted by the researcher and amended in consultation with the research team (author and two academic supervisors). Data collected included authors, year and country of publication, study aims, setting, intervention aims, number of participants, study design, intervention components and delivery methods, comparison groups and outcome measures, notes and follow-up questions for the authors. Studies were quality assessed using the PRISMA criteria for randomised controlled trials, Mays et al. (Moher et al. 2009; Moher, Liberati et al. 2009, 154, 153; Mays et al. 2005) for the action research and qualitative studies and the Critical Skills Appraisal programme for cohort studies. This was also applied to randomised controlled trials and qualitative studies. All studies were cohort studies.

References

Mays N, Pope C, Popay J. Systematically reviewing qualitative and quantitative evidence to inform management and policy-making in the health field. J Health Serv Res Policy. 2005;10(Suppl. 1):6–20.

Moher D, Liberati A, Tetzlaff J, Altman DG. Preferred reporting items for systematic reviews and meta-analyses: the prisma statement. BMJ. 2009;339(7716):332–6.

Chapter 63
Systematic Review Results on Bladder Cancer and Female Gender

63.1 Female Gender Impact on Presentation of Bladder Cancer

Sex, race, and age at diagnosis have a significant impact on mortality from bladder cancer (BC) (Scosyrev et al. 2009). The Surveillance, Epidemiology, and End Results (SEER) database was reviewed for the presentations and outcomes from BC between 1990 and 2005 (Scosyrev et al. 2009). Excess hazard of death from BC was present during the first 2 to 3 years of follow-up among women and during the first 4 years of follow-up (Scosyrev et al. 2009). Significant differences in tumor characteristics and age at presentation did not fully account for the excess hazard of death from BC among women (Scosyrev et al. 2009).

Aziz analyzed gender-specific differences regarding clinical symptoms, referral patterns and tumor biology prior to initial diagnosis of urothelial carcinoma of the bladder (UCB) (Aziz et al. 2015). In total, 68 patients (50 men, 18 women) with newly diagnosed UCB at admission for transurethral resection of bladder tumors were recruited. Dysuria was more often observed in women (55.6% vs. 38.0%, $p = 0.001$) (Aziz et al. 2015). Direct consultation of the urologist was conducted by 84.0% of males and 66.7% of females ($p = 0.120$). One third of the women saw their general practitioner and/or gynecologist once or twice ($p = 0.120$) before referral to the urologist (Aziz et al. 2015). Furthermore, women were significantly more often treated for urinary tract infections than men (61.1% vs. 20.0%, $p = 0.005$). Cystoscopy at first presentation to the urologist was more often performed in men than women (88.0% vs. 66.7%, $p = 0.068$), with a more favorable tumor detection rate at first cystoscopy in men (96.0% vs. 50.0%, $p < 0.001$) (Aziz et al. 2015).

Henning evaluated gender-dependent disparities regarding clinical symptoms, referral patterns or treatments before diagnosis of urothelial carcinoma of the bladder (UCB) (Henning et al. 2013). In men ($n = 130$) the distribution of tumour

© Springer Nature Switzerland AG 2020
S. S. Goonewardene et al., *Management of Non-Muscle Invasive Bladder Cancer*,
https://doi.org/10.1007/978-3-030-28646-0_63

stages was pTa 62.3%, pT1 23.1% and pT ≥2 12.3%. The respective percentages in women ($n = 38$) were pTa 57.9%, pT1 23.7% and pT ≥2 18.4% ($p > 0.05$) (Henning et al. 2013). A total of 78% of men versus 55% of women directly consulted a urologist ($p < 0.05$) (Henning et al. 2013). Symptomatic treatment for voiding disorders/pain was given without further evaluation to 19% of men versus 47% of women 1 year before the diagnosis of UCB ($p < 0.05$) (Henning et al. 2013). A total of 3.8% of men versus 15.8% of women received three or more treatments for urinary tract infections (UTIs) within the same time period ($p < 0.05$) (Henning et al. 2013). Women were more likely to be treated for voiding complaints or alleged UTIs without further evaluation or referral to urology than men (Henning et al. 2013). Gender-dependent disparities in referral patterns exist and might delay definitive diagnosis of UCB in women.

Garg assessed gender differences in hematuria evaluation in older adults with bladder cancer (Garg et al. 2014). Of 35,646 patients with a hematuria claim in the year preceding bladder cancer diagnosis 97% had a urology visit claim (Garg et al. 2014). Mean time to urology visit was 27 days (range 0 to 377). Time to urology visit was longer for women than for men (adjusted HR 0.9, 95% CI 0.87–0.92). Women were more likely to undergo delayed (after greater than 30 days) hematuria evaluation (adjusted OR 1.13, 95% CI 1.07–1.21) (Garg et al. 2014).

63.2   Prognostic Factors on Female Bladder Cancer

Tracey, investigated factors that most influenced survival from bladder cancer in New South Wales, Australia (NSW) (Tracey et al. 2009). The likelihood of death was 11% (95% confidence interval, CI 5–18%) higher in females than in males, with case fatality most influenced by age at diagnosis, extent of disease, and histological type) (Tracey et al. 2009). The likelihood of death was 13% (95% CI 5–21%) higher in females than in males (Tracey et al. 2009). The analysis shows significantly lower survival from bladder cancer in NSW women compared with men, with no improvement in survival from 1980 to 2003 (Tracey et al. 2009).

63.3   Female Gender and Advanced Bladder Cancer Outcomes

Women with advanced bladder cancer have inferior survival compared with men. However, women treated on clinical trials do not appear to have a survival disadvantage (Rose et al. 2016). Less frequent administration of systemic chemotherapy in women with advanced bladder cancer may contribute to their inferior survival (Rose et al. 2016). A total of 23,981 patients were identified (35% of whom were female). Compared with men, women were older, more likely to be black, and less likely to be insured ($p < 0.01$ for all). The Charlson-Deyo comorbidity score did not differ between men and women (Rose et al. 2016). Women were less likely to receive systemic chemotherapy than men (45% vs. 52%; adjusted relative risk, 0.91 [95% confidence interval (95% CI), 0.88–0.94]) . Women had a lower median OS compared with men (8.0 months [95% CI, 7.7–8.3 months] vs. 9.8 months [95% CI, 9.5–10.0 months]; $p<0.001$) (Rose et al. 2016). OS remained lower for women on multivariable analysis, even after adjusting for the administration of systemic chemotherapy (hazard ratio for death, 1.11 [95% CI, 1.08–1.15]) (Rose et al. 2016). Women are less likely than men to receive systemic chemotherapy for advanced bladder remains lower in women independent of chemotherapy use, and may be related to unmeasured comorbidities, functional status, or tumor biology. Cancer 2016; 122:2012–20. © 2016 American Cancer Society.

63.4   Management of Bladder Cancer in Females

Thorstenson reviewed treatments and survival in patients with urinary bladder cancer (UBC) in a national population-based cohort, with special reference to gender-related differences (Thorstenson et al. 2016). A larger proportion of women than men had stage T2–T4 ($p < 0.001$), and women also had more G1 tumours ($p < 0.001$) (Thorstenson et al. 2016). However, compared to women, a larger proportion of men with carcinoma in situ or T1G3 received intravesical treatment with bacillus Calmette-Guérin or intravesical chemotherapy, and a larger proportion of men with stage T2–T4 underwent radical cystectomy (38% men vs. 33% women, $p < 0.0001$) (Thorstenson et al. 2016). The cancer-specific survival at 5 years was 77% for men and 72% for women ($p < 0.001$), and the relative survival at 5 years was 72% for men and 69% for women ($p < 0.001$) (Thorstenson et al. 2016). In this population-based cohort comprising virtually all patients diagnosed with UBC in Sweden between 1997 and 2011, female gender was associated with inferior cancer-specific and relative survival (Thorstenson et al. 2016). Although women had a higher rate of aggressive tumours, a smaller proportion of women than men received optimal treatment (Thorstenson et al. 2016).

63.5   Female Gender Impact on Post Operative Radical Cystectomy Recovery

The oncological basis behind the observation that females experience worse outcomes following radical cystectomy for urothelial carcinoma of the bladder (UCB) is unclear (Mitra et al. 2014). Mitra examined the impact of gender on postcystectomy UCB outcomes and identifying potential factors (Mitra et al. 2014). Median follow-up for cases, controls, and independent control cohort was 12.2, 8.6, and

13.5 years, respectively. Females were matched to male controls for tumor and nodal stages ($p = 1.00$), lymphovascular invasion and surgical margin status, age, prior intravesical treatment, and neoadjuvant and adjuvant chemotherapy administration ($p = 0.61–1.00$) (Mitra et al. 2014). When compared with an independent unmatched male control cohort, females had significantly poorer outcomes ($p \leq 0.006$). In this comparison, females presented with higher tumor ($p < 0.001$) and nodal ($p = 0.049$) stages and a lesser proportion received precystectomy intravesical therapy ($p = 0.032$) (Mitra et al. 2014). Females have similar UCB outcomes to males when matched for demographic, clinicopathologic, and management characteristics. However, they present with more advanced tumors, thus explaining the observation of poor outcomes.

63.6   Complications from Urinary Diversion in Females

Gschliesser analysed an online database was developed that included patient demographics, intra/perioperative data, surgical data and in-house complications (Gschliesser et al. 2017). Four hundred fifty-eight patients (112 [24.5%] women and 346 [75.5%] men) were analysed. Men and women were comparable regarding age (mean 68 years), body mass index (mean 26.5) and the mean Charlson score (4.8). Women had more advanced tumour-stages (pT3/pT4; women: 57.1%; men: 48.1%) (Gschliesser et al. 2017). The rate of incontinent urinary diversion was higher in women (83.1%) than in men (60.2%) and in a multivariate analysis, the strongest predictors were M+status (OR 11.2), female gender (OR 6.9) and age (OR 6.5). Women had a higher intraoperative blood transfusion rate (Gschliesser et al. 2017). The overall rate of in-house complications was similar in both genders (men: 32.0%, women: 32.6%). Severe (Clavien-Dindo grade >2) medical (women: 6.3%; men: 5.2%) and surgical (women: 21.5%; men: 14.4%) in-house complications, however, were more frequent in women (Gschliesser et al. 2017). This multicentre registry demonstrates several gender-related differences in patients undergoing radical cystectomy. The higher transfusion rate, the rare use of orthotopic bladder substitutes and the higher in-house complication rate underline the higher complexity of this procedure in women.

63.7   Bladder Cancer Outcomes and Female Gender

May assessed the impact of detailed clinical and histopathological criteria on gender-dependent cancer-specific survival (CSS) in a large consecutive series of patients following radical cystectomy (RCE) for muscle-invasive bladder cancer (MIBC) (May et al. 2012). Among clinical and histopathological parameters, only type of urinary diversion differed between men and women (May et al. 2012). In multivariable Cox-regression analysis, advanced pT-stage (HR = 2.12; $p < 0.001$), lymphovascular invasion (LVI) (HR = 3.47; $p < 0.001$), time interval between diagnosis of MIBC and RCE exceeding 90 days (HR = 2.07; $p < 0.001$) and female gender (HR = 1.35; $p = 0.048$) were related to reduced CSS. In separate multivariable Cox-models for time period of surgery between 1992 an 1999 (HR = 1.52; $p = 0.050$), age ≤ 55 years (HR = 3.00; $p = 0.022$), presence of LVI (HR = 1.45; $p = 0.031$) and female gender were associated with independent reduced CSS (May et al. 2012). Established clinical and histopathological parameters do not differ significantly between both genders in the present series. Reduced CSS in women is present in historic cohorts possibly suggesting improvement in management over the last years (May et al. 2012). In particular, female gender has a significant negative impact on CSS in patients younger of age and with positive LVI status possibly suggesting different clinical phenotypes (May et al. 2012).

63.8 Mortality Outcomes in Female Bladder Cancer

Noon, 2013 determined the bladder cancer-specific mortality (CSM) rate and other-cause mortality (OCM) rate for patients with newly diagnosed BC (Noon et al. 2013). At 5 years after diagnosis, 1246 (40%) patients were dead: 617 (19%) from BC and 629 (19%) from other causes (Noon et al. 2013). The 5-year BC mortality rate varied between 1 and 59%, and OCM rate between 6 and 90%, depending primarily on the tumour type and patient age (Noon et al. 2013). Cancer-specific mortality was highest in the oldest patient groups. Few elderly patients received radical treatment for invasive cancer (52% vs. 12% for patients <60 vs. >80 years, respectively). Female patients with high-risk non-muscle-invasive BC had worse CSM than equivalent males (Gray's $p < 0.01$) (Noon et al. 2013). Bladder CSM is highest among the elderly. Female patients with high-risk tumours are more likely to die of their disease compared with male patients. Clinicians should consider offering more aggressive treatment interventions among older patients.

References

Aziz A, Madersbacher S, Otto W, Mayr R, Comploj E, Pycha A, Denzinger S, Fritsche HM, Burger M, Gierth M. Comparative analysis of gender-related differences in symptoms and referral patterns prior to initial diagnosis of urothelial carcinoma of the bladder: a prospective cohort study. Urol Int. 2015;94(1):37–44.

Garg T, Pinheiro LC, Atoria CL, Donat SM, Weissman JS, Herr HW, Elkin EB. Gender disparities in hematuria evaluation and bladder cancer diagnosis: a population based analysis. J Urol. 2014;192(4):1072–7.

Gschliesser T, Eredics K, Berger I, Szelinger M, Klingler HC, Colombo T, Ponholzer A, Plas E, Grubmüller K, Dunzinger M, Jeschke K, Würnschimmel E, Krause FS, Shariat S, Leeb K, Pelzer A, Riedl C, Rauchenwald M, Hübner W, Brössner C, Madersbacher S, Cystectomy Registry of the Austrian Society of Urology. The impact of gender on tumour stage in in-house complications and choice of urinary diversion: results of the Austrian cystectomy registry. Urol Int. 2017;99(4):429–35.

Henning A, Wehrberger M, Madersbacher S, Pycha A, Martini T, Comploj E, Jeschke K, Tripolt C, Rauchenwald M. Do differences in clinical symptoms and referral patterns contribute to the gender gap in bladder cancer? BJU Int. 2013;112(1):68–73.

May M, Stief C, Brookman-May S, Otto W, Gilfrich C, Roigas J, Zacharias M, Wieland WF, Fritsche HM, Hofstädter F, Burger M. Gender-dependent cancer-specific survival following radical cystectomy. World J Urol. 2012;30(5):707–13.

Mitra AP, Skinner EC, Schuckman AK, Quinn DI, Dorff TB, Daneshmand S. Effect of gender on outcomes following radical cystectomy for urothelial carcinoma of the bladder: a critical analysis of 1,994 patients. Urol Oncol. 2014;32(1):52.e1–9.

Noon AP, Albertsen PC, Thomas F, Rosario DJ, Catto JW. Competing mortality in patients diagnosed with bladder cancer: evidence of undertreatment in the elderly and female patients. Br J Cancer. 2013;108(7):1534–40.

Rose TL, Deal AM, Nielsen ME, Smith AB, Milowsky MI. Sex disparities in use of chemotherapy and survival in patients with advanced bladder cancer. Cancer. 2016;122(13):2012–20.

Scosyrev E, Noyes K, Feng C, Messing E. Sex and racial differences in bladder cancer presentation and mortality in the US. Cancer. 2009;115(1):68–74.

Thorstenson A, Hagberg O, Ljungberg B, Liedberg F, Jancke G, Holmäng S, Malmström PU, Hosseini A, Jahnson S. Gender-related differences in urothelial carcinoma of the bladder: a population-based study from the Swedish National Registry of Urinary Bladder Cancer. Scand J Urol. 2016;50(4):292–7.

Tracey E, Roder D, Luke C, Bishop J. Bladder cancer survivals in New South Wales, Australia: why do women have poorer survival than men? BJU Int. 2009;104(4):498–504.

Chapter 64
Reviews on Female Gender and Bladder Cancer

Women are generally less likely to develop bladder cancer compared with men; however, once they acquire this disease, they have a less favorable prognosis (Scosyrev et al. 2010). Scosyrev et al. (2010) reviewed the relationship between sex and bladder cancer incidence. Despite some evidence suggesting involvement of hormonal factors in bladder cancer carcinogenesis, the exact mechanisms responsible for increased bladder cancer incidence in men are still incompletely understood (Scosyrev et al. 2010). The causes of increased mortality in women are also unclear. It has been hypothesized that women present with more advanced stages (and thus have inferior survival) than men because early signs of bladder cancer in women are often attributed to more common benign conditions (Scosyrev et al. 2010). However, recent studies have shown that excess mortality in women persists after adjustment for stage and other tumor characteristics. Women also do not appear to be significantly undertreated for bladder cancer (Scosyrev et al. 2010). Despite considerable research efforts, both increased incidence in men and decreased survival in women remain somewhat of a mystery. The causes of these phenomena may include poorly understood biological factors or environmental influences, which may become a subject of future research.

Fajkovic reviewed the literature on the effect of gender on bladder cancer incidence, biology, mortality, and treatment (Fajkovic et al. 2011). Although men are nearly 3–4 times more likely to develop bladder cancer than women, women present with more advanced disease and have worse survival (Fajkovic et al. 2011). Recently, a number of population-based and multicenter collaborative studies have shown that female gender is associated with a significantly higher rate of cancer-specific recurrence and mortality after radical cystectomy (Fajkovic et al. 2011). The disparity between genders is proposed to be the result of a differences exposure to carcinogens (i.e., tobacco and chemicals) as well as reflective of genetic, anatomic, hormonal, societal, and environmental factors (Fajkovic et al. 2011). Explanations for the differential behavior of bladder cancer between genders include sex steroids and their receptors as well as inferior quality of care

© Springer Nature Switzerland AG 2020
S. S. Goonewardene et al., *Management of Non-Muscle Invasive Bladder Cancer*,
https://doi.org/10.1007/978-3-030-28646-0_64

for women (inpatient length of stay, referral patterns, and surgical outcomes) (Fajkovic et al. 2011). It is imperative that health care practitioners and researchers from disparate disciplines collectively focus efforts to appropriately develop gender-specific evidence-based guidelines for bladder cancer patients. MDT collaborative efforts to provide tailored gender-specific care for bladder cancer patients must be developed.

Dobruch reviewed the literature on potential biologic mechanisms underlying differential gender risk for bladder cancer, and evidence regarding gender disparities in bladder cancer presentation, management, and outcomes (Dobruch et al. 2016). It has been shown that the gender difference in bladder cancer incidence is independent of differences in exposure risk, including smoking status. Potential molecular mechanisms include disparate metabolism of carcinogens by hepatic enzymes between men and women, resulting in differential exposure of the urothelium to carcinogens (Dobruch et al. 2016). In addition, the activity of the sex steroid hormone pathway may play a role in bladder cancer development, with demonstration that both androgens and estrogens have biologic effects in bladder cancer in vitro and in vivo. Importantly, gender differences exist in the timeliness and completeness of hematuria evaluation, with women experiencing a significantly greater delay in urologic referral and undergoing guideline-concordant imaging less frequently (Dobruch et al. 2016). Correspondingly, women have more advanced tumors at the time of bladder cancer diagnosis. Interestingly, higher cancer-specific mortality has been noted among women even after adjusting for tumor stage and treatment modality (Dobruch et al. 2016).

References

Dobruch J, Daneshmand S, Fisch M, Lotan Y, Noon AP, Resnick MJ, Shariat SF, Zlotta AR, Boorjian SA. Gender and bladder cancer: a collaborative review of etiology, biology, and outcomes. Eur Urol. 2016;69(2):300–10.
Fajkovic H, Halpern JA, Cha EK, Bahadori A, Chromecki TF, Karakiewicz PI, Breinl E, Merseburger AS, Shariat SF. Impact of gender on bladder cancer incidence, staging, and prognosis. World J Urol. 2011;29(4):457–63.
Scosyrev E, Trivedi D, Messing E. Female bladder cancer: incidence, treatment, and outcome. Curr Opin Urol. 2010;20(5):404–8.

Part IX
Bladder Cancer Survivorship

Chapter 65
Definition of Bladder Cancer Survivorship

The definition of cancer survivorship is varied. Survivorship is defined by Macmillan Cancer Support (Maher 2013), as 'someone who has completed initial cancer management with no evidence of apparent disease'. According to the National Cancer Institute in the USA, cancer survivorship encompasses the "physical, psychosocial, and economic issues of cancer from diagnosis until the end of life". The National Coalition of Cancer Survivors defines being a survivor as 'from diagnosis of cancer onwards'. This has been extended to include 'the experience of living with, through and beyond a diagnosis'.

Bladder cancer (BC) is a common disease with a variety of treatment options and a range of outcomes (Edmondson et al. 2017). Despite the disease's high prevalence, not much is known of Survivorship patient experience in bladder cancer (Edmondson et al. 2017). National patient experience surveys suggest patients with bladder cancer have poorer experiences than those with other common cancers (Edmondson et al. 2017). Delays may occur in diagnosis, many do not present in a timely manner. Additionally, learning how to cope with a 'post-surgery body', changing sexuality and incontinence are distressing (Edmondson et al. 2017). Much less is known about survivorship in patients receiving Bacillus Calmette-Guerin (BCG).

Seo and Langabeer (2018), discovered survivorship disparities were ubiquitous across age, sex, race/ethnicity, and marital status groups (Seo and Langabeer 2018). Non-white, unmarried, and elderly patients had significantly shorter survivorship time periods (Seo and Langabeer 2018). This highlights the need for focus on specific groups.

Survivors of muscle invasive bladder cancer (MIBC) experience physical and psychosocial side effects (Rammant et al. 2017). There is significant research lacking into this region. This impacts significantly on patient reported outcome measures. To date, there is evidence that rehabilitation interventions such as physical activity and psychosocial support have a positive effect on the HRQoL of cancer survivors (Rammant et al. 2017). Unfortunately, there are no specific guidelines for rehabilitation or survivorship programmes for MIBC survivors (Rammant et al. 2017).

© Springer Nature Switzerland AG 2020
S. S. Goonewardene et al., *Management of Non-Muscle Invasive Bladder Cancer*,
https://doi.org/10.1007/978-3-030-28646-0_65

References

Edmondson AJ, Birtwistle JC, Catto JWF, Twiddy M. The patients' experience of a bladder cancer diagnosis: a systematic review of the qualitative evidence. J Cancer Surviv. 2017;11(4):453–61.

Maher EJ. Managing the consequences of cancer treatment and the English National Cancer Survivorship Initiative. Acta Oncol. 2013;52(2):225–32.

Rammant E, Bultijnck R, Sundahl N, Ost P, Pauwels NS, Deforche B, Pieters R, Decaestecker K, Fonteyne V. Rehabilitation interventions to improve patient-reported outcomes and physical fitness in survivors of muscle invasive bladder cancer: a systematic review protocol. BMJ Open. 2017;7(5):e016054.

Seo M, Langabeer II JR. Demographic and survivorship disparities in non-muscle-invasive bladder cancer in the United States. J Prev Med Public Health. 2018;51(5):242–7.

Chapter 66
The Impact of Bladder Cancer Survivorship

Cystectomy has advanced to the point where, at its most sophisticated level, the procedure is robotic with intra-corporeal ileal conduit formation or even neobladder formation. Minimally invasive approaches have advantages such as reduced blood loss, postoperative pain, quicker recovery of bowel function and earlier convalescence. As such they contribute favourably interns of survivorship in bladder cancer. Firstly, patient time spent in hospital is reduced to allow greater enjoyment of slier return to health in the community. Secondly, long term complications with wound pain, herniation, incontinence etc. are less likely to occur with a lowered readmission and clinical intervention rate leading to better quality of (remaining) life and survivorship outside of a clonal environment.

In the same way, we think of the trifecta of post radical prostatectomy as oncological outcomes, erectile function and continence, we should think of the 'trifecta,' of bladder cancer outcomes similarly encompassing oncological outcome, continence/urinary diversion complications and sexual function.

Health-related quality of life and self-esteem have been improved following orthotopic bladder substitutions. These are the preferred method for urinary reconstruction post-cystectomy in younger, motivated and informed patients. Both in men and in women, orthotopic neobladder should be considered as often, the preferred choice, with excellent long-term oncologic and functional outcome. Now we can offer this procedure entirely minimally invasively and intracorporeally we should embrace the opportunity in terms of improving health related quality of life as well as survival.

Additionally, because bladder cancer patients tend to be of an older age group sexual counselling, is not often offered, but is an 'ageist' phenomenon that we can be potentially criticised for as urologists. These considerations should be taken forward by upcoming generations of surgeons who should embrace the new technology hand in hand with the principles of Survivorship.

© Springer Nature Switzerland AG 2020
S. S. Goonewardene et al., *Management of Non-Muscle Invasive Bladder Cancer*,
https://doi.org/10.1007/978-3-030-28646-0_66

Chapter 67
Unmet Needs in Bladder Cancer Survivorship

Bladder cancer is a large and unmet need. A bladder cancer think tank identified areas for development including (1) the development of a survivorship care plan for early and late-stage bladder cancer; (2) the development of consensus criteria for eligibility and endpoints for bladder cancer clinical trials; (3) an improved understanding of current practice patterns regarding the use of perioperative chemotherapy in an effort to standardize care; (4) creation of a comprehensive handbook to assist researchers with developing bladder cancer databases; and (5) identification of response to therapy of high-grade non muscle invasive disease through a collaborative exchange of expertise and resources (Svatek et al. 2013).

Little is known about the unmet supportive care needs of patients affected by muscle invasive bladder cancer (MIBC) (Paterson et al. 2018). Paterson examined individual unmet needs: patient-clinician communication, daily living needs, health system/information needs, practical needs, family-related needs, social needs, psychological needs, physical needs and intimacy needs (Paterson et al. 2018). Patients reported high unmet needs at diagnosis and into survivorship. Existing studies indicated needs commonly related to intimacy, informational, physical and psychological needs (Paterson et al. 2018).

Assessing the unmet needs of cancer patients can help providers tailor health care services to patients' specific needs (Mohammed et al. 2016). Mohammed examined whether the unmet informational and supportive care needs of the patients with muscle-invasive bladder cancer vary by the patients' age, sex, or individual treatment choices (Mohammed et al. 2016). This study demonstrated unmet informational and supportive needs of patients with muscle-invasive bladder cancer during survivorship (Mohammed et al. 2016). This also demonstrated survivorship care needs vary by age, sex, and treatment choices (Mohammed et al. 2016). Educational and psychological assessments as well as clinical interventions should individually tailored.

Brearley identified four main gaps in knowledge relating to the practical and physical problems (Brearley et al. 2011). These are key symptoms, unmet

© Springer Nature Switzerland AG 2020
S. S. Goonewardene et al., *Management of Non-Muscle Invasive Bladder Cancer*,
https://doi.org/10.1007/978-3-030-28646-0_67

supportive care needs, employment and older cancer survivors, and should be addressed by future research and systematic literature reviews (Brearley et al. 2011). Work is also needed to address the nomenclature of survivorship and to improve the methodology of research into cancer survivors (including standardised measures, theoretical frameworks, longitudinal design, inclusion of older survivors and age-matched controls for comparison) (Brearley et al. 2011). The review highlighted the need for better research within the identified areas in order to improve the experiences of cancer survivors (Brearley et al. 2011).

References

Brearley SG, Stamataki Z, Addington-Hall J, Foster C, Hodges L, Jarrett N, Richardson A, Scott I, Sharpe M, Stark D, Siller C, Ziegler L, Amir Z. The physical and practical problems experienced by cancer survivors: a rapid review and synthesis of the literature. Eur J Oncol Nurs. 2011;15(3):204–12.

Mohamed NE, Pisipati S, Lee CT, Goltz HH, Latini DM, Gilbert FS, Wittmann D, Knauer CJ, Mehrazin R, Sfakianos JP, McWilliams GW, Quale DZ, Hall SJ. Unmet informational and supportive care needs of patients following cystectomy for bladder cancer based on age, sex, and treatment choices. Urol Oncol. 2016;34(12):531.

Paterson C, Jensen BT, Jensen JB, Nabi G. Unmet informational and supportive care needs of patients with muscle invasive bladder cancer: a systematic review of the evidence. Eur J Oncol Nurs. 2018;35:92–101.

Svatek RS, Rosenberg JE, Galsky MD, Lee CT, Latini DM, Bochner BH, Weizer AZ, et al. Summary of the 6th annual bladder cancer think tank: new directions in urologic research. Urol Oncol. 2013;31(7):968–73.

Chapter 68
Systematic Review—Bladder Cancer Survivorship—Unmet Needs

A systematic review relating to literature on survivorship programmes for men with bladder cancer and screening was conducted. This was to identify the role of screening in bladder cancer and also the components of a survivorship programme. The search strategy aimed to identify all references related to bladder cancer AND Survivorship and Unmet needs. Search terms used were as follows: (Bladder cancer) AND (unmet needs) and survivorship. The following databases were screened from 1989 to June 2019:

- CINAHL
- MEDLINE (NHS Evidence)
- Cochrane
- AMed
- EMBASE
- PsychINFO
- SCOPUS
- Web of Science.

In addition, searches using Medical Subject Headings (MeSH) and keywords were conducted using Cochrane databases. Two UK-based experts in bladder cancer were consulted to identify any additional studies.

Studies were eligible for inclusion if they reported primary research focusing on bladder cancer and screening. Papers were included if published after 1984 and had to be in English. Studies that did not conform to this were excluded. Only primary research was included. The overall aim was to identify the role and components of bladder cancer screening.

Abstracts were independently screened for eligibility by two reviewers and disagreements resolved through discussion or third party opinion. Agreement level was calculated using Cohen's Kappa to test the intercoder reliability of this screening process. Cohens' Kappa allows comparison of inter-rater reliability between papers using relative observed agreement. This also takes account of

© Springer Nature Switzerland AG 2020
S. S. Goonewardene et al., *Management of Non-Muscle Invasive Bladder Cancer*,
https://doi.org/10.1007/978-3-030-28646-0_68

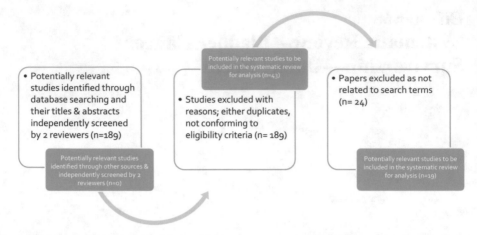

Fig. 68.1 Flow chart of studies identified through the systematic review (adapted from PRISMA)

the comparison occurring by chance. The first reviewer agreed all 19 papers to be included, the second, agreed on 19 (Fig. 68.1).

Data extraction was piloted by the researcher and amended in consultation with the research team (author and two academic supervisors). Data collected included authors, year and country of publication, study aims, setting, intervention aims, number of participants, study design, intervention components and delivery methods, comparison groups and outcome measures, notes and follow-up questions for the authors. Studies were quality assessed using the PRISMA criteria for randomised controlled trials, Mays et al. (Moher et al. 2009; Moher, Liberati et al. 2009, 154, 153; Mays et al. 2005) for the action research and qualitative studies and the Critical Skills Appraisal programme for cohort studies. This was also applied to randomised controlled trials and qualitative studies.

References

Mays N, Pope C, Popay J. Systematically reviewing qualitative and quantitative evidence to inform management and policy-making in the health field. J Health Serv Res Policy. 2005;10 Suppl 1:6–20.

Moher D, Liberati A, Tetzlaff J, Altman DG. Preferred reporting items for systematic reviews and meta-analyses: the prisma statement. BMJ. 2009;339(7716):332–6.

Chapter 69
Systematic Review Search Results—Bladder Cancer Survivorship and Unmet Need

69.1 Bladder Cancer Survivivorship—Support Required

Over half of the patients (56.67%) found the information they received from physicians to be insufficient (Mohamed et al. 2014). Of these patients, 26.67% had searched the Internet, joined support groups, or read on-line patients' blogs for more information about treatment options and side effects. Other unmet needs that were mentioned more than a few times included worries about survival, pain, change in body image, and reduced sexual function after surgery (Mohamed et al. 2012). Only 20% of patients reported that their physicians mentioned possible changes in sexual function during the discussion about treatment options (Mohamed et al. 2012). One-third of patients (33.33%) reported feeling severely depressed at the time of diagnosis but did not receive referrals for care.

An Internet-based survey reviewed institutional resources and support systems devoted to bladder cancer survivors (Lee et al. 2012). Although 63% of respondent institutions had a National Cancer Institute designation, only 33% had an active bladder cancer support group (Lee et al. 2012). Survivorship clinics were available in 29% of institutions, and peer support networks, community resources for education, and patient navigation were available in 58%, 13%, and 25% of respondent institutions, respectively (Lee et al. 2012). This paper demonstrated resources for bladder cancer survivors vary widely and are lacking at several academic centers with high-volume bladder cancer populations.

69.2 Bladder Cancer Survivorship and Risk Factors

Cancer survivors who continue to smoke following diagnosis are at increased risk for recurrence. Yet, smoking prevalence among survivors is similar to the general population (Kowalkowski et al. 2014). Compared to non-smokers, current smokers

© Springer Nature Switzerland AG 2020
S. S. Goonewardene et al., *Management of Non-Muscle Invasive Bladder Cancer*,
https://doi.org/10.1007/978-3-030-28646-0_69

reported increased fear of recurrence and psychological distress ($p < 0.05$). Research assessing survivorship needs and designing and evaluating educational programs for NMIBC survivors should be a high priority. Identifying unmet needs among NMIBC survivors and developing programs to address these needs may increase compliance with cystoscopic monitoring, improve outcomes, and enhance quality of life (Kowalkowski et al. 2014).

Wakai et al. examined the prognostic significance of lifestyle factors in urinary bladder cancer.

Univariate analyses revealed significant associations of 5-year survivorship with educational attainment, marital status, drinking habits and consumption of green tea in males, and age at first consultation, histological type and grade of tumor, stage and distant metastasis in both sexes. After adjustment for age, stage, histology (histological type and grade) and distant metastasis by means of a proportional hazards model, drinking of alcoholic beverages was significantly associated with the prognosis of bladder cancer in males. No prognostic significance was found for such lifestyle factors as smoking habit, uses of artificial sweeteners and hair dye, and consumption of coffee, black tea, matcha (powdered green tea) and cola.

Approximately 30% of all cancer deaths in the United States are caused by tobacco use and smoking (Karam-Hage et al. 2014). While quit rates and quit attempt rates are relatively high shortly after a cancer diagnosis, the recidivism rates are also high. Therefore, screening, treating, and preventing relapse to tobacco use is imperative among patients with and survivors of cancer. To date, research has consistently shown that a combination of pharmacologic and behavioral interventions is needed to achieve the highest smoking cessation rates, with a recent emphasis on individualized treatment as a most promising approach. Challenges in health care systems, including the lack of appropriate resources and provider training, have slowed the progress in addition to important clinical considerations relevant to the treatment of tobacco dependence (e.g., a high degree of comorbidity with psychiatric disorders and other substance use disorders).

69.3   Bladder Cancer Survivorship and Non Muscle Invasive Bladder Cancer

More than 70,000 new cases of bladder cancer are diagnosed in the United States annually; with 75% being non-muscle-invasive (NMIBC) (Kowalkowski et al. 2014).

In non muscle invasive bladder cancer, participants reported sexual inactivity (38.8%) (Kowalkowski et al. 2014). Sexually active participants reported erectile difficulties (60.0%), vaginal dryness (62.5%), and worry about contaminating partner with treatment agents (23.2%) (Kowalkowski et al. 2014). While almost one-half reported the usefulness of talking with partners about sexual function, only one-fifth of participants reported sharing all concerns with their partners. One-half of interviewees reported sexual dysfunction (Kowalkowski et al. 2014). Two-thirds reported negative impacts on their relationships, including perceived loss of intimacy and divorce; over one-third were sexually inactive for fear of contaminating their partner or spreading NMIBC (Kowalkowski et al. 2014). This highlights how further work is still needed on this region.

Mohammed et al., looked at unmet needs in the survivorship population. Half the study sample (50%) reported difficulties with post-surgical recovery and almost half (46.67%) reported difficulties related to medical complication. These include urinary tract infections, incisional hernia, deep vein thrombosis, and kidney-related problems (Mohamed et al. 2012). Incontinence was a major concern for patients treated with neobladder and lack of urine control and leakage with ileal conduit (Mohamed et al. 2012).

Koo et al. examined discomfort, anxiety, and preferences for decision making in patients undergoing surveillance cystoscopy for non-muscle-invasive bladder cancer (NMIBC) (Koo et al. 2016). Twelve patients participated in 3 focus groups. Based on survey responses, two-thirds of participants (64%) experienced some degree of procedural discomfort or worry, and all participants reported improvement in at least 2 dimensions of overall well-being following cystoscopy (Koo et al. 2016). Although many participants did not perceive themselves as having a defined role in decision making surrounding their surveillance care, their preferences to be involved in decision making varied widely, ranging from acceptance of the physician's recommendation, to uncertainty, to dissatisfaction with not being involved more in determining the intensity of surveillance care (Koo et al. 2016). Many patients with NMIBC experience discomfort, anxiety, and worry related to disease progression and not only cystoscopy. Although some patients are content to defer surveillance decisions to their physicians, others prefer to be more involved. Future work should focus on defining patient-centered approaches to surveillance decision making.

Although approximately 75% of bladder cancers are non-muscle invasive (NMIBC) at diagnosis, most research tends to focus on invasive disease (e.g., experiences related to radical cystectomy and urinary diversion) (Garg et al. 2007). There is a lack of studies on quality of life, and especially qualitative research, in bladder cancer generally. As a result, relatively little is known about the experiences and needs of NMIBC patients (Garg et al. 2007). Gard et al. (2007) examined patient experience, define care priorities, and identify targets for care improvement in NMIBC across the cancer continuum.

Twenty patients (16 male, 4 female, all white) participated in three focus groups. Five primary themes emerged: access to care, provider characteristics and communication, quality of life, goals of care/influences on decision-making, and role of social support (Gard et al. 2007). Patients with NMIBC desired timely access to care and honest and caring provider communication. They described urinary function and emotional quality of life changes resulting from diagnosis and treatment. Avoiding cystectomy and being alive for family were the major decision influencers (Garg et al. 2007).

Access to care, provider characteristics and communication, quality of life, values/influences on decision-making, and social support as priority areas to improve patient experience in NMIBC Garg et al. (2007). Care redesign efforts should focus on improving access, enhancing provider communication, reducing side effects, and supporting caregiver roles (Garg et al. 2007).

69.4 Muscle Invasive Bladder Cancer

Bladder cancer is the fifth most commonly diagnosed cancer and the most expensive adult cancer in average healthcare costs incurred per patient in the USA (Mohammed et al. 2012). However, little is known about factors influencing patients' treatment decisions, quality of life, and responses to treatment impairments (Mohammed et al. 2012).

Mohammed et al. (2016) assessed the unmet needs of cancer patients can help providers tailor health care services to patients' specific needs. Younger patients (<60y) were less satisfied with the treatment information received presurgery and more likely to report posttreatment complications, choose a neobladder, and seek and receive professional support regarding sexual function, than were older patients ($p<0.05$) (Mohammed et al. 2016). More women than men reported difficulties with self-care and relied on themselves in disease self-management as opposed to relying on spousal support ($p<0.05$). Patients with neobladder were more likely to report difficulties with urinary incontinence and deterioration in sexual function, whereas patients with ileal conduit were more likely to require spousal help with self-care (Mohammed et al. 2016). Patients who received chemotherapy were significantly more likely to report changes in everyday life ($p<0.05$). Lastly, regardless of age, sex, or treatment choice, up to 50% of patients reported feeling depressed before or after treatment.

This demonstrates unmet informational and supportive needs of patients with muscle-invasive bladder cancer during survivorship, and vary by age, sex, and treatment choices. Educational and psychological assessments as well as clinical interventions should be tailored to a patient's specific unmet needs, and to specific clinical and demographic characteristics.

To improve care for patients after radical cystoprostatectomy (RCP), focus on survivorship issues such as sexual function needs to increase (Chippidi et al. 2017). Chippidi et al. (2017) determined the rates of ED treatment use (phosphodiesterase type 5 inhibitors, injectable therapies, urethral suppositories, vacuum erection devices, and penile prosthetics) in patients with bladder cancer before and after RCP to better understand current patterns of care (Chippidi et al. 2017). At baseline, 6.5% of patients (77 of 1,176) used ED treatments. The rates of ED treatment use at 0–6, 7–12, 13–18, and 19–24 months after RCP were 15.2%, 12.7%, 8.1%, and 10.1% respectively (Chippidi et al. 2017). While the burden of ED following RCP is known to be high, overall ED treatment rates are low. This demonstrates ED treatment use after RCP is quite low. The strongest predictor of ED treatment use after RCP was baseline treatment use. These findings suggest ED treatment is a low priority for patients with RCP or education about potential ED therapies might not be commonly discussed with patients after RCP. Urologists should consider discussing sexual function more frequently with their patients undergoing RCP.

Sun et al. examined the impact of survival probability according to duration of survivorship following radical cystectomy (RC) in patients diagnosed with urothelial carcinoma of the urinary bladder (UCUB) (Sun et al. 2012). Overall, 4991 UCUB patients who underwent RC were included (Sun et al. 2012). CSM-free survival rate was 63.9% at RC, and increased to 71.0, 77.5, 81.7, 85.9 and 86.3% in patients who survived ≥ 1, 2, 3, 4 and 5 years, respectively (Sun et al. 2012). Patients with pT2-4 disease benefitted from the highest increase in survivorship two years after RC. The same findings were recorded according to patients' nodal status. The survival of the first two years after RC markedly improves individual patient prognosis. The prognostic gains differ according to patient and tumour characteristics (Sun et al. 2012).

Informational needs during this period included a lack of information about recovery and post-treatment self-care. Many patients reported a lack of adequate training on the use of stomal appliances and catheters (i.e., stoma pouch changing, tailoring, cleaning, emptying, and choice of appliances, Mohamed et al. 2012).

69.5 Bladder Cancer Survivorship and the Older Patient—What Do We Need to Be Ready For?

Smith et al. (2018) identified changes in health-related quality of life (HRQoL) after diagnosis of bladder cancer in older adults in comparison with a group of adults without bladder cancer (controls) (Smith et al. 2018). After matching, 535 patients with bladder cancer (458 non-muscle-invasive bladder cancer [NMIBC] and 77 with muscle-invasive bladder cancer [MIBC]) and 2 770 control subjects without cancer were identified. Both patients with NMIBC and those with MIBC reported significant declines in HRQoL scores over time versus controls (Smith et al. 2018). After diagnosis, patients with bladder cancer experienced significant declines in physical, mental and social HRQoL relative to controls. Decrements were most pronounced among individuals with MIBC. Methods to better understand and address HRQoL decrements among patients with bladder cancer are needed.

Overall, consistent positive outcomes have been reported across studies showing that exercise is beneficial to reduce a number of treatment-related toxicities and improve symptoms (Galvão et al. 2011). Additional studies are needed in genitourinary cancers other than prostate to establish specific physical activity requirements and implementation strategies.

Physical activity has been shown to significantly improve health-related quality of life (HRQOL) and survivorship in a variety of patients with cancer (Gopalakrishna et al. 2017). However, little is known about the physical activity patterns of bladder cancer survivors. In a cross-sectional study, long-term bladder cancer survivors database were mailed a survey that included the Functional Assessment of Cancer Therapy Bladder Cancer (FACT-BL) and the International Physical Activity Questionnaire (IPAQ) (Gopalakrishna et al. 2017). A total of 472 subjects (49% response rate) completed the survey. Subjects reporting "high" physical activity had a median FACT-BL score of 129 compared with 119 among those reporting "low" physical activity, a statistically and clinically significant difference. Similarly, subjects reporting "high" physical activity had a 2.2-fold increased odds of reporting higher global HRQOL compared with subjects reporting "low" physical activity (Gopalakrishna et al. 2017). This large cohort of bladder cancer survivors reported high levels of physical activity. Physical activity was positively associated with HRQOL.

Monfardini et al. (2017) investigated a comprehensive geriatric assessment (CGA) to verify the usefulness of the incorporation of geriatric principles in future care plans. CGA was performed in 126 patients with bladder cancer. 21% were fit, 42% were vulnerable, and 37% were frail. During follow-up, 60% of patients with cardiac diseases, 42% of those with diabetes/other metabolic disorders, 35% of those with hypertension, and 35% of those with respiratory diseases were followed by a specialist (for these severe/extremely severe comorbidities). Of 16 patients with ADL impairment and 63 with IADL impairment, only 4 (25%) and 6 (10%), respectively, were referred to a rehabilitation service. Only one case was referred to a geriatrician. Appropriate clinical care patterns are advisable to improve quality of survivorship in older patients with urological cancers.

Physical exercises offer a variety of health benefits to cancer survivors during and post-treatment (Jensen et al. 2016). A prospective randomized controlled clinical trial investigated efficacy of a multidisciplinary rehabilitation program on length of stay following RC. A total of 107 patients were included in the intension-to-treat population revealing 50 patients in the intervention group and 57 patients in the standard group (Jensen et al. 2016). A total of 66% (95% confidence interval (CI) 51; 78) adhered more than 75% of the recommended progressive standardized exercise program. In the intervention group, a significant improvement in muscle power of 18% ($p < 0.002$) was found at time for surgery. Moreover, muscle power was significantly improved compared to that in the standard group with 0.3 W/kg (95% CI 0.08; 0.5%) ($p < 0.006$) (Jensen et al. 2016). In patients awaiting RC, a short-term exercise-based pre-habilitation intervention is feasible and effective and should be considered in future survivorship strategies.

69.6 Bladder Cancer Survivorship—Conclusions from Other Reviews

Bladder cancer (BC) is a common disease with disparate treatment options and variable outcomes (Edmondson et al. 2017). Despite the disease's high prevalence, little is known of the lived experience of affected patients. National patient experience surveys suggest that those with BC have poorer experiences than those with other common cancers (Edmondson et al. 2017). The inconsistent nature of symptoms contributes to delays in diagnosis. Post-diagnosis, many patients are not actively engaged in the treatment decision-making process and rely on their doctor's expertise (Edmondson et al. 2017). This can result in patients not adequately exploring the consequences of these decisions. Learning how to cope with a 'post-surgery body', changing sexuality and incontinence are distressing. Much less is known about the quality of life of patients receiving conservative treatments such as Bacillus Calmette-Guerin (BCG). Collective knowledge of the patients' self-reported experience of the cancer care pathway will facilitate understanding of the outcomes following treatment.

Four main gaps in knowledge relating to the practical and physical problems associated with cancer survivorship have been identified (Brearley et al. 2011). These are key symptoms, unmet supportive care needs, employment and older cancer survivors. Work is also needed to address the nomenclature of survivorship and to improve the methodology of research into cancer survivors (including standardised measures, theoretical frameworks, longitudinal design, inclusion of older survivors and age-matched controls for comparison).

New models of survivorship care are required to address the needs of genitourinary (GU) cancer survivors (Bender et al. 2011). Current approaches do not effectively engage cancer survivors or advocacy groups. A group of clinicians in collaboration with the Canadian Urologic Association held a forum for GU cancer survivors, advocacy groups, and health professionals to explore ways to collaboratively enhance survivorship care (Bender et al. 2011). Strategies to facilitate collaboration reflected a need to: (1) raise awareness of the shared and unique needs of GU cancer survivors and the expertise of cancer advocacy groups, (2) facilitate communication and collaborative opportunities among clinicians/researchers and cancer survivors/advocacy groups, (3) facilitate collaborative programming and fund-raising among GU advocacy groups, and (4) synthesize and facilitate access to GU cancer survivorship resources and services (Bender et al. 2011).

References

Bender JL, Wiljer D, Matthew A, Canil CM, Legere L, Loblaw A, Jewett MA. Fostering partnerships in survivorship care: report of the 2011 Canadian genitourinary cancers survivorship conference. J Cancer Surviv. 2012;6(3):296–304.
Brearley SG, Stamataki Z, Addington-Hall J, Foster C, Hodges L, Jarrett N, Richardson A, Scott I, Sharpe M, Stark D, Siller C, Ziegler L, Amir Z. The physical and practical problems experienced by cancer survivors: a rapid review and synthesis of the literature. Eur J Oncol Nurs. 2011;15(3):204–12.
Chippidi MR, Kates M, Sopko NA, et al. Erectile dysfunction treatment following radical cystoprostatectomy: analysis of a nationwide insurance claims database. J Sex Med. 2017;14:810–7.

Edmondson AJ, Birtwistle JC, Catto JWF, Twiddy M. The patients' experience of a bladder cancer diagnosis: a systematic review of the qualitative evidence. J Cancer Surviv. 2017;11(4):453–61.

Galvão DA, Taaffe DR, Spry N, Newton RU. Physical activity and genitourinary cancer survivorship. Recent Results Cancer Res. 2011;186:217–36.

Garg T, Connors JN, Ladd IG, Bogaczyk TL, Larson SL. Defining priorities to improve patient experience in non-muscle invasive bladder cancer. Cancer. 2007;109(1):1–12.

Gopalakrishna A, Longo TA, Fantony JJ, Harrison MR, Inman BA. Physical activity patterns and associations with health-related quality of life in bladder cancer survivors. Urol Oncol. 2017;35(9):540.

Jensen BT, Laustsen S, Jensen JB, Borre M, Petersen AK. Exercise-based pre-habilitation is feasible and effective in radical cystectomy pathways-secondary results from a randomized controlled trial. Support Care Cancer. 2016;24(8):3325–31.

Karam-Hage M, Cinciripini PM, Gritz ER. Tobacco use and cessation for cancer survivors: an overview for clinicians. CA Cancer J Clin. 2014;64(4):272–90.

Koo K, Zubkoff L, Sirovich BE, Goodney PP, Robertson DJ, Seigne JD, Schroeck FR. The burden of cystoscopic bladder cancer surveillance: anxiety, discomfort, and patient preferences for decision making. Urol Oncol. 2016;34(12):531.

Kowalkowski MA, Chandrashekar A, Amiel GE, Lerner SP, Wittmann DA, Latini DM, Goltz HH. Examining sexual dysfunction in non-muscle-invasive bladder cancer: results of cross-sectional mixed-methods research. Sex Med. 2014;2:141–51.

Lee CT, Mei M, Ashley J, Breslow G, O'Donnell M, Gilbert S, Lemmy S, Saxton C, Sagalowsky A, Sansgiry S, Latini DM, Bladder Cancer Think Tank, Bladder Cancer Advocacy Network. Patient resources available to bladder cancer patients: a pilot study of healthcare providers. Urology. 2012;79(1):172–7.

Mohamed NE, Diefenbach MA, Goltz HH, Lee CT, Latini D, Kowalkowski M, Philips C, Hassan W, Hall SJ. Muscle invasive bladder cancer: from diagnosis to survivorship. Adv Urol. 2012;2012:135–42.

Mohamed NE, Chaoprang Herrera P, Hudson S, Revenson TA, Lee CT, Quale DZ, Zarcadoolas C, Hall SJ, Diefenbach MA. Muscle invasive bladder cancer: examining survivor burden and unmet needs. J Urol. 2014;191(1):48–53.

Mohamed NE, Pisipati S, Lee CT, Goltz HH, Latini DM, Gilbert FS, Wittmann D, Knauer CJ, Mehrazin R, Sfakianos JP, McWilliams GW, Quale DZ, Hall SJ. Unmet informational and supportive care needs of patients following cystectomy for bladder cancer based on age, sex, and treatment choices. Urol Oncol. 2016;34(12):531.e7–14. https://doi.org/10.1016/j.urolonc.2016.06.010 Epub 2016 Jul 19.

Monfardini S, Morlino S, Valdagni R, Catanzaro M, Tafa A, Bortolato B, Petralia G, Bonetto E, Villa E, Picozzi S, Locatelli MC, Galetti G Millul A, Albanese Y, Bianchi E, Panzarino C, Gerardi F, Beghi E. Follow-up of elderly patients with urogenital cancers: evaluation of geriatric care needs and related actions. J Geriatr Oncol. 2017;8(4):289–95.

Smith AB, Jaeger B, Pinheiro LC, Edwards LJ, Tan HJ, Nielsen ME, Reeve BB. Impact of bladder cancer on health-related quality of life. BJU Int. 2018;121(4):549–557. https://doi.org/10.1016/j.ejon.2018.05.006 Epub 2018 Jun 30, Eur J Oncol Nurs. 2018;35:92–101.

Sun M, Abdollah F, Bianchi M, Trinh QD, Shariat SF, Jeldres C, Tian Z, Hansen J, Briganti A, Graefen M, Montorsi F, Perrotte P, Karakiewicz PI. Conditional survival of patients with urothelial carcinoma of the urinary bladder treated with radical cystectomy. Eur J Cancer. 2012;48(10):1503–11.

Chapter 70
Survivorship Challenges in Non-Muscle Invasive Bladder Cancer

Non-muscle-invasive bladder cancer (NMIBC) accounts for approximately 75% of incident bladder cancers (Sexton et al. 2010) yet research tends to focus on muscle invasive disease (e.g., experiences related to radical cystectomy and urinary diversion) (Garg et al. 2018). There is a lack of studies on quality of life, and especially qualitative research, in bladder cancer, especially related to women. As a result, not much is known about survivorship care for these patients.

Any malignancy of the pelvis, including BlCa, may lead to sexual dysfunction among men or women, defined as a decrease in sexual desire or variability of the sexual response cycle (i.e., excitement, plateau, orgasm, resolution) due to psychogenic or organic causes (Kowalkowski et al. 2014)

Intravesical therapy is known to increased sexual dysfunction side effects. Bacillus Calmette–Guérin (BCG) treatment may cause pain, dysuria, and urinary frequency (Koya et al. 2006). This can also lead to erectile dysfunction. This was reviewed by (Sighinolfi et al. 2007). Baseline ED and the association with lower urinary tract symptoms are variables significantly connected with post-treatment results ($p = 0.016$ and 0.00 respectively) whereas the age seems not to be related to ED ($p = 0.256$). It is concluded that BCG treatment is effective for prophylaxis of non-muscle invasive bladder cancer; however, it may induce a high incidence of ED. Although this effect is transient and reversible, erectile failure is another source of psychological distress that adversely affects the quality of life of men undergoing BCG treatment (Sighinolfi et al. 2007).

Sexual dysfunction is more prevalent for women (43%) than men (31%) and is associated with various demographic characteristics, including age and educational attainment (Laumann et al. 1999). Women of different racial groups demonstrate different patterns of sexual dysfunction. Differences among men are not as marked but generally consistent with women (Laumann et al. 1999). Experience of sexual dysfunction is more likely among women and men with poor physical and emotional health. Moreover, sexual dysfunction is highly associated with negative experiences in sexual relationships and overall well-being.

© Springer Nature Switzerland AG 2020
S. S. Goonewardene et al., *Management of Non-Muscle Invasive Bladder Cancer*,
https://doi.org/10.1007/978-3-030-28646-0_70

Stav et al., looked at outcomes from cystoscopy in non-muscle invasive bladder cancer. The pre-cystoscopy anxiety level was 2.01 (Stav et al. 2004). The mean IPSS increased following cystoscopy (6.75 vs. 5.43, $p = 0.001$) and returned to baseline 2 weeks later. A decline in libido was reported by 55.6% (25/45) and 50% (3/6) of the sexually active men and women, respectively (Stav et al. 2004). Cystoscopy was associated with a decreased Erectile Dysfunction Intensity Score, from 15.6 to 9.26 during the first 2 weeks ($p = 0.04$). The overall complication rate was 15% and included urethrorrhagia and dysuria, None of the patients had fever or urinary retention and none was hospitalized. The complication rate was higher in patients with benign prostatic hyperplasia (24% vs. 9.7%, $p = 0.001$). This demonstrated the rigid cystoscopy is well tolerated by most patients and has only a minor impact on quality of life. However, cystoscopy transiently impairs sexual performance and libido transiently.

This was further investigated by van der Aa et al. (2009). In a randomised controlled trial, they evaluated two surveillance schemes. The response rate was 95% (142/150); 61% (87/142) of the respondents were sexually active in the previous 4 weeks after diagnosis, 66% (70/105) of men and 46% (17/37) of women. Although libido was not negatively affected, 54% (47/87) of the patients had a sexual dysfunction, and 23% (17/73) were afraid to inflict harm on their partner by sexual contact. Sexually active patients perceived a higher state of general health ($p = 0.03$) (van der Aa et al. 2009). This demonstrated the prevalence of sexual dysfunction in patients with NMI UC is very high (54%) compared with an age- and gender-matched healthy population (20–45%). No predictors for sexual dysfunction were found. These patients and partners would benefit from proper sexual information in the outpatient clinic (van der Aa et al. 2009).

Garg et al. (2018) identified five primary themes: access to care, provider characteristics and communication, quality of life, goals of care/influences on decision-making, and role of social support. This study identified, patients with NMIBC desired timely access to care and honest and caring provider communication. They described urinary function and emotional quality of life changes resulting from diagnosis and treatment (Garg et al. 2018). Avoiding cystectomy and being alive for family were the major decision influencers. This highlights important factors such as access to care, provider characteristics and communication, quality of life, values/influences on decision-making, and social support as priority areas to improve patient experience in NMIBC (Garg et al. 2018).

Barocas et al. found an unmet need exists for new treatment options associated with fewer complications, better patient compliance, and decreased healthcare costs. Increased prevention of recurrence through greater adherence to evidence-based guidelines and the development of novel therapies could therefore result in substantial savings to the healthcare system (Barocas et al. 2012).

References

Barocas DA, Globe DR, Colayco DC, Onyenwenyi A, Bruno AS, Bramley TJ, Spear RJ. Surveillance and treatment of non-muscle-invasive bladder cancer in the USA. Adv Urol. 2012;2012:421709.

Garg T, Connors JN, Ladd IG, Bogaczyk TL, Larson SL. Defining priorities to improve patient experience in non-muscle invasive bladder cancer. Bladder Cancer. 2018;4(1):121–8.

Kowalkowski MA, Chandrashekar A, Amiel GE, Lerner SP, Wittmann DA, Latini DM, Goltz HH. Examining sexual dysfunction in non-muscle-invasive bladder cancer: results of cross-sectional mixed-methods research. Sex Med. 2014;2(3):141–51.

Koya MP, Simon MA, Soloway MS. Complications of intravesical therapy for urothelial cancer of the bladder. J Urol. 2006;175:2004–10.

Laumann EO, Paik A, Rosen RC. Sexual dysfunction in the United States: prevalence and predictors. JAMA. 1999;281:537–44.

Sexton WJ, Wiegand LR, Correa JJ, Politis C, Dickinson SI, Kang LC. Bladder cancer: a review of non-muscle invasive disease. Cancer Control. 2010;17:256–68.

Sighinolfi MC, Micali S, De Stefani S, Mofferdin A, Ferrari N, Giacometti M, Bianchi G. Bacille Calmette-Guerin intravesical instillation and erectile function: is there a concern? Andrologia. 2007;39:51–4.

Stav K, Leibovici D, Goren E, Livshitz A, Siegel YI, Lindner A, Zisman A. Adverse effects of cystoscopy and its impact on patients' quality of life and sexual performance. Isr Med Assoc J. 2004;6:474–8.

van der Aa MN, Bekker MD, van der Kwast TH, Essink-Bot ML, Steyerberg EW, Zwarthoff EC, Sen FE, Elzevier HW. Sexual function of patients under surveillance for bladder cancer. BJU Int. 2009;104:35–40.

Chapter 71
Bladder Cancer Survivorship Care Plans

There are currently more than 12 million cancer survivors in the USA (Smith et al. 2013). Survivors face many issues related to cancer and treatment that are outside the purview of the clinical care system (Smith et al. 2013). Therefore, understanding the needs of cancer survivors and supplementing them with survivorship care plans are key to management of bladder cancer patients in the survivorship phase.

In 2004, the Centers for Disease Control and Prevention and the Lance Armstrong Foundation, now the Livestrong Foundation, partnered with national cancer survivorship organizations to develop the National Action Plan for Cancer Survivorship (NAPCS) (Smith et al. 2013). Strategies associated with surveillance and applied research; communication, education, and training; and programs, policy, and infrastructure represent a large amount of the organizational efforts (Smith et al. 2013). However, there are gaps in research on preventive interventions, evaluation of implemented activities, and translation.

Increased recognition of cancer survivorship as a distinct and important phase that follows the diagnosis and treatment of cancer has contributed to the development of public health-related strategies and plans to address those strategies (Fairley et al. 2009). CDC's Division of Cancer Prevention and Control (DCPC) uses an interdisciplinary public health approach to address the needs of cancer survivors through applied research, public health surveillance and data collection, education, and health promotion, especially among underserved populations that may be at risk for health disparities (Fairley et al. 2009).

Bender et al. identified new models of survivorship care are required to address the needs of genitourinary (GU) cancer survivors (Bender et al. 2012). Current approaches do not effectively engage cancer survivors or advocacy groups (Bender et al. 2012). A group of clinicians in collaboration with the Canadian Urologic Association held a forum for GU cancer survivors, advocacy groups, and health professionals to explore ways to collaboratively enhance survivorship care. They identified strategies to facilitate collaboration reflected a need to: (1) raise awareness of the shared and unique needs of GU cancer survivors and the expertise of

© Springer Nature Switzerland AG 2020   345
S. S. Goonewardene et al., *Management of Non-Muscle Invasive Bladder Cancer*,
https://doi.org/10.1007/978-3-030-28646-0_71

cancer advocacy groups, (2) facilitate communication and collaborative opportunities among clinicians/researchers and cancer survivors/advocacy groups, (3) facilitate collaborative programming and fund-raising among GU advocacy groups, and (4) synthesize and facilitate access to GU cancer survivorship resources and services (Bender et al. 2012). This demonstrated there is strong support for formal collaboration to enhance survivorship care for all stakeholders (Bender et al. 2012). Strategies to foster such partnerships should employ integrated knowledge translation approaches that actively engage all parties throughout the entire research to practice process (Bender et al. 2012).

Alfano et al. identified it is essential to accelerate the translation of survivorship research into evidence-based interventions (Alfano et al. 2014). To better understand this problem and identify strategies to encourage the translation of survivorship research findings into practice, four agencies (American Cancer Society, Centers for Disease Control and Prevention, LIVE STRONG: Foundation, National Cancer Institute) hosted a meeting where participants concluded that accelerating science into care will require a coordinated, collaborative effort by individuals from diverse settings, including researchers and clinicians, survivors and families, public health professionals, and policy makers (Alfano et al. 2014).

Campbell et al. identified Survivorship models of care from LIVESTRONG Survivorship Center of Excellence (COE) Network sites and to identify barriers and facilitators influencing survivorship care (Campbell et al. 2011). System barriers include reimbursement issues, lack of space, and the need for leadership commitment to support changes in clinical practices as well as having program "champions" among clinical staff (Campbell et al. 2011). Self-managembent support was largely limited to health promotion provided in clinic-based education and counseling sessions, with few centres providing patients with self-management tools and interventions. This demonstrates a requirement for a quality survivorship program designed to meet patient needs.

Grant et al. demonstrated, health care institutions focused on developing survivorship care programs and educating staff, in an effort to prepare colleagues to provide and coordinate survivorship care, in cancer settings across the country (Grant et al. 2015). Goal-directed education provided insight into survivorship activities occurring across the nation (Grant et al. 2015). Researchers were able to identify survivorship care programs and activities, as well as the barriers to developing these programs (Grant et al. 2015).

As cancer survivorship care becomes an important part of quality cancer care oncology professionals need education to prepare themselves to provide this care (Grant et al. 2012). Survivorship care requires a varied approach depending on the survivor population, treatment regimens and care settings. An NCI-funded educational program: Survivorship Education for Quality Cancer Care provided multidiscipline two-person teams an opportunity to gain this important knowledge using a goal-directed, team approach. Educational programs were funded for yearly courses from 2006 to 2009 (Grant et al. 2012). Institutional assessments found improvement in seven domains of care that related to institutional change.

This course provided education to participants that led to significant changes in survivorship care in their settings.

Morgan et al. reviewed survivorship care plans (CSCPs) (Morgan et al. 2009). A cancer survivor is an individual who has been diagnosed with cancer, regardless of when that diagnosis was received, who is still living (Morgan et al. 2009). Cancer survivorship is complex and involves many aspects of care. Major areas of concern for survivors are recurrence, secondary malignancies, and long-term treatment sequelae that affect quality of life (Morgan et al. 2009). Four essential components of survivorship care are prevention, surveillance, intervention, and coordination (Morgan et al. 2009). A CSCP should address the survivor's long-term care, such as type of cancer, treatments received, potential side effects, and recommendations for follow-up (Morgan et al. 2009). It should include preventive practices, how to maintain health and well-being, information on legal protections regarding employment and health insurance, and psychosocial services in the community (Morgan et al. 2009). Survivorship care for patients with cancer requires a multidisciplinary effort and team approach. Enhanced knowledge of long-term complications of survivorship is needed for healthcare providers. Further research on evidence-based practice for cancer survivorship care also is necessary.

References

Alfano CM, Smith T, de Moor JS, Glasgow RE, Khoury MJ, Hawkins NA, Stein KD, Rechis R, Parry C, Leach CR, Padgett L, Rowland JH. An action plan for translating cancer survivorship research into care. J Natl Cancer Inst. 2014;106(11).
Bender JL, Wiljer D, Matthew A, Canil CM, Legere L, Loblaw A, Jewett MA. Fostering partnerships in survivorship care: report of the 2011 Canadian genitourinary cancers survivorship conference. J Cancer Surviv. 2012;6(3):296–304.
Campbell MK, Tessaro I, Gellin M, Valle CG, Golden S, Kaye L, Ganz PA, McCabe MS, Jacobs LA, Syrjala K, Anderson B, Jones AF, Miller K. Adult cancer survivorship care: experiences from the LIVESTRONG centers of excellence network. J Cancer Surviv. 2011;5(3):271–82.
Fairley TL, Pollack LA, Moore AR, Smith JL. Addressing cancer survivorship through public health: an update from the Centers for Disease Control and Prevention. J Womens Health (Larchmt). 2009;18(10):1525–31. https://doi.org/10.1089/jwh.2009.1666.
Grant M, Economou D, Ferrell B, Uman G. Facilitating survivorship program development for health care providers and administrators. J Cancer Surviv. 2015;9(2):180–7.
Morgan MA. Cancer survivorship: history, quality-of-life issues, and the evolving multidisciplinary approach to implementation of cancer survivorship care plans. Oncol Nurs Forum. 2009;36(4):429–36.
Smith JL, Pollack LA, Rodriguez JL, Hawkins NA, Smith T, Rechis R, Miller A, Willis A, Miller H, Hall IJ, Fairley TL, Stone-Wiggins B. Assessment of the status of a National Action Plan for Cancer Survivorship in the USA. J Cancer Surviv. 2013;7(3):425–38. https://doi.org/10.1007/s11764-013-0276-8 Epub 2013 Apr 23.
TvGrant M, Economou D, Ferrell B, Uman G. Educating health care professionals to provide institutional changes in cancer survivorship care. J Cancer Educ. 2012;27(2):226–32.

Chapter 72
Research Summary—A New Model of Care for Patients with Bladder Cancer (MODA)

Radical cystectomy is the most extensive operation within urology. There are a wide range of side effects experienced. Very often, there is no standardised pathway as part of follow-up. Patient reported outcome measures in bladder cancer are reviewed. This chapter covers the research summary (Figs. 72.1 and 72.2).

© Springer Nature Switzerland AG 2020   349
S. S. Goonewardene et al., *Management of Non-Muscle Invasive Bladder Cancer*,
https://doi.org/10.1007/978-3-030-28646-0_72

	Aim: To develop a new model of care forpatientswith emotional and sexual concerns after curative surgery for bladder cancer Objectives: For this population: (i) To assess the evidence on unmetneeds (ii) To assess patient views on psychosexual care, to determine standard care management and to determine the optimal pathway, from patients (iii) To develop a psychosexual pathway, develop recommendations for psychosexual care, implementation of pathway and future research
Study design methods	Design: Participatory research (i) Systematic Literature Review to explore psychosexual needs. (ii) Telephonised interviews with anonymised patients
Inclusion criteria:	• Patients from 6 weeks up to 6 months, post surgery for bladder cancer • Able and willing to give informed consent
Exclusion criteria:	(i) Patients with disease that is not potentially cured (ii) Patients who are unable to speak or understand English
Outcomes:	(i) Psychosexual care needs from the literature (ii) Psychosexual care needs of patients, Standard Care Pathway, Optimal psychosexual pathway, according to patients Standard care pathway, according to healthcare professionals (iii) Development of optimal psychosexual pathway
Sample size and selection	Sample size 5paitents Selection: Purposive patient sample and purposive healthcare professional sample, both from Southend University Hospital
Analysis	(i) Critical Appraisal of systematic reviews using Critical Appraisal Skills Programme Tool (ii) Telephone interviews- thematic analysis will be conducted

Fig. 72.1 A new model of care for patients with bladder cancer (MODA)

Fig. 72.2 A new model of
care for patients with bladder
cancer (MODA)

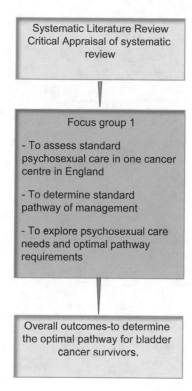

Chapter 73
What Is the Impact of Sexual and Emotional Concerns on Patients Post Surgery for Patients with Bladder Cancer?

73.1 Introduction

Radical cystectomy is the most extensive operation within urology. There are a wide range of side effects experienced. Very often, there is no standardised pathway as part of follow-up. Patient reported outcome measures for radical cystectomy are reviewed.

73.2 Methods

This was registered at Southend University Hospital. 5 patients were contacted via telephone and asked their opinion on the operation and support as part of a quality improvement project. Codes and themes were then analysed via a framework approach.

73.3 Results

The codes and themes generated were as follows:

Codes	Themes generated
Erectile dysfunction	National Pathway—opt in needed
Age related	Young patient input
Side effects post op	CNS needed to help manage and peer support group

© Springer Nature Switzerland AG 2020   353
S. S. Goonewardene et al., *Management of Non-Muscle Invasive Bladder Cancer*,
https://doi.org/10.1007/978-3-030-28646-0_73

Psychological impact from ED	Counselling and support needed
Support needed with impact of operation on general health	Early start to pathway and dietician needed

73.4   Conclusions

This quality improvement project clearly demonstrates a lack of patient care, related to radical cystectomy. Based on these results a pathway was drawn up aswell as bladder survivorship tool, to further patient care.

Chapter 74
Results—Telephone Interviews with Thematic Analyses

A framework analysis approach was used to analyse tabulated results (Guest 2012). Transcripts were reviewed several times by the research team and using a highlighter in a tabulated approach, codes and recurrent themes were identified before the final analysis was drawn. After research team familiarization with data and transcripts, the initial codes were generated manually, using a framework analysis (Braun 2006). All codes relating to the topic of surgery and bladder cancer were identified. Within these codes the over-arching themes were identified and named.

Transcripts were then reviewed for evidence for and against these codes:

Erectile dysfunction
Age related
Side effects post op
Psychological impact from ED
Support needed with impact of operation on general health

References

Braun V. Using thematic analysis in psychology. In: Clarke V, editor. Qualitative research in psychology; 2006.
Guest G, Macqueen K, Namey E. Applied thematic analyis. London: SAGE Publications; 2012.

Chapter 75
Bladder Cancer Survivorship and Patient Reported Outcome Measures—Code 1 Erectile Dysfunction

Post TURBT, seven patients were involved. Comments made were as followed:

Table code (1) Erectile dysfunction	Comments made were as followed
Age related disease	'ED does apply to elderly'
No requirement for treatment	'Op docs not affect erectile problem'
Side effects of surgery and requirement for a pathway	'ED afterwards—1 month—age dependant—would initially try to see if it resolved, then seek cns help—an opt in pathway would help'
Side effects of surgery	

This clearly indicates, that ED is an age-related problem, which would be of more concern to younger patients. There clearly needs to be a pathway in place to support this.

Post MMC instillation, 5 patients were involved there were no side effects experienced.

Post cystectomy, there were 10 patients involved. Comments made were as follows:

© Springer Nature Switzerland AG 2020

S. S. Goonewardene et al., *Management of Non-Muscle Invasive Bladder Cancer*,
https://doi.org/10.1007/978-3-030-28646-0_75

Table code (1) Erectile Dysfunction	Comments made as follows
Side effects of treatment	Problems getting erections, prolonged time to get prescription, have to order in caverject
Psychological impact	Biggest psychological effect from lack of erections
Requirement for pathway	Specialised pathway would make a difference, with CNS, and counsellor, but needs to start 6 months after cystectomy
Requirement for pathway	Lack of support in a timely manner
Age related disease	ED present, age related as to whether it is treated
Requirement for pathway	No erections—not prepared—pathway few months after

Chapter 76
Bladder Cancer Survivorship and Patient Reported Outcome Measures—Code 2 Age Related Disease

Post TURBT, seven patients were involved. Comments made were as followed:

Table Code (2) Age related disease	Comments made were as followed
Age related disease	'ED does apply to elderly'
Age related disease	'ED afterwards –1 month—age dependant—would initially try to see if it resolved, then seek cns help—an opt in pathway would help'
Side effects of surgery	

Post BCG/MMC there were 7 patients involved, there were no age related effects experienced

Post radical cystectomy, there were 10 patients involved, the comments made were as follows:

Table Code (2) Age related disease	Comments made were as followed
Age related disease	Operation went well, not ready for prolonged healing process. Not prepared for hernia
Age related disease	Not prepared for length of rehabilitation
Side effects of surgery	Nutritionist needed. Taken erections away, but age related

This demonstrates, there is a clear requirement for a pathway, and to specific individualised age related focus for treatment.

© Springer Nature Switzerland AG 2020
S. S. Goonewardene et al., *Management of Non-Muscle Invasive Bladder Cancer*,
https://doi.org/10.1007/978-3-030-28646-0_76

Chapter 77
Bladder Cancer Survivorship and Patient Reported Outcome Measures—Code 3 Side Effects Post Operatively

Post TURBT, seven patients were involved. Comments made were as followed:

Table Code (3) Side effects post operatively	Comments made were as followed
Age related disease	No side effects
Age related disease	Op does not affect erectile problem
Side effects of surgery	Recurrent problems with chest and uti—managed medically—really happy

Post BCG/ MMC there were 7 patients involved, there were no age related effects experienced

Table Code (3) Side effects post surgery	Comments made were as followed
Side effects post surgery	Prepared for side effects
Education pre op	Shock at diagnosis but well supported
Side effects of surgery	No side effects experienced

Post radical cystectomy, there were 10 patients involved, the comments made were as follows:

Table Code (3) Side effects post surgery	Comments made were as followed
Side effects post surgery	Operation went well, not ready for prolonged healing process. Not prepared for hernia
Requirement for pathway	Specialised pathway would make a difference, with CNS, and counsellor, but needs to start 6 months after cystectomy

© Springer Nature Switzerland AG 2020
S. S. Goonewardene et al., *Management of Non-Muscle Invasive Bladder Cancer*,
https://doi.org/10.1007/978-3-030-28646-0_77

Side effects of surgery	Minor infection post op—wound infection
	Not fully prepared for operation or side effects
	Not prepared for length of rehabilitation
Side effects of surgery	Lymphoedema-currently present. Pathway needed with CNS, but difficult to get a time as to when to start-pt dependant

This demonstrates, there is a clear requirement for a pathway, more so to address side effects of surgery and age related diseases.

Chapter 78
Bladder Cancer Survivorship and Patient Reported Outcome Measures—Code 4 Psychological Impact

There were no psychological issues experienced in either the TURBT/MMC/BCG groups.

There were 10 patients who underwent radical cystectomy. Comments made were as follows.

Table Code (4) Psychological impact from ED	Comments made were as followed
Impact of operation	Biggest psychological effect from lack of erections
Impact of operation	Operation went well, not ready for prolonged healing process
Impact of operation	Not fully prepared for operation or side effects

All of these issues could be dealt with by a bladder cancer survivorship pathway.

© Springer Nature Switzerland AG 2020
S. S. Goonewardene et al., *Management of Non-Muscle Invasive Bladder Cancer*,
https://doi.org/10.1007/978-3-030-28646-0_78

Chapter 79
Bladder Cancer Survivorship and Patient Reported Outcome Measures—Code 5 Impact of Operation on General Health

There were 7 patients involved with TURBTs.

Table Code (5) Impact of operation on general health	Comments made were as followed
Impact of operation	No side effects
Impact of operation	ED afterwards—1 month—age dependant— would initially try to see if it resolved, then seek CNS help—an opt in pathway would help
Impact of operation	Recurrent problems with chest and uti—managed medically—really happy

There was no impact of procedure experience for BCG/MMC patients.

There were 10 patients who underwent radical cystectomy. Comments made were as follows:

Table Code (5) Impact of operation on general health	Comments made were as followed
Requirement for pathway	Peer support group with CNS beforehand would have helped
Nutritionist requirement	Nutritionist needed. Taken erections away, but age related
	Lymphoedema-currently present. Pathway needed with CNS, but difficult to get a time as to when to start-pt dependant
Impact of operation	Problem post op-hernia post op

© Springer Nature Switzerland AG 2020
S. S. Goonewardene et al., *Management of Non-Muscle Invasive Bladder Cancer*,
https://doi.org/10.1007/978-3-030-28646-0_79

Chapter 80
Bladder Cancer Survivorship Tool

80.1 Introduction

Bladder Cancer is the 7th most common cancer worldwide in men and the 17th most common cancer worldwide in women (Burger et al. 2013). In contrast, bladder cancer survivorship is poorly addressed within contemporary research. Patients within this cohort, both with NMIBC and MIBC have significant unmet needs, often unaddressed in todays healthcare world. This study aims to determine the unmet needs of bladder cancer survivorship patients via systematic review, then develop a bladder cancer survivorship care assessment tool (Fig. 80.1).

80.2 Conclusion

From the systematic review, unmet needs were found in patient information, requirement for patient support groups an active bladder cancer support group are required. Access to healthcare to management side effects of surgery, erectile dysfunction and fatigue, are also important. Survivorship clinics are needed as are community resources for education, and patient navigation are needed. Based on these results a bladder cancer survivorship tool is developed, which highlights a requirement for healthcare resources to change, based on patient requirement (Fig. 80.2).

© Springer Nature Switzerland AG 2020

S. S. Goonewardene et al., *Management of Non-Muscle Invasive Bladder Cancer*,
https://doi.org/10.1007/978-3-030-28646-0_80

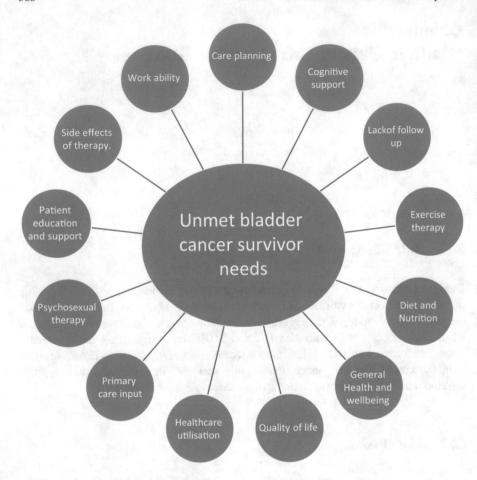

Fig. 80.1 Unmet needs from systematic review

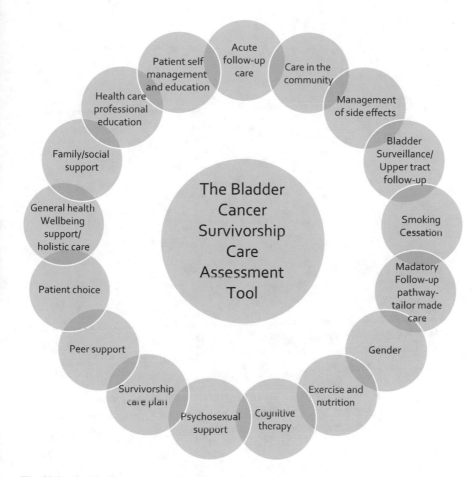

Fig. 80.2   The bladder cancer survivorship care assessment tool

Reference

Burger M, Oosterlinck W, Konety B, Chang S, Gudjonsson S, Pruthi R, Soloway M, et al. ICUD-EAU international consultation on bladder cancer 2012: non-muscle-invasive urothelial carcinoma of the bladder. Eur Urol. 2013;63(1):36–44.

Chapter 81
Health Related Quality of Life Measurements in Bladder Cancer Survivorship

Health-related quality of life (HRQOL) has not been adequately measured in bladder cancer (Gilbert et al. 2007). A recently developed reliable and disease-specific quality of life instrument (Bladder Cancer Index, BCI) was used to measure urinary, sexual, and bowel function and bother domains in patients with bladder cancer managed with several different interventions, including cystectomy and endoscopic-based procedures. In all, 315 bladder cancer patients treated at the University of Michigan completed the BCI in 2004 (Gilbert et al. 2007). Significant differences were seen in mean BCI function and bother scores between cystectomy and native bladder treatment groups (Gilbert et al. 2007). In addition, urinary function scores were significantly lower among cystectomy patients treated with continent neobladder compared with those treated with ileal conduit (all pairwise $p < 0.05$).

This demonstrated the BCI is responsive in patients with bladder cancer and with urinary, bowel, and sexual domains (Gilbert et al. 2007).

A 36-item short-form (SF-36) was constructed to survey health status in the Medical Outcomes Study (Ware and Sherbourne 1992). The SF-36 was designed for use in clinical practice and research, health policy evaluations, and general population surveys. The SF-36 includes one multi-item scale that assesses eight health concepts: (1) limitations in physical activities because of health problems; (2) limitations in social activities because of physical or emotional problems; (3) limitations in usual role activities because of physical health problems; (4) bodily pain; (5) general mental health (psychological distress and well-being); (6) limitations in usual role activities because of emotional problems; (7) vitality (energy and fatigue); and (8) general health perceptions (Ware and Sherbourne 1992). This questionnaire has a role in bladder cancer survivorship.

Radical cystectomy for bladder cancer is associated with many changes in bodily function with sexual and urinary dysfunction most prevalent. However, little research has been done on how efforts to improve erectile function relate to quality of life (Fujisawa et al. 2000). Also, the psychological benefits associated with

© Springer Nature Switzerland AG 2020
S. S. Goonewardene et al., *Management of Non-Muscle Invasive Bladder Cancer*,
https://doi.org/10.1007/978-3-030-28646-0_81

continent urinary diversion have not been fully explored. Fujisawa et al. compared long-term quality of life outcomes among 3 urinary diversion groups, and between patients who had and had not received an inflatable penile prosthesis.

Regardless of type of urinary diversion the majority of patients reported good overall quality of life, little emotional distress and few problems with social, physical or functional activities (Fujisawa et al. 2000). Problems with urinary diversion and sexual functioning were identified as most common. Findings suggest that physicians may wish to discuss urinary diversion problems and sexual dysfunction as long-term correlates of radical cystectomy for bladder cancer (Fujisawa et al. 2000). Furthermore, they may also wish to discuss the option of erectile aids in men with erectile dysfunction after cystectomy.

Kikuchi et al. assessed and compare quality of life (QOL) of patients followed for a long time who underwent an ileal conduit (IC), continent reservoir (CR) or ileal neobladder (NB) using FACT-BL, a bladder-cancer-specific questionnaire (Kikuchi et al. 2006). One hundred and forty-seven patients underwent radical cystectomy and urinary diversion for bladder cancer from 1987 to 2002 at our institution (Kikuchi et al. 2006). Four categories (physical, social/familial, emotional and functional well-being) in FACT-G were equally favorable in these groups. Patients with IC had less trouble controlling urine but had a worse image on altered body appearance compared with NB patients (Kikuchi et al. 2006). Interest in sex was extremely low in all patients and capability of maintaining an erection was also low in 39 male patients. Ten (77%) of 13 IC, seven (78%) of nine CR and six (86%) of seven NB patients answered that they would choose the same type of diversion if they had the choice again (Kikuchi et al. 2006). The type of urinary diversion does not appear to be associated with a different QOL by general cancer-related assessment. Urinary function and body image are affected and related to the method used to reconstruct the urinary system.

Gilbert et al. developed and validated a reliable, responsive multidimensional instrument to measure disease specific health related quality of life in bladder cancer survivors treated with local cancer therapy (Gilbert et al. 2010). Draft items were piloted and revised, resulting in the 36-item Bladder Cancer Index consisting of urinary, bowel and sexual health domains. Internal consistency, test-retest reliability, convergent validity, concurrent validity and criterion validity were then assessed. Moderate correlation was observed with existing external measures, indicating that the Bladder Cancer Index detects aspects of health related quality of life related to bladder cancer treatments that are not recorded by more general measures (Gilbert et al. 2010). The Bladder Cancer Index is a robust, multidimensional measure of bladder cancer specific health related quality of life and to our knowledge is the first available validated instrument to assess health outcomes across a range of local treatments commonly used for bladder cancer (Gilbert et al. 2010).

Cookson et al. reviewed the impact of treatment on the health related quality of life (HRQOL) in patients with urological conditions (Cookson et al. 2003). However, a validated disease and treatment specific instrument to assess HRQOL following radical cystectomy (RC) and urinary diversion (UD) is currently lacking (Cookson et al. 2003). A 45-item questionnaire consisting of the Functional Assessment of Cancer Therapy (FACT)-General and 17 additional items designed to measure disease and treatment specific health outcomes were combined to form the Vanderbilt Cystectomy Index (FACT-VCI) (Cookson et al. 2003). Overall FACT-VCI was found to have adequate internal consistency (Cronbach's alpha>0.70). A prospective longitudinal study of FACT-VCI is currently ongoing (Cookson et al. 2003).

In 1986, the European Organization for Research and Treatment of Cancer (EORTC) initiated a research program to develop an integrated, modular approach for evaluating the quality of life of patients participating in international clinical trials (Aaronson et al. 1993). The QLQ-C30 incorporates nine multi-item scales: five functional scales (physical, role, cognitive, emotional, and social); three symptom scales (fatigue, pain, and nausea and vomiting); and a global health and quality-of-life scale. Several single-item symptom measures are also included. These results support the EORTC QLQ-C30 as a reliable and valid measure of the quality of life of cancer patients in multicultural clinical research settings (Aaronson et al. 1993).

The quality of life (QOL) of long-term survivors of bladder cancer in a population-based registry was assessed by using The Functional Assessment of Cancer Therapy (FACT-BL) instrument was used to evaluate QOL in a population-based sample of bladder cancer patients (Allareddy et al. 2006). QOL scores were compared between those undergoing radical cystectomy (RC) or those with an intact bladder (BI) and between continent and conduit urinary diversion groups (Allareddy et al. 2006).

A total of 259 patients participated in the study who had undergone RC ($n = 82$) or other therapy (BI) ($n = 177$). There were no differences in general QOL scores between RC and BI groups and between the 2 urinary diversion groups, but patients undergoing RC had worse sexual function scores (Allareddy et al. 2006). QOL scores for BI patients tended to decrease with increasing age ($p = 0.01$). Presence of comorbid conditions lowered QOL ($p < 0.05$). General QOL does not vary among long-term bladder cancer survivors regardless of treatment, but sexual functioning can be adversely affected in those undergoing cystectomy (Allareddy et al. 2006). Long-term QOL declines even in those with intact bladders, particularly in those with comorbidities.

References

Aaronson NK, Ahmedzai S, Bergman B, et al. The European organization for research and treatment of cancer QLQ-C30: a quality-of-life instrument for use in international clinical trials in oncology. J Natl Cancer Inst. 1993;85(5):365–76.
Allareddy V, Kennedy J, West MM, Konety BR. Quality of life in long-term survivors of bladder cancer. Cancer. 2006;106(11):2355–62.

Cookson MS, Dutta SC, Chang SS, Clark T, Smith JA Jr, Wells N. Health related quality of life
    in patients treated with radical cystectomy and urinary diversion for urothelial carcinoma
    of the bladder: development and validation of a new disease specific questionnaire. J Urol.
    2003;170(5):1926–30.
Fujisawa M, Isotani S, Gotoh A, Okada H, Arakawa S, Kamidono S. Health-related quality of
    life with orthotopic neobladder versus ileal conduit according to the SF-36 survey. Urology.
    2000;55(6):862–5.
Gilbert SM, Wood DP, Dunn RL, et al. Measuring health-related quality of life outcomes in blad-
    der cancer patients using the Bladder Cancer Index (BCI). Cancer. 2007;109(9):1756–62.
Gilbert SM, Dunn RL, Hollenbeck BK, et al. Development and validation of the Bladder Cancer
    Index: a comprehensive, disease specific measure of health related quality of life in patients
    with localized bladder cancer. J Urol. 2010;183(5):1764–70.
Kikuchi E, Horiguchi Y, Nakashima J, et al. Assessment of long-term quality of life using the
    FACT-BL questionnaire in patients with an ileal conduit, continent reservoir, or orthotopic
    neobladder. Jpn J Clin Oncol. 2006;36(11):712–6.
Ware JE Jr, Sherbourne CD. The MOS 36-item short-form health survey (SF-36). I. Conceptual
    framework and item selection. Med Care. 1992;30(6):473–83.

Bibliography

Abaza R. Robotic ureteroileal anastomosis revision. J Endourol. 2009;23:A386.

Abdel-Rahman O. Squamous cell carcinoma of the bladder: a seer database analysis. Clin Genitourin Cancer. 2017;15(3):e463–8.

Adding C, Collins JW, Laurin O, Hosseini A, Wiklund NP. Enhanced recovery protocols (Erp) in robotic cystectomy surgery. Review of current status and trends. Curr Urol Rep. 2015;16(5).

Ajili F, Manai M, Darouiche A, Chebil M, Boubaker S. Tumor multiplicity is an independent prognostic factor of non-muscle-invasive bladder cancer treated with Bacillus Calmette-Guerin Immunotherapy. Ultrastruct Pathol. 2012;36(5):320–4.

Ajili F, Darouiche A, Chebil M, Boubaker S. The efficiency of the corte scoring system for the prediction of recurrence and progression of non-muscle-invasive bladder cancer treated by Bacillus Calmette-Guerin Immunotherapy. Ultrastruct Pathol. 2013a;37(4):249–53.

Ajili F, Darouiche A, Chebil M, Boubaker S. The efficacy of intravesical bacillus Calmette-Guerin in the treatment of patients with pT1 stage non-muscle-invasive bladder cancer. Ultrastruct Pathol. 2013b;37(4):278–83.

Akbal C, Tinay I, Simsek F, Turkeri LN. Erectile dysfunction following radiotherapy and brachytherapy for prostate cancer: pathophysiology, prevention and treatment.. Int Urol Nephrol. 2008;40(2):355–63.

Al-Zalabani AH, Stewart KF, Wesselius A, Schols AM, Zeegers MP. Modifiable risk factors for the prevention of bladder cancer: a systematic review of meta-analyses. Eur J Epidemiol. 2016;31(9):811–51.

Albersen M, Orabi H, Lue TF. Evaluation and treatment of erectile dysfunction in the aging male: a mini-review. Gerontology. 2012;58(1):3–14.

Alexandrov A, Kassabov B, Buse S. Robot-assisted intracorporal radical cystectomy, lymph node dissection, and fully intracorporal ileal conduit reconstruction. Eur Urol Suppl. 2011;10(8):559.

Altobelli E, Buscarini M, Gill H, Skinner E. Readmission rate after radical cystectomy in patients managed following the enhanced recovery after surgery protocols. J Urol. 2015;1:e855–56.

Aminsharifi A, Brousell SC, Chang A, Leon J, Inman BA. Heat-targeted drug delivery: a promising approach for organsparing treatment of bladder cancer. Thermodox(R). Arch Esp Urol. 2018;71(4):447–52.

Athanasiadis G, Soares R, Swinn M, Perry M, Jones C, Patil K. Setting up a new robot assisted radical cystectomy service. Eur Urol Suppl. 2014;13(3):31.

Bae SU, Min BS, Kim NK. Robotic Low ligation of the inferior mesenteric artery with real-time identification of the vascular system for rectal cancer using the firefly technique. Surg Endosc Other Interv Tech. 2015;29:S374.

Bandura A. Health promotion by social cognitive means. Health Educ Behav. 2004a;31(2):143–64.

Bandura A. Swimming against the mainstream: the early years from chilly tributary to transformative mainstream. Behav Res Ther. 2004b;42(6):613–30.

Bandura A, Caprara GV, Barbaranelli C, Gerbino M, Pastorelli C. Role of affective self-regulatory efficacy in diverse spheres of psychosocial functioning. Child Dev. 2003;74(3):769–82.

Bandura A, Caprara GV, Barbaranelli C, Pastorelli C, Regalia C. Sociocognitive self-regulatory mechanisms governing transgressive behavior. J Pers Soc Psychol. 2001;80(1):125–35.

Banerjee S, Manley K, Shaw B, Lewis L, Cucato G, Mills R, Rochester M, Clark A, Saxton JM. Vigorous intensity aerobic interval exercise in bladder cancer patients prior to radical cystectomy: a feasibility randomised controlled Trial. Support Care Cancer. 2018;26(5):1515–23.

Bannowsky A, Schulze H, Uckert S, Junemann KP. Rehabilitation of erectile function two years after nerve-sparing radical prostatectomy: is there a real significant effect with nightly low-dose sildenafil (25 Mg)? J Fur Urol Und Urogynakologie. 2014;21(3):16–21.

Barbour RS. Making sense of focus groups. Med Educ. 2005;39(7):742–50.

Barnett C, Kumar P, Challacombe B, Dasgupta P. Robot assisted laparoscopic prostatectomy. Striving for trifecta outcomes in localised prostate cancer. Minerva Med. 2011;102(4):333–38.

Bashir U, Ahmed I, Bashir O, Azam M, Faruqui ZS, Uddin N. Diagnostic accuracy of high resolution MR imaging in local staging of bladder tumors. J Coll Physicians Surg Pak. 2014;24(5):314–7.

Baten E, Joniau S, Van Poppel H, Van Der Aa F. When is a conservative management recommended for ureterointestinal strictures following radical cystectomy with ileal conduit? Eur Urol Suppl. 2014;13(1):e284.

Becker A, Tennstedt P, Hansen J, Trinh QD, Kluth L, Atassi N, Schlomm T, et al. Functional and oncological outcomes of patients aged <50 years treated with radical prostatectomy for localised prostate cancer in a european population. BJU Int. 2014;114(1):38–45.

Benight CC, Bandura A. Social cognitive theory of posttraumatic recovery: the role of perceived self-efficacy. Behav Res Ther. 2004;42(10):1129–48.

Benson MC, Olsson CA. Continent urinary diversion. Urol Clin North Am. 1999;26(1):125–47, ix.

Benzo R, Kelley GA, Recchi L, Hofman A, Sciurba F. Complications of lung resection and exercise capacity: a meta-analysis. Respir Med. 2007;101(8):1790–97.

Berger MM, Marazzi A, Freeman J, Chiolero R. Evaluation of the consistency of acute physiology and chronic health evaluation (Apache Ii) scoring in a surgical intensive care unit. Crit Care Med. 1992;20(12):1681–87.

Berry DL, Blumenstein BA, Halpenny B, Wolpin S, Fann JR, Austin-Seymour M, Bush N, et al. Enhancing patient-provider communication with the electronic self-report assessment for cancer: a randomized trial. J Clin Oncol. 2011;29(8):1029–35.

Bhindi B, Mamdani M, Kulkarni GS, Finelli A, Hamiton RJ, Trachtenberg J, Zlotta AR, et al. Prostate biopsy trends in relation to U.S. preventative task for recommendations against routine psa-based screening: a time-series analysis. Eur Urol Suppl. 2014;13(1):e852.

Bjerre BD, Johansen C, Steven K. Health-related quality of life after cystectomy: bladder substitution compared with ileal conduit diversion. A questionnaire survey. Br J Urol. 1995;75(2):200–5.

Blanco Lanzillotti T. Plan for sexual function rehabilitation post radical prostatectomy (interdisciplinary work). J Sex Med. 2014;11:247.

Bober SL, Sanchez Varela V. Sexuality in adult cancer survivors: challenges and intervention. J Clin Oncol. 2012;30(30):3712–19.

Bogdan RC. Qualitative research for education: an introduction to theory and methods. Edited by S Biklen. Boston: Allyn and Bacon. 1982.

Bohle A, Leyh H, Frei C, Kuhn M, Tschada R, Pottek T, Wagner W, et al. Single postoperative instillation of gemcitabine in patients with non-muscle-invasive transitional cell carcinoma of the bladder: a randomised, double-blind, placebo-controlled phase III multicentre study. Eur Urol. 2009;56;(3):495–503.

Bosschieter J, Nieuwenhuijzen JA, Vis AN, van Ginkel T, Lissenberg-Witte BI, Beckers GMA, van Moorselaar RJA. An Immediate, single intravesical instillation of mitomycin C is of benefit in patients with non-muscle-invasive bladder cancer irrespective of prognostic risk groups. Urol Oncol. 2018.

Boyd SD, Feinberg SM, Skinner DG, Lieskovsky G, Baron D, Richardson J. Quality of life survey of urinary diversion patients: comparison of ileal conduits versus continent kock ileal reservoirs. J Urol. 1987;138(6):1386–9.

Braun V. Using thematic analysis in psychology. In: Clarke V, editor. Qualitative research in psychology, vol. 82. 2006.

Brechin A. Developing your practice. Nurs Manag (Harrow, London, England: 1994). 2002;9(3):36–9.

Bronner G, Shefi S, Raviv G. Sexual dysfunction after radical prostatectomy: treatment failure or treatment delay? J Sex Marital Ther. 2010;36(5):421–9.

Brown LD. Ideology and Political Economy in Inquiry: action research and participatory action research. Edited by Tandon R, 277–94: J Appl Behav Sci. 1983.

Burger M, van der Aa MN, van Oers JM, Brinkmann A, van der Kwast TH, Steyerberg EC, Stoehr R, et al. Prediction of progression of non-muscle-invasive bladder cancer by who 1973 and 2004 grading and by FGFR3 mutation status: a prospective study. Eur Urol. 2008;54(4):835–43.

Campain N, McGrath J, Jackson L, Batchelor N, Daugherty M, Waine E. The robot alone is not enough-how to to provide a comprehensive enhanced recovery service. Eur Urol Suppl. 2014;13(3):14–15.

Canada AL, Neese LE, Sui D, Schover LR. Pilot Intervention to enhance sexual rehabilitation for couples after treatment for localized prostate carcinoma. Cancer. 2005;104(12):2689–700.

Cantiello F, Cicione A, Autorino R, Salonia A, Briganti A, Ferro M, De Domenico R, Perdona S, Damiano R. Visceral obesity predicts adverse pathological features in urothelial cell carcinomapatients undergoing radical cystectomy: a retrospective cohort study. World J Urol. 2014;32(2):559–64.

Cappelleri JC, Rosen RC. The sexual health inventory for men (shim): A 5-Year review of research and clinical experience. Int J Impot Res. 2005;17(4):307–19.

Carneiro A, Dovirak O, Kaplan J, Chang P, Wagner AA. Robot-assisted ureteroileal reimplantation for post-cystectomy anastomotic stricture. J Urol. 2015;(1):e848.

Cerantola Y, Valerio M, Persson B, Jichlinski P, Ljungqvist O, Hubner M, Kassouf W, et al. Guidelines for perioperative care after radical cystectomy for bladder cancer: enhanced recovery after surgery (Eras) society recommendations. Clin Nutr. 2013;32(6):879–87.

Challacombe B, Dasgupta P. Reconstruction of the lower urinary tract by laparoscopic and robotic surgery. Curr Opin Urol. 2007;17(6):390–95.

Chambers SK, Occhipinti S, Schover L, Nielsen L, Zajdlewicz L, Clutton S, Halford K, Gardiner RA, Dunn J. A randomised controlled trial of a couples-based sexuality intervention for men with localised prostate cancer and their female partners. Psychooncology. 2004;8.

Charles Osterberg E, Ramasamy R, Greenwood E, Dubin J, Ng CK, Lee RK, Shariat SF, Scherr DS. Robotic radical cystectomy is feasible and safe in the treatment of adequately selected octogenarians. J Urol. 2011;1:e196.

Cheng B, Qiu X, Li H, Yang G. The safety and efficacy of front-firing green-light laser endoscopic en bloc photoselective vapo-enucleation of non-muscle-invasive bladder cancer. Ther Clin Risk Manag. 2017;13:983–88.

Chevalier JM. A guide to collaborative inquiry and social engagement. Edited by DJ Buckles. Ottawa: Sage; 2008.

Clark JA, Inui TS, Silliman RA, Bokhour BG, Krasnow SH, Robinson RA, Spaulding M, Talcott JA. Patients' perceptions of quality of life after treatment for early prostate cancer. J Clin Oncol: Off J Am Soc Clin Oncol. 2003;21(20):3777–84.

Clark PE. Urinary diversion after radical cystectomy. Curr Treat Options Oncol. 2002;3(5):389–402.

Clayton RA, Bannard-Smith JP, Washington SJ, Wisely N, Columb M, Rees L. Cardiopulmonary exercise testing and length of stay in patients undergoing major surgery. Anaesthesia. 2011;66(5):393–4.

Cobo M, Delgado R, Gil S, Herruzo I, Baena V, Carabante F, Moreno P, et al. Conservative treatment with transurethral resection, neoadjuvant chemotherapy followed by radiochemotherapy in stage T2-3 transitional bladder cancer. Clin Transl Oncol. 2006;8(12):903–11.

Cohen J. Weighted kappa: nominal scale agreement with provision for scaled disagreement or partial credit. Psychol Bull. 1968;70(4):213–20.

Collins J. Letter from the editor: what is the US preventive services task force? Semin Roentgenol. 2015;50(2):65–6.

Collins JW, Tyritzis S, Nyberg T, Schumacher MC, Laurin O, Adding C, Jonsson M, et al. Robot-assisted radical cystectomy (Rarc) with intracorporeal neobladder—what is the effect of the learning curve on outcomes? BJU Int. 2014;113(1):100–7.

Collins JW, Wiklund NP. Totally intracorporeal robot-assisted radical cystectomy: optimizing total outcomes. BJU Int. 2014;114(3):326–33.

Conde Redondo C, Estebanez Zarranz J, Rodriguez Tovez A, Amon Sesmero J, Alonso Fernandez D, Martinez Sagarra JM. Quality of life in patients treated with orthotopic bladder substitution versus cutaneous ileostomy. Actas Urol Esp. 2001;25(6):435–44.

Connelly J, Gnanasegaran G, Schilling C, McGurk M. 99mtc-Nanocolloid SPECT/CT and a portable gamma camera for image-guided sentinel node biopsy in head and neck malignancy: science & practice. Nucl Med Commun. 2013;34(4):386.

Cookson MS, Herr HW, Zhang ZF, Soloway S, Sogani PC, Fair WR. The treated natural history of high risk NMI bladder cancer: 15-year outcome. J Urol. 1997;158(1):62–7.

Copeland LA, Elshaikh MA, Jackson J, Penner LA, Underwood W, 3rd. Impact of brachytherapy on regional, racial, marital status, and age-related patterns of definitive treatment for clinically localized prostate carcinoma. Cancer. 2005;104(7):1372–80.

Cormie P, Chambers SK, Newton RU, Gardiner RA, Spry N, Taaffe DR, Joseph D, et al. Improving Sexual health in men with prostate cancer: randomised controlled trial of exercise and psychosexual therapies. BMC Cancer. 2014;14(1).

Crofts M, Jeal N. Improving quality through service user involvement: focus groups with street-based sex workers. HIV Med. 2014;15:21–2.

D'Amico AV, Whittington R, Bruce Malkowicz S, Schultz D, Blank K, Broderick GA, Tomaszewski JE, et al. Biochemical outcome after radical prostatectomy, external beam radiation therapy, or interstitial radiation therapy for clinically localized prostate cancer. J Am Med Assoc. 1998a;280(11):969–74.

D'Amico AV, Whittington R, Malkowicz SB, Fondurulia J, Chen MH, Tomaszewski JE, Wein A. The combination of preoperative prostate specific antigen and postoperative pathological findings to predict prostate specific antigen outcome in clinically localized prostate cancer. J Urol. 1998b;160(6 Pt 1):2096–101.

Dabi Y, Rouscoff Y, Anract J, Delongchamps NB, Sibony M, Saighi D, Zerbib M, Peyraumore M, Xylinas E. Impact of body mass index on the oncological outcomes of patients treated with radical cystectomy for muscle-invasive bladder cancer. World J Urol. 2017;35(2):229–35.

Daneshmand S, Ahmadi H, Huynh LN, Dobos N. preoperative staging of invasive bladder cancer with dynamic gadolinium-enhanced magnetic resonance imaging: results from a prospective study. Urology. 2012;80(6):1313–8.

Danesi DT, Arcangeli G, Cruciani E, Altavista P, Mecozzi A, Saracino B, Orefici F. Conservative treatment of invasive bladder carcinoma by transurethral resection, protracted intravenous infusion chemotherapy, and hyperfractionated radiotherapy: long term results. Cancer. 2004;101(11):2540–8.

Das Nair R, Orr KS, Vedhara K, Kendrick D. Exploring recruitment barriers and facilitators in early cancer detection trials: the use of pre-trial focus groups. Trials. 2014;15(1).

Davis JW, Dasgupta P. A case-mix-adjusted comparison of early oncological outcomes of open and robotic prostatectomy performed by experienced high volume surgeons. BJU Int. 2013;111(2):184–5.

Davison BJ, Elliott S, Ekland M, Griffin S, Wiens K. Development and evaluation of a prostate sexual rehabilitation clinic: a pilot project. BJU Int. 2005;96(9):1360–64.

Davison BJ, So AI, Goldenberg SL. Quality of life, sexual function and decisional regret at 1 year after surgical treatment for localized prostate cancer. BJU Int. 2007;100(4):780–5.

Day JR, Rossiter HB, Coats EM, Skasick A, Whipp BJ. The maximally attainable Vo2 during exercise in humans: the peak vs. maximum issue. J Appl Physiol. 2003;95(5):1901–7.

Desai MM, Berger AK, Brandina RR, Zehnder P, Simmons M, Aron M, Skinner EC, Gill IS. Robotic and laparoscopic high extended pelvic lymph node dissection during radical cystectomy: technique and outcomes. Eur Urol. 2012;61(2):350–5.

Desai MM, de Abreu AL, Goh AC, Fairey A, Berger A, Leslie S, Xie HW, et al. Robotic intracorporeal urinary diversion: technical details to improve time efficiency. J Endourol/Endourol Soc. 2014;28(11):1320–7.

Desai MM, Gill IS, de Castro Abreu AL, Hosseini A, Nyberg T, Adding C, Laurin O, et al. Robotic intracorporeal orthotopic neobladder during radical cystectomy in 132 patients. J Urol. 192(6):1734–40.

Descazeaud A, Zerbib M, Hofer MD, Chaskalovic J, Debre B, Peyromaure M. Evolution of health-related quality of life two to seven years after retropubic radical prostatectomy: evaluation by Ucla prostate cancer index. World J Urol. 2005;23(4):257–62.

Domes T, Chung E, Deyoung L, MacLean N, Al-Shaiji T, Brock G. Clinical outcomes of intracavernosal injection in postprostatectomy patients: a single-center experience. Urology. 2012;79(1):150–5.

Duffty J, Hilditch G. Anaesthesia for urological surgery. Anaesth Intensiv Care Med. 2009;10(6):307–12.

Dutta SC, Chang SC, Coffey CS, Smith JA, Jr, Jack G, Cookson MS. Health related quality of life assessment after radical cystectomy: comparison of ileal conduit with continent orthotopic neobladder. J Urol. 2002;168(1):164–7.

Eden CG, Moon DA. Laparoscopic radical prostatectomy: minimum 3-year follow-up of the first 100 patients in the UK. BJU Int. 2006;97(5):981–4.

Eden CG, Zacharakis E, Bott S. The learning curve for laparoscopic extended pelvic lymphadenectomy for intermediate- and high-risk prostate cancer: implications for compliance with existing guidelines. BJU Int. 2013;112(3):346–54.

Eisenberg M, Dorin R, Bartsch G, Cai J, Miranda G, Skinner E. Cystectomy after high dose pelvic radiation: does type of urinary diversion affect late complications? J Urol. 2010;1:e297.

Fahmy O, Khairul-Asri MG, Schubert T, Renninger M, Malek R, Kubler H, Stenzl A, Gakis G. A systematic review and meta-analysis on the oncological long-term outcomes after trimodality therapy and radical cystectomy with or without neoadjuvant chemotherapy for muscle-invasive bladder cancer. Urol Oncol. 2018;36(2):43–53.

Fereday J. Demonstrating rigor using thematic analysis: a hybrid approach of inductive and deductive coding development. Int J Qual Methods. 2006.

Ferrell BR, Winn R. Medical and nursing education and training opportunities to improve survivorship care. J Clin Oncol. 2006;24(32):5142–8.

Ferro M, Vartolomei MD, Russo GI, Cantiello F, Farhan ARA, Terracciano D, Cimmino A, et al. An increased body mass index is associated with a worse prognosis in patients administered BCG immunotherapy for T1 bladder cancer. World J Urol. 2018.

Ficarra V, Borghesi M, Suardi N, De Naeyer G, Novara G, Schatteman P, De Groote R, Carpentier P, Mottrie A. Long-term evaluation of survival, continence and potency (Scp) outcomes after robot-assisted radical prostatectomy (Rarp). BJU Int. 2013;112(3):338–45.

Ficarra V, Novara G, Fracalanza S, D'Elia C, Secco S, Iafrate M, Cavalleri S, Artibani W. A prospective, non-randomized trial comparing robot-assisted laparoscopic and retropubic radical prostatectomy in one European institution. BJU Int. 2009;104(4):534–9.

Fisher RA, Dasgupta P, Mottrie A, Volpe A, Khan MS, Challacombe B, Ahmed K. An overview of robot assisted surgery curricula and the status of their validation. Int J Surg. 2015;13:115–23.

Fitch MI, Miller D, Sharir S, McAndrew A. Radical cystectomy for bladder cancer: a qualitative study of patient experiences and implications for practice. Can Oncol Nurs J. 2010;20(4):177–87.

Flynn KE, Jeffery DD, Keefe FJ, Porter LS, Shelby RA, Fawzy MR, Gosselin TK, Reeve BB, Weinfurt KP. Sexual functioning along the cancer continuum: focus group results from the patient-reported outcomes measurement information system (promis). Psycho Oncol. 2011;20(4):378–86.

Fode M, Borre M, Ohl DA, Lichtbach J, Sonksen J. Penile vibratory stimulation in the recovery of urinary continence and erectile function after nerve-sparing radical prostatectomy: a randomized, controlled trial. BJU Int. 2014a;114(1):111–7.

Fode M, Borre M, Ohl D, Lichtbach J, Sonksen J. Penile vibratory stimulation in the recovery of erectile function and urinary continence after nerve sparing radical prostatectomy: a randomized, controlled trial. J Sex Med. 2014b;11:20.

Forbat L, White I, Marshall-Lucette S, Kelly D. Discussing the sexual consequences of treatment in radiotherapy and urology consultations with couples affected by prostate cancer. BJU Int. 2012;109(1):98–103.

French R, Kurup V. Targetted axillary node sampling- is there a role in the era of sentinal node biopsy? Eur J Surg Oncol. 2012;38(5):426.

French S, Swain J. Changing disability research: participating and emancipatory research with disabled people. Physiotherapy. 1997;83(1):26–32.

Frew G, Dashfield E. Testing care pathways for prostate cancer survivors. Nurs Times. 2012;108(13):30–1.

Galbraith ME, Arechiga A, Ramirez J, Pedro LW. Prostate cancer survivors' and partners' self-reports of health-related quality of life, treatment symptoms, and marital satisfaction 2.5–5.5 years after treatment. Oncol Nurs Forum. 2005;32(2):E30–41.

Gan C, Stephenson W, Rottenberg G, Thomas K, Khan MS, O'Brien T. A prospective study of the utility of a routine 'Loopogram' 3 months after surgery for the detection of anastomotic stricture post cystectomy and ileal conduit formation. Eur Urol Suppl. 2015;14(2):e473.

Garcia-Perdomo HA, Montes-Cardona CE, Guacheta M, Castillo DF, Reis O. Muscle-invasive bladder cancer organ-preserving therapy: systematic review and meta-analysis. World J Urol. 2018.

Garg T, Connors JN, Ladd IG, Bogaczyk TL, Larson SL. defining priorities to improve patient experience in non-muscle invasive bladder cancer. Bladder Cancer. 2018;4(1):121–8.

Gerharz EW, Weingartner K, Dopatka T, Kohl UN, Basler HD, Riedmiller HN. Quality of life after cystectomy and urinary diversion: results of a retrospective interdisciplinary study J Urol.1997;158(3 Pt 1):778–85.

Gerson MC, Hurst JM, Hertzberg VS, Baughman R, Rouan GW, Ellis K, Fischer EE, Colthar MS, Burwinkle PM. Prediction of cardiac and pulmonary complications related to elective abdominal and noncardiac thoracic surgery in geriatric patients. Am J Med. 1990;88(2):101–7.

Gierth M, Zeman F, Denzinger S, Vetterlein MW, Fisch M, Bastian PJ, Syring I, et al. Influence of body mass index on clinical outcome parameters, complication rate and survival after radical cystectomy: evidence from a prospective european multicentre study. Urol Int. 2018;101(1):16–24.

Girgis A, Lambert S, Lecathelinais C. The supportive care needs survey for partners and caregivers of cancer survivors: development and psychometric evaluation. Psychooncology. 2011;20(4):387–93.

Girish M, Trayner E Jr, Dammann O, Pinto-Plata V, Celli B. Symptom-limited stair climbing as a predictor of postoperative cardiopulmonary complications after high-risk surgery. Chest. 2001;120(4):1147–51.

Given BA, Given CW, Sherwood PR. Family and caregiver needs over the course of the cancer trajectory. J Support Oncol. 2012;10(2):57–64.

Goel A, Gupta A, Khanna S, Vashishtha S, Rawal S. Surgical technique of staplerless total intra-corporeal robot assisted laparoscopic ileal conduit for transitional cell carcinoma of bladder. J Urol. 2014;1:e551–2.

Golijanin J, Amin A, Moshnikova A, Brito JM, Tran TY, Adochite RC, Andreev GO, et al. Targeted imaging of urothelium carcinoma in human bladders by an Icg phlip peptide ex vivo. Proc Natl Acad Sci USA. 2016;113(42):11829–34.

Gontero P. The not-infrequent story of a NMI bladder carcinoma...Discussion of clinical case no. 2. Arch Ital Urol Androl. 2006;78(4, Suppl. 1):11–2.

Gontero P, Bohle A, Malmstrom PU, O'Donnell MA, Oderda M, Sylvester R, Witjes F. The role of bacillus Calmette-Guerin in the treatment of non-muscle-invasive bladder cancer. Eur Urol. 2010;57(3):410–29.

Goonewardene SS, Nanton V, Young A, Makar A. The worcestershire prostate cancer survivorship programme: a new concept for holistic long term care and follow-up. BJU Int. 2014;113:116–7.

Goonewardene SS, Persad R, Young A, Makar A, Bourke L, Gilbert S, Hooper R, et al. Lifestyle changes for improving disease-specific quality of life in sedentary men on long-term androgen-deprivation therapy for advanced prostate cancer: a randomised controlled trial. Eur Urol. 2014a;65:865–72. Eur Urol. 2014;66(3):e51–2.

Goonewardene SS, Rowe E. Radical robotic assisted laparoscopic prostatectomy: a day case procedure. BJU Int. 2014b;113:116.

Goonewardene SS, Young A, Symons M, Sullivan A, McCormack G, Milner V, Makar A. The prostate cancer survivorship program: a new concept for holistic long-term support and follow-up. J Clin Oncol. 2012;1.

Gore JL, Kwan L, Lee SP, Reiter RE, Litwin MS. Survivorship beyond convalescence: 48-month quality-of-life outcomes after treatment for localized prostate cancer. J Natl Cancer Inst. 2009;101(12):888–92.

Graham J, Kirkbride P, Cann K, Hasler E, Prettyjohns M. Prostate cancer: summary of updated nice guidance. BMJ. 2014;348(f7524).

Graziottin A, Trombetta C, Ciciliato S, Wiesenfeld U. Psychosexual outcomes after radical prostatectomy. Urodinamica. 2001;11(2):60–65.

Green HJ, Steinnagel G, Morris C. Using the commonsense and transtheoretical models to understand health behaviours after diagnosis with prostate or breast cancer. Psycho Oncol. 2011;20:271–2.

Grov EK, Valeberg BT. Does the cancer patient's disease stage matter? a comparative study of caregivers' mental health and health related quality of life. Palliat Support Care. 2012;10(3):189–96.

Guest, G, Macqueen KM, Namey E. Applied thematic analyis. Edited by Elizabeth Namey. London: Sage; 2012.

Gutierrez, C, Hernansanz S, Rubiales AS, Del Valle ML, Cuadrillero Rodriguez F, Flores LA, Garcia C. Clinical manifestations and care in tumors with pelvic involvement: is there a pelvic syndrome in palliative care? Med Paliativa. 2006;13(1):32–6.

Gutnick D, Reims K, Davis C, Gainforth H, Jay M, Cole S. Brief action planning to facilitate behavior change and support patient self-management. J Clin Outcomes Manag. 2014;21(1):17–29.

Hafron J, Mitra N, Dalbagni G, Bochner B, Herr H, Donat SM. Does body mass index affect survival of patients undergoing radical or partial cystectomy for bladder cancer? J Urol. 2005;173(5):1513–7.

Hagen S, Glazener C, Boachie C, Buckley B, Cochran C, Dorey G, Grant A, et al. Urinary incontinence and erectile dysfunction after radical prostatectomy: association with route and technique of operation. Int Urogynecol J Pelvic Floor Dysfunct. 2010;21:S25–7.

Hall, BL. Participatory action research; an approach for change. 2 Vols. Vol. 8: Convergence; 1975.

Han M, Trock BJ, Partin AW, Humphreys EB, Bivalacqua TJ, Guzzo TJ, Walsh PC. The impact of preoperative erectile dysfunction on survival after radical prostatectomy. BJU Int. 2010;106(11):1612–17.

Hanly N, Juraskova I. Sexual adjustment and self-perception in men following prostate cancer. Supportive Care in Cancer. 2011;1:S332.

Hanly N, Mireskandari S, Juraskova I. The struggle towards 'the new normal': a qualitative insight into psychosexual adjustment to prostate cancer. BMC Urol. 2014a;14(1).

Hanly N, Mireskandari S, Juraskova I. The struggle towards 'the new normal': a qualitative insight into psychosexual adjustment to prostate cancer. BMC Urol. 2014b;14:56.

Hara I, Miyake H, Hara S, Gotoh A, Nakamura I, Okada H, Arakawa S, Kamidono S. Health-related quality of life after radical cystectomy for bladder cancer: a comparison of ileal conduit and orthotopic bladder replacement. BJU Int. 2002;89(1):10–3.

Harrington A, Bradley S, Jeffers L, Linedale E, Kelman S, Killington G. The implementation of intentional rounding using participatory action research. Int J Nurs Pract. 2013;19(5):523–9.

Harris CJ, Anderson CB, Dietrich MS, Barocas DA, Chang SS, Cookson MS, Smith JA Jr, et al. Recovery of erectile function after radical prostatectomy: identification of trajectory cluster groups. J Urol. 2014;1:e337.

Harris CR, Punnen S, Carroll PR. Men with low preoperative sexual function may benefit from nerve sparing radical prostatectomy. J Urol. 2013;190(3):981–6.

Hedgepeth RC, Gilbert SM, He C, Lee CT, Wood DP, Jr. Body image and bladder cancer specific quality of life in patients with ileal conduit and neobladder urinary diversions. Urology. 2010;76(3):671–5.

Heidenreich A, Epplen R, Thuer D, Van Erps T, David D. Eau guideline on clinically localized prostate cancer: compliance among urologists concerning diagnosis, staging and treatment. Eur Urol. 2011;2(Suppl. 10):113.

Heldenbrand SD, Turnbow LE, Payakachat N. Patient self-efficacy and satisfaction after medication education following solid organ transplantation. Pharmacotherapy. 2010;30(10):425e.

Hellenthal NJ, Hussain A, Andrews PE, Carpentier P, Castle E, Dasgupta P, Kaouk J, et al. Surgical margin status after robot assisted radical cystectomy: results from the international robotic cystectomy consortium. J Urol. 2010;184(1):87–91.

Herrell SD, Webster R, Simaan N. Future robotic platforms in urologic surgery: recent developments. Curr Opin Urol. 2014;24(1):18–26.

Hlatky MA, Boineau RE, Higginbotham MB, Lee KL, Mark DB, Califf RM, Cobb FR, Pryor DB. A brief self-administered questionnaire to determine functional capacity (the duke activity status index). Am J Cardiol. 1989;64(10):651–4.

Hobisch A, Tosun K, Kinzl J, Kemmler G, Bartsch G, Holtl L, Stenzl A. Life after cystectomy and orthotopic neobladder versus Ileal conduit urinary diversion. Semin Urol Oncol. 2001;19(1):8–23.

Hockenberry MS, Smith ZL, Mucksavage P. A novel use of near-infrared fluorescence imaging during robotic surgery without contrast agents. J Endourol. 2014;28(5):509–12.

Hofbauer SL, Shariat SF, Chade DC, Sarkis AS, Ribeiro-Filho LA, Nahas WC, Klatte T. The Moreau strain of Bacillus Calmette-Guerin (Bcg) for high-risk non-muscle invasive bladder cancer: an alternative during worldwide Bcg shortage? Urol Int. 2016;96(1):46–50.

Horovitz D, Meng Y, Joseph JV, Feng C, Wu G, Rashid H, Messing EM. The role of urinary cytology when diagnostic workup is suspicious for upper tract urothelial carcinoma but tumour biopsy is nonconfirmatory. Can Urol Assoc J. 2017;11(7):E285–e90.

Horstmann M, Banek S, Gakis G, Todenhofer T, Aufderklamm S, Hennenlotter J, Stenzl A, Schwentner C. Prospective evaluation of fluorescence-guided cystoscopy to detect bladder cancer in a high-risk population: results from the uroscreen-study. Springerplus. 2014;3:24.

Horton M, Freire P. We Make the road by walking. Conversations on education and social change. Edited by Horton M. Philadelphia: Temple University Press; 1990.

Hours M, Cardis E, Marciniak A, Quelin P, Fabry J. Mortality of a cohort in a polyamide-polyester factory in lyon: a further follow up. Br J Ind Med. 1989;46(9):665–70.

Houskova L, Zemanova Z, Babjuk M, Melichercikova J, Pesl M, Michalova K. Molecular cytogenetic characterization and diagnostics of bladder cancer. Neoplasma. 2007;54(6):511–6.

Hoyland, K., N. Vasdev, J. M. Adshead, and A. Thorpe. "Cardiopulmonary Exercise Testing in Patients Undergoing Radical Cystectomy (Open, Laparoscopic and Robotic)." [In English]. *Journal of Clinical Urology* 7, no. 6 (29 Nov 2014): 374-79.

Huguet J, Crego M, Sabate S, Salvador J, Palou J, Villavicencio H. Cystectomy in patients with high risk NMI bladder tumors who fail intravesical Bcg therapy: pre-cystectomy prostate involvement as a prognostic factor. Eur Urol. 2005;48(1):53–9; discussion 59.

Iida S, Kondo T, Kobayashi H, Hashimoto Y, Goya N, Tanabe K. Clinical outcome of high-grade non-muscle-invasive bladder cancer: a long-term single center experience. Int J Urol. 2009;16(3):287–92.

Inoue K, Ota U, Ishizuka M, Kawada C, Fukuhara H, Shuin T, Okura I, Tanaka T, Ogura S. Porphyrins as urinary biomarkers for bladder cancer after 5-aminolevulinic acid (ala) administration: the potential of photodynamic screening for tumors. Photodiagnosis Photodyn Ther. 2013a;10(4):484–9.

Inoue S, Shiina H, Mitsui Y, Yasumoto H, Matsubara A, Igawa M. Identification of lymphatic pathway involved in the spread of bladder cancer: evidence obtained from fluorescence navigation with intraoperatively injected indocyanine green. Can Urol Assoc J. 2013b;7(5–6):E322–8.

Inoue T, Ohyama C, Horikawa Y, Togashi H, Matsuura S, Tsuchiya N, Satoh S, et al. Active chemotherapy with gemcitabine, carboplatin and docetaxel for three patients with mvac-resistant liver metastasis of urothelial carcinoma. Hinyokika Kiyo. 2004;50(4):273–7.

Isbarn H, Budaus L, Pichlmeier U, Conrad S, Huland H, Friedrich MG. Comparison of the effectiveness between long-term instillation of mitomycin C and short-term prophylaxis with Mmc or Bacille Calmette-Guerin. Study of patients with non-muscle-invasive urothelial cancer of the urinary bladder. Urologe A. 2008;47(5):608–15.

Jafari M, Carmichael J, Pigazzi A. Robotic-assisted low anterior resection with transanal extraction: single stapling technique and fluorescence evaluation of bowel perfusion. Dis Colon Rectum. 2015;58(5):e137.

Jarvinen R, Kaasinen E, Sankila A, Rintala E. Long-term efficacy of maintenance bacillus Calmette-Guerin versus maintenance mitomycin C instillation therapy in frequently recurrent Tat1 tumours without carcinoma in situ: a subgroup analysis of the prospective, randomised finnbladder I study with a 20-year follow-up. Eur Urol. 2009;56(2):260–5.

Jensen BT, Petersen AK, Jensen JB, Laustsen S, Borre M. Efficacy of a multiprofessional rehabilitation programme in radical cystectomy pathways: a prospective randomized controlled trial. Scand J Urol. 2015;49(2):133–41.

Jensen TK, Holt P, Gerke O, Riehmann M, Svolgaard B, Marcussen N, Bouchelouche K. Preoperative lymph-node staging of invasive urothelial cell carcinomawith 18f-fluorodeoxyglucose positron emission tomography/computed axial tomography and magnetic resonance imaging: correlation with histopathology. Scand J Urol Nephrol. 2011;45(2):122–8.

Jochems SHJ, van Osch FHM, Reulen RC, van Hensbergen M, Nekeman D, Pirrie S, Wesselius A, et al. Fruit and vegetable intake and the risk of recurrence in patients with non-muscle invasive bladder cancer: a prospective cohort study. Cancer Causes Control. 2018;29(6):573–79.

Johnen G, Gawrych K, Bontrup H, Pesch B, Taeger D, Banek S, Kluckert M, et al. Performance of survivin Mrna as a biomarker for bladder cancer in the prospective study uroscreen. PLoS One. 2012;7(4):e35363.

Johnson RB. Mixed methods research: a research paradigm whose time has come. Edited by WJ Onuwegbuzie, p. 14–26: Educational Researcher; 2004.

Jones LW, Hornsby WE, Freedland SJ, Lane A, West MJ, Moul JW, Ferrandino MN, et al. Effects of nonlinear aerobic training on erectile dysfunction and cardiovascular function following radical prostatectomy for clinically localized prostate cancer. Eur Urol. 2014;65(5):852–55.

Jonsson MN, Schumacher MC, Hosseini A, Adding C, Nilsson A, Carlsson S, Wiklund NP. Oncological outcome after robot-assisted radical cystectomy with intracorporeal urinary diversion technique. Eur Urol Suppl. 2011;10(2):273–74.

Kaasinen E, Wijkstrom H, Malmstrom PU, Hellsten S, Duchek M, Mestad O, Rintala E. Alternating mitomycin C and Bcg instillations versus Bcg alone in treatment of carcinoma in situ of the urinary bladder: a nordic study. Eur Urol. 2003;43(6):637–45.

Kabat GC, Kim MY, Luo J, Hou L, Cetnar J, Wactawski-Wende J, Rohan TE. Menstrual and reproductive factors and exogenous hormone use and risk of transitional cell bladder cancer in postmenopausal women. Eur J Cancer Prev. 2013;22(5):409–16.

Kaimakliotis HZ, Monn MF, Cheng L, Masterson TA, Cary KC, Pedrosa JA, Foster RS, Koch MO, Bihrle R. Plasmacytoid bladder cancer: variant histology with aggressive behavior and a new mode of invasion along fascial planes. Urology. 2014;83(5):1112–6.

Kamat AM, Flaig TW, Grossman HB, Konety B, Lamm D, O'Donnell MA, Uchio E, Efstathiou JA, Taylor JA, 3rd. Expert consensus document: consensus statement on best practice management regarding the use of intravesical immunotherapy with Bcg for bladder cancer. Nat Rev Urol. 2015;12(4):225–35.

Kamboj M, Gandhi JS, Gupta G, Sharma A, Pasricha S, Mehta A, Chandragouda D, Sinha R. Neuroendocrine carcinoma of gall bladder: a series of 19 cases with review of literature. J Gastrointest Cancer. 2015;46(4):356–64.

Karam-Hage M, Cinciripini PM, Gritz ER. Tobacco use and cessation for cancer survivors: an overview for clinicians. CA Cancer J Clin. 2014;64(4):272–90.

Kardas P, Mazurkiewicz M. Patients' assessment of point-of-care sensors for a telemedicine system for type 2 diabetes mellitus management: a focus-group study. Diabetes Technol Ther. 2013;15:A106–A07.

Karvinen KH, Courneya KS, Venner P, North S. Exercise programming and counseling preferences in bladder cancer survivors: a population-based study. J Cancer Surviv. 2007;1(1):27–34.

Kassouf W, Spiess PE, Siefker-Radtke A, Swanson D, Grossman HB, Kamat AM, Munsell MF, et al. Outcome and patterns of recurrence of nonbilharzial pure squamous cell carcinoma of the bladder: a contemporary review of the University of Texas MD Anderson Cancer center experience. Cancer. 2007;110(4):764–9.

Kendirci M, Bejma J, Hellstrom WJG. Update on erectile dysfunction in prostate cancer patients. Curr Opin Urol. 2006;16(3):186–95.

Kenney DM, Geschwindt RD, Kary MR, Linic JM, Sardesai NY, Li ZQ. Detection of newly diagnosed bladder cancer, bladder cancer recurrence and bladder cancer in patients with hematuria using quantitative Rt-Pcr of urinary survivin. Tumour Biol. 2007;28(2):57–62.

Kim HS, Jeong CW, Kwak C, Kim HH, Ku JH. Adjuvant chemotherapy for muscle-invasive bladder cancer: a systematic review and network meta-analysis of randomized clinical trials. Oncotarget. 2017;8(46):81204–14.

Kim SH, Song SG, Paek OJ, Lee HJ, Park DH, Lee JK. Nerve-stimulator-guided pudendal nerve block by pararectal approach. Colorectal Dis. 2012;14(5):611–5.

Kimura M, Banez LL, Polascik TJ, Bernal RM, Gerber L, Robertson CN, Donatucci CF, Moul JW. Sexual bother and function after radical prostatectomy: predictors of sexual bother recovery in men despite persistent post-operative sexual dysfunction. Andrology. 2013;1(2):256–61.

King AJ, Evans M, Moore TH, Paterson C, Sharp D, Persad R, Huntley AL. Prostate cancer and supportive care: a systematic review and qualitative synthesis of men's experiences and unmet needs. Eur J Cancer Care (Engl). 2015.

Kinsella J, Acher P, Ashfield A, Chatterton K, Dasgupta P, Cahill D, Popert R, O'Brien T. Demonstration of erectile management techniques to men scheduled for radical prostatectomy reduces long-term regret: a comparative cohort study. BJU Int. 2012;109(2):254–58.

Kirby CN, Piterman L, Giles C. Gp management of erectile dysfunction: the impact of clinical audit and guidelines. Aust Fam Physician. 2009;38(8):637–41.

Kluth LA, Xylinas E, Crivelli JJ, Passoni N, Comploj E, Pycha A, Chrystal J, et al. Obesity is associated with worse outcomes in patients with t1 high grade urothelial carcinoma of the bladder. J Urol. 2013;190(2):480–6.

Koebnick C, Michaud D, Moore SC, Park Y, Hollenbeck A, Ballard-Barbash R, Schatzkin A, Leitzmann MF. Body mass index, physical activity, and bladder cancer in a large prospective study. Cancer Epidemiol Biomarkers Prev. 2008;17(5):1214–21.

Kok HP, Ciampa S, de Kroon-Oldenhof R, Steggerda-Carvalho EJ, van Stam G, Zum Vorde Sive Vording PJ, Stalpers LJ, et al. Toward online adaptive hyperthermia treatment planning: correlation between measured and simulated specific absorption rate changes caused by phase steering in patients. Int J Radiat Oncol Biol Phys. 2014;90(2):438–45.

Kollarik B, Zvarik M, Bujdak P, Weibl P, Rybar L, Sikurova L, Hunakova L. Urinary fluorescence analysis in diagnosis of bladder cancer. Neoplasma. 2018;65(2):234–41.

Kollberg P, Almquist H, Blackberg M, Cronberg C, Garpered S, Gudjonsson S, Kleist J, et al. [(18)F]Fluorodeoxyglucose—positron emission tomography/computed tomography improves staging in patients with high-risk muscle-invasive bladder cancer scheduled for radical cystectomy. Scand J Urol. 2015;49(4):296–301.

Koya MP, Simon MA, Soloway MS. complications of intravesical therapy for urothelial cancer of the bladder. J Urol. 2006;175(6):2004–10.

Krabbe LM, Svatek RS, Shariat SF, Messing E, Lotan Y. Bladder cancer risk: use of the Plco and Nlst to identify a suitable screening cohort. Urol Oncol. 2015;33(2):65.e19–25.

Krahn M, Ritvo P, Irvine J, Tomlinson G, Bezjak A, Trachtenberg J, Naglie G. Construction of the patient-oriented prostate utility scale (porpus): a multiattribute health state classification system for prostate cancer. J Clin Epidemiol. 2000;53(9):920–30.

Krege S, Giani G, Meyer R, Otto T, Rubben H. A randomized multicenter trial of adjuvant therapy in NMI bladder cancer: transurethral resection only versus transurethral resection plus mitomycin C versus transurethral resection plus bacillus Calmette-Guerin. Participating clinics. J Urol. 1996;156(3):962–6.

Kreshover J, Richstone L, Kavoussi L. Acute bleeding requiring re-operation in minimally invasive urologic surgery. J Endourol. 2014;28:A11.

Krupski T, Theodorescu D. Orthotopic neobladder following cystectomy: indications, management, and outcomes. J Wound Ostomy Continence Nurs. 2001;28(1):37–46.

Kukreja JB, Kiernan M, Schempp B, Hontar A, Ghazi A, Rashid H, Wu G, Messing E. Cystectomy enhanced recovery pathway: reduction in length of stay without increased morbidity or readmissions. J Urol. 2015;1:e813–e14.

Kulkarni GS, Alibhai SM, Finelli A, Fleshner NE, Jewett MA, Lopushinsky SR, Bayoumi AM. Cost-effectiveness analysis of immediate radical cystectomy versus intravesical bacillus Calmette-Guerin therapy for high-risk, high-grade (T1g3) bladder cancer. Cancer. 2009;115(23):5450–9.

Kulkarni GS, Finelli A, Fleshner NE, Jewett MA, Lopushinsky SR, Alibhai SM. Optimal management of high-risk T1g3 bladder cancer: a decision analysis. PLoS Med. 2007;4(9):e284.

Kulkarni GS, Hakenberg OW, Gschwend JE, Thalmann G, Kassouf W, Kamat A, Zlotta A. An updated critical analysis of the treatment strategy for newly diagnosed high-grade T1 (previously T1g3) bladder cancer. Eur Urol. 2010;57(1):60–70.

Kulkarni GS, Klaassen Z. Trimodal therapy is inferior to radical cystectomy for muscle-invasive bladder cancer using population-level data: is there evidence in the (lack of) details? Eur Urol. 2017;72(4):488–9.

Kwon T, Jeong IG, You D, Han KS, Hong S, Hong B, Hong JH, Ahn H, Kim CS. Obesity and prognosis in muscle-invasive bladder cancer: the continuing controversy. Int J Urol. 2014;21(11):1106–12.

Kyrdalen AE, Dahl AA, Hernes E, Smastuen MC, Fossa SD. A national study of adverse effects and global quality of life among candidates for curative treatment for prostate cancer. BJU Int. 2013;111(2):221–32.

Larré S, Catto JW, Cookson MS, Messing EM, Shariat SF, Soloway MS, Svatek RS, et al. Screening for bladder cancer: rationale, limitations, whom to target, and perspectives. Eur Urol. 2013;63(6):1049–58.

Latini, D. M., S. P. Lerner, S. W. Wade, D. W. Lee, and D. Z. Quale. "Bladder Cancer Detection, Treatment and Outcomes: Opportunities and Challenges." [In eng]. *Urology* 75, no. 2 (Feb 2010): 334-9.

Laumann EO, Paik A, Rosen RC. Sexual dysfunction in the united states: prevalence and predictors. JAMA. 1999;281(6):537–44.

Lee CT, Hafez KS, Sheffield JH, Joshi DP, Montie JE. orthotopic bladder substitution in women: nontraditional applications. J Urol. 2004;171(4):1585–8.

Lee CT, Mei M, Ashley J, Breslow G, O'Donnell M, Gilbert S, Lemmy S, et al. Patient resources available to bladder cancer patients: a pilot study of healthcare providers. Urology. 2012;79(1):172–7.

Lee CY, Yang KL, Ko HL, Huang RY, Tsai PP, Chen MT, Lin YC, et al. Trimodality bladder-sparing approach without neoadjuvant chemotherapy for node-negative localized muscle-invasive urinary bladder cancer resulted in comparable cystectomy-free survival. Radiat Oncol. 2014;9:213.

Lee JT, Chaloner EJ, Hollingsworth SJ. The role of cardiopulmonary fitness and its genetic influences on surgical outcomes. Br J Surg. 2006;93(2):147–57.

Lehmann K, Eichlisberger R, Gasser TC. Lack of diagnostic tools to prove erectile dysfunction: consequences for reimbursement? J Urol. 2000;163(1):91–4.

Levinson AW, Lavery HJ, Ward NT, Su LM, Pavlovich CP. Is a return to baseline sexual function possible? An analysis of sexual function outcomes following laparoscopic radical prostatectomy. World J Urol. 2011;29(1):29–34.

Lewin K. Action research and minority problems. In: Action research and minority problems. USA, Tavistock Institute: Tavist; 1946.

Li S, Li L, Zeng Q, Zhang Y, Guo Z, Liu Z, Jin M, et al. Characterization and noninvasive diagnosis of bladder cancer with serum surface enhanced raman spectroscopy and genetic algorithms. Sci Rep. 2015;5:9582.

Liedberg F, Bendahl PO, Davidsson T, Gudjonsson S, Holmer M, Mansson W, Wallengren NO. Preoperative staging of locally advanced bladder cancer before radical cystectomy using 3 tesla magnetic resonance imaging with a standardized protocol. Scand J Urol. 2013;47(2):108–12.

Lim YW, Cheng C, Lee LS. Eras enhances perioperative outcomes after open radical cystectomy for bladder cancer. BJU Int. 2015;115:23.

Lindof TR. Qualitative communication research methods. Edited by BC Taylor. Caluforniia: Sage; 2002.

Lipsker, A., Y. Hammoudi, B. Parier, J. Drai, R. Bahi, T. Bessede, J. J. Patard, and G. Pignot. "[Should We Propose a Systematic Second Transurethral Resection of the Bladder for All High-Risk Non-Muscle Invasive Bladder Cancers?]." [In fre]. *Prog Urol* 24, no. 10 (Sep 2014): 640-5.

Litwin MS, Hays RD, Fink A, Ganz PA, Leake B, Brook RH. The ucla prostate cancer index: development, reliability, and validity of a health-related quality of life measure. Med Care. 1998;36(7):1002–12.

Llewellyn MA, Gordon NS, Abbotts B, James ND, Zeegers MP, Cheng KK, Macdonald A, et al. Defining the frequency of human papillomavirus and polyomavirus infection in urothelial bladder tumours. Sci Rep. 2018;8(1):11290.

Luchey AM, Lin H-Y, Yue B, Agarwal G, Gilbert SM, Lockhart J, Poch MA, et al. Implications of definitive prostate cancer therapy on soft tissue margins and survival in patients undergoing radical cystectomy for bladder urothelial cancer. J Urol. 194(5):1220–25.

Lum BL, Torti FM. Adjuvant intravesicular pharmacotherapy for NMI bladder cancer. J Natl Cancer Inst. 1991;83:682–94.

Ma F, Fleming LE, Lee DJ, Trapido E, Gerace TA, Lai H, Lai S. Mortality in florida professional firefighters, 1972 to 1999. Am J Ind Med. 2005;47(6):509–17.

Ma P, Navaran P, Eghbalieh B. Glowing green: case report of indocyanine green uptake in gastro-intestinal stromal tumors. Surg Endosc Other Interv Tech. 2015;29:S543.

Maarouf AM, Khalil S, Salem EA, ElAdl M, Nawar N, Zaiton F. Bladder preservation multimo-dality therapy as an alternative to radical cystectomy for treatment of muscle invasive bladder cancer. BJU Int. 2011;107(10):1605–10.

MacIntosh J, MacKay E, Mallet-Boucher M, Wiggins N. Discovering co-learning with students in distance education sites. Nurse Educator. 2002;27(4):182–86.

Mactaggart R. The action research planner. Edited by Nixon R, p. 15–20. Spinger; 2014.

Maddams J, Brewster D, Gavin A, Steward J, Elliott J, Utley M, Moller H. Cancer prevalence in the United Kingdom: estimates for 2008. Br J Cancer. 2009;101(3):541–47.

Maddams J, Utley M, Moller H. Projections of cancer prevalence in the United Kingdom, 2010–2040. Br J Cancer. 2012;107(7):1195–202.

Makela VJ, Kotsar A, Tammela TL, Murtola TJ. Bladder cancer survival in men using 5-alpha-re-ductase inhibitors. J Urol. 2018.

Malkowicz SB, Nichols P, Lieskovsky G, Boyd SD, Huffman J, Skinner DG. The role of radi-cal cystectomy in the management of high grade NMI bladder cancer (Pa, P1, Pis and P2). J Urol. 1990;144(3):641–5.

Malmstrom PU, Wijkstrom H, Lundholm C, Wester K, Busch C, Norlen BJ. 5-year followup of a randomized prospective study comparing mitomycin c and bacillus Calmette-Guerin in patients with NMI bladder carcinoma. Swedish-Norwegian Bladder Cancer Study Group. J Urol. 1999;161(4):1124–7.

Mangiarotti B, Trinchieri A, Del Nero A, Montanari E. A randomized prospective study of intra-vesical prophylaxis in non-musle invasive bladder cancer at intermediate risk of recurrence: mitomycin chemotherapy Vs Bcg immunotherapy. Arch Ital Urol Androl. 2008;80(4):167–71.

Manne SL, Kissane DW, Nelson CJ, Mulhall JP, Winkel G, Zaider T. Intimacy-enhancing psy-chological intervention for men diagnosed with prostate cancer and their partners: a Pilot study. J Sex Med. 2011;8(4):1197–209.

Manny TB, Hemal AK. Fluorescence-enhanced robotic radical cystectomy using unconjugated indocyanine green for pelvic lymphangiography, tumor marking, and mesenteric angiogra-phy: the initial clinical experience. Urology. 2014;83(4):824–9.

Manoharan M, Katkoori D, Kishore TA, Antebie E. Robotic-assisted radical cystec-tomy and orthotopic ileal neobladder using a modified pfannenstiel incision. Urology. 2011;77(2):491–3.

Mansour AM, Abol-Enein H, Manoharan M. Exploring the marcille triangle during robot-as-sisted pelvic lymphadenectomy for bladder cancer: replicating the open surgical technique. J Endourol. 2013;27:A308–A09.

Mansson A, Johnson G, Mansson W. Quality of life after cystectomy. comparison between patients with conduit and those with continent caecal reservoir urinary diversion. Br J Urol. 1988;62(3):240–5.

Mathieu R, Lucca I, Klatte T, Babjuk M, Shariat SF. Trimodal therapy for invasive bladder can-cer: is it really equal to radical cystectomy? Curr Opin Urol. 2015;25(5):476–82.

Maurer T, Eiber M, Krause BJ. Molecular multimodal hybrid imaging in prostate and bladder cancer. Urologe A. 2014;53(4):469–83.

May M, Braun KP, Richter W, Helke C, Vogler H, Hoschke B, Siegsmund M. Radical cystec-tomy in the treatment of bladder cancer always in due time? Urologe A. 2007;46(8):913–9.

May M, Burger M, Brookman-May S, Stief CG, Fritsche HM, Roigas J, Zacharias M, et al. Eortc progression score identifies patients at high risk of cancer-specific mortality after radical cystectomy for secondary muscle-invasive bladder cancer. Clin Genitourin Cancer. 2014;12(4):278–86.

May M, Stief C, Brookman-May S, Otto W, Gilfrich C, Roigas J, Zacharias M, et al. Gender-dependent cancer-specific survival following radical cystectomy. World J Urol. 2012;30(5):707–13.

McCammon KA, Kolm P, Main B, Schellhammer PF. Comparative quality-of-life analysis after radical prostatectomy or external beam radiation for localized prostate cancer. Urology. 1999;54(3):509–16.

McCombie S, Nack T, Willmott J, Hayne D. The development of a radical cystectomy enhanced recovery pathway at fremantle hospital. BJU Int. 2015;115:98–99.

McGuire MS, Grimaldi G, Grotas J, Russo P. The type of urinary diversion after radical cystectomy significantly impacts on the patient's quality of life. Ann Surg Oncol. 2000;7(1):4–8.

McHorney CA, Ware JE Jr, Raczek AE. The Mos 36-Item short-form health survey (Sf-36): Ii. Psychometric and clinical tests of validity in measuring physical and mental health constructs. Med Care. 1993;31(3):247–63.

Meade CD, Calvo A, Rivera MA, Baer RD. Focus groups in the design of prostate cancer screening information for hispanic farmworkers and african American men. Oncology Nursing Forum. 2003;30(6):967–75.

Megas G, Papadopoulos G, Stathouros G, Moschonas D, Gkialas I, Ntoumas K. Comparison of efficacy and satisfaction profile, between penile prosthesis implantation and oral Pde5 inhibitor Tadalafil therapy, in men with nerve-sparing radical prostatectomy erectile dysfunction. BJU Int. 2013;112(2):E169–E76.

Mertens LS, Mir MC, Scott AM, Lee ST, Fioole-Bruining A, Vegt E, Vogel WV, et al. 18f-Fluorodeoxyglucose–positron emission tomography/computed tomography aids staging and predicts mortality in patients with muscle-invasive bladder cancer. Urology. 2014;83(2):393–8.

Messing EM, Madeb R, Young T, Gilchrist KW, Bram L, Greenberg EB, Wegenke JD, et al. Long-term outcome of hematuria home screening for bladder cancer in men. Cancer. 2006;107(9):2173–9.

Miller DC, Wei JT, Dunn RL, Montie JE, Pimentel H, Sandler HM, McLaughlin PW, Sanda MG. Use of medications or devices for erectile dysfunction among long-term prostate cancer treatment survivors: potential influence of sexual motivation and/or indifference. Urology. 2006;68(1):166–71.

Milne DJ, Mulder LL, Beelen HC, Schofield P, Kempen GI, Aranda S. Patients' self-report and family caregivers' perception of quality of life in patients with advanced cancer: how do they compare? Eur J Cancer Care (Engl). 2006;15(2):125–32.

Milowsky MI, Kim WY. The geriatrics and genetics behind bladder cancer. Am Soc Clin Oncol Educ Book. 2014:e192–5.

Miner MM. Erectile dysfunction: a harbinger for cardiovascular events and other comorbidities, thereby allowing a 'window of curability'. Int J Clin Pract. 2009;63(8):1123–26.

Minervini A, Serni S, Vittori G, Masieri L, Siena G, Lanciotti M, Lapini A, Gacci M, Carini M. Current indications and results of orthotopic ileal neobladder for bladder cancer. Expert Rev Anticancer Ther. 2014;14(4):419–30.

Mitra AP, Skinner EC, Schuckman AK, Quinn DI, Dorff TB, Daneshmand S. Effect of gender on outcomes following radical cystectomy for urothelial carcinoma of the bladder: a critical analysis of 1,994 patients. Urol Oncol. 2014;32(1):52.e1–9.

Mohamed NE, Diefenbach MA, Goltz HH, Lee CT, Latini D, Kowalkowski M, Philips C, Hassan W, Hall SJ. Muscle invasive bladder cancer: from diagnosis to survivorship. Adv Urol. 2012;(2012):142135.

Mohamed NE, Gilbert F, Lee CT, Sfakianos J, Knauer C, Mehrazin R, Badr H, et al. Pursuing quality in the application of bladder cancer quality of life research. Bladder Cancer. 2016;2(2):139–49.

Molton IR, Siegel SD, Penedo FJ, Dahn JR, Kinsinger D, Traeger LN, Carver CS, et al. Promoting recovery of sexual functioning after radical prostatectomy with group-based stress management: the role of interpersonal sensitivity. J Psychosom Res. 2008;64(5):527–36.

Moore BW, Giusto LL, Lee Z, Sterious SN, Mydlo JH, Eun DD. Use of indocyanine green (Icg) for complex robotic reconstruction involving bowel urinary diversions. J Urol. 2014;1:e735.

Morales-Olivas FJ, Estan L. Solifenacin pharmacology. Arch Esp Urol. 2010;63(1):43–52.

Morales A, Cohen Z. Mycobacterium phlei cell wall-nucleic acid complex in the treatment of nonmuscle invasive bladder cancer unresponsive to Bacillus Calmette-Guerin. Expert Opin Biol Ther. 2016;16(2):273–83.

Morgan MA. Cancer survivorship: history, quality-of-life issues, and the evolving multidisciplinary approach to implementation of cancer survivorship care plans. Oncol Nurs Forum. 2009;36(4):429–36.

Mukesh M, Cook N, Hollingdale AE, Ainsworth NL, Russell SG. Small cell carcinoma of the urinary bladder: a 15-year retrospective review of treatment and survival in the Anglian cancer Network. BJU Int. 2009;103(6):747–52.

Muller-Mattheis V, Schulz C, Schmelzer R, Mortsiefer A, Rotthoff T, Albers P, Karger A. Evaluation of a new course on teaching of erectile dysfunction following pelvic surgery in men with prostate or bladder cancer in undergraduate medical education. J Cancer Res Clin Oncol. 2012;138:124.

Muto G, Collura D, Giacobbe A, D'Urso L, Muto GL, Demarchi A, Coverlizza S, Castelli E. Thulium:Yttrium-aluminum-garnet laser for en bloc resection of bladder cancer: clinical and histopathologic advantages. Urology. 2014;83(4):851–5.

Mr-conditional pacemaker means big changes for Mr providers. Health Devices. 2012;41(2):63–4.

Naccarato AMEP, Souto SC, Moreira M, Heckler P, Ferreira U, Souza EAP, Denardi F. Effects of phosphodiesterase inhibitors on erectile function and performance, and impacts of psychotherapy on the quality of life of patients submitted to radical prostatectomy for prostate cancer. J Sex Med. 2014;11:244.

Naccarato A, Reis L, Mendonca G, Denardi F. Post radical prostatectomy erectile dysfunction rehabilitation is couple dependent: a missing piece in the puzzle. Urology. 2013;1:S184.

Nagao K, Hara T, Nishijima J, Shimizu K, Fujii N, Kobayashi K, Kawai Y, et al. The efficacy of trimodal chemoradiotherapy with cisplatin as a bladder-preserving strategy for the treatment of muscle-invasive bladder cancer. Urol Int. 2017;99(4):446–52.

Nagele U, Kugler M, Nicklas A, Merseburger AS, Walcher U, Mikuz G, Herrmann TR. Waterjet hydrodissection: first experiences and short-term outcomes of a novel approach to bladder tumor resection. World J Urol. 2011;29(4):423–7.

Namiki S, Ishidoya S, Ito A, Arai Y. The impact of sexual desire on sexual health related quality of life following radical prostatectomy: a 5-year follow up study in Japan. Eur Urol, Suppl. 2012;11(1):e671–c71a.

Nayak B, Dogra PN, Naswa N, Kumar R. Diuretic 18f-Fdg Pet/Ct imaging for detection and locoregional staging of urinary bladder cancer: prospective evaluation of a novel technique. Eur J Nucl Med Mol Imaging. 2013;40(3):386–93.

Nelson CJ, Kenowitz J. Communication and intimacy-enhancing interventions for men diagnosed with prostate cancer and their partners. J Sex Med. 2013;10:127–32.

Nelson CJ, Mulhall JP, Roth AJ. The association between erectile dysfunction and depressive symptoms in men treated for prostate cancer. J Sex Med. 2011;8(2):560–66.

Nelson C, Kenowitz J, Pessin H, Lacey S, Mulhall J. Acceptance and commitment therapy for adherence to an erectile rehabilitation program after radical prostatectomy: preliminary results from a randomized control trial. Psycho-Oncol. 2013;22:34.

Neuzillet Y, Roupret M, Wallerand H, Pignot G, Larre S, Irani J, Davin JL, et al. Diagnosis and management of adverse events occurring during Bcg therapy for non-muscle invasive bladder cancer (Nmibc): review of the cancer committee of the French association of urology. Prog Urol. 2012;22(16):989–98.

Nguyen-Huu Y, Delorme G, Lillaz J, Bedgedjian I, Le Ray-Ferrieres I, Chabannes E, Bernardini S, et al. muscularis mucosae invasion: prognostic factor for intravesical Bcg immunotherapy failure for T1 bladder carcinoma. Prog Urol. 2012;22(5):284–90.

Nguyen HT, Pohar KS, Jia G, Shah ZK, Mortazavi A, Zynger DL, Wei L, et al. Improving bladder cancer imaging using 3-t functional dynamic contrast-enhanced magnetic resonance imaging. Invest Radiol. 2014;49(6):390–5.

Nielsen ME, Smith AB, Pruthi RS, Guzzo TJ, Amiel G, Shore N, Lotan Y. Reported use of intra-vesical therapy for non-muscle-invasive bladder cancer (nmibc): results from the bladder cancer advocacy Network (Bcan) survey. BJU Int. 2012;110(7):967–72.

Nizamova RS. occupational hazards and bladder cancer. Urol Nefrol (Mosk). 1991;(5):35–8.

Noguchi JL, Liss MA, Parsons JK. Obesity, physical activity and bladder cancer. Curr Urol Rep. 2015;16(10):74.

Northouse LL, Mood DW, Schafenacker A, Montie JE, Sandler HM, Forman JD, Hussain M, et al. Randomized clinical trial of a family intervention for prostate cancer patients and their spouses. Cancer. 2007;110(12):2809–18.

Northouse L, Williams AL, Given B, McCorkle R. Psychosocial care for family caregivers of patients with cancer. J Clin Oncol. 2012;30(11):1227–34.

Nyame Y, Babbar P, Greene D, Shoshtari HZ, Krishnamurthi V, Haber GP. Robotic anterior pelvic exenteration with intracorporeal ileal conduit in a patient with history of kidney pancreas transplantation. J Urol. 2015;1:e718.

O'Brien R, Rose PW, Campbell C, Weller D, Neal RD, Wilkinson C, Watson EK. Experiences of follow-up after treatment in patients with prostate cancer: a qualitative study. BJU Int. 2010;106(7):998–1003.

O'Shaughnessy PT, Laws TA, Pinnock C, Moul JW, Esterman A. Differences in self-reported outcomes of open prostatectomy patients and robotic prostatectomy patients in an international web-based survey. Eur J Oncol Nurs. 2013;17(6):775–80.

O'Brien R, Rose P, Campbell C, Weller D, Neal RD, Wilkinson C, McIntosh H, Watson E. "I Wish I'd Told Them": a qualitative study examining the unmet psychosexual needs of prostate cancer patients during follow-up after treatment. Patient Educ Couns. 2011;84(2):200–07.

Oberoi S, Barchowsky A, Wu F. The global burden of disease for skin, lung, and bladder cancer caused by Arsenic in food. Cancer Epidemiol Biomarkers Prev. 2014;23(7):1187–94.

Ohgiya Y, Suyama J, Sai S, Kawahara M, Takeyama N, Ohike N, Sasamori H, et al. Preoperative T staging of urinary bladder cancer: efficacy of stalk detection and diagnostic performance of diffusion-weighted imaging at 3t. Magn Reson Med Sci. 2014;13(3):175–81.

Older P, Hall A, Hader R. Cardiopulmonary exercise testing as a screening test for perioperative management of major surgery in the elderly. Chest. 1999;116(2):355–62.

Olfert SM, Felknor SA, Delclos GL. An updated review of the literature: risk factors for bladder cancer with focus on occupational exposures. South Med J. 2006;99(11):1256–63.

Orsola A, Werner L, de Torres I, Martin-Doyle W, Raventos CX, Lozano F, Mullane SA, et al. Reexamining treatment of high-grade t1 bladder cancer according to depth of lamina propria invasion: a prospective trial of 200 patients. Br J Cancer. 2015;112(3):468–74.

Ouellet-Hellstrom R, Rench JD. Bladder cancer incidence in arylamine workers. J Occup Environ Med. 1996;38(12):1239–47.

Ouzaid I, Diaz E, Autorino R, Samarasekera D, Ganesan V, Stein R, Kaouk J, Haber GP. Ileal conduit revision and ureteral stenosis repair: robot assisted laparoscopic technique. J Endourol. 2013;27:A439.

Pagano MJ, Badalato G, McKiernan JM. Optimal treatment of non-muscle invasive urothelial carcinoma including perioperative management revisited. Curr Urol Rep. 2014;15(11):450.

Palou J, Breda A, Gausa L, Gaya JM, Rodriguez-faba O, Villavicencio HM. Lymphadenectomy at the time of robotassisted radical cystectomy: procedure and performance. J Endourol. 2010;24:A357.

Pansadoro V, Emiliozzi P, de Paula F, Scarpone P, Pansadoro A, Sternberg CN. Long-term follow-up of G3t1 transitional cell carcinoma of the bladder treated with intravesical Bacille Calmette-Guerin: 18-year experience. Urology. 2002;59(2):227–31.

Pansadoro V, Emiliozzi P, depaula F, Scarpone P, Pizzo M, Federico G, Martini M, Pansadoro A, Sternberg CN. High grade NMI (G3t1) transitional cell carcinoma of the bladder treated with intravesical Bacillus Calmette-Guerin (Bcg). J Exp Clin Cancer Res. 2003;22(4):223–7.

Park RM, Mirer FE. A survey of mortality at two automotive engine manufacturing plants. Am J Ind Med. 1996;30(6):664–73.

Parker GB, Arvela O, Braye S, Edwards M, French P, Leung A, Parsons J, Smiley M. Letter: the economy, social integration and utilization of health services. Med J Aus. 1974;2(12):464.

Parker PA, Pettaway CA, Babaian RJ, Pisters LL, Miles B, Fortier A, Wei Q, Carr DD, Cohen L. The effects of a presurgical stress management intervention for men with prostate cancer undergoing radical prostatectomy. J Clin Oncol. 2009;27(19):3169–76.

Patschan O, Sjodahl G, Chebil G, Lovgren K, Lauss M, Gudjonsson S, Kollberg P, et al. A molecular pathologic framework for risk stratification of stage T1 urothelial carcinoma. Eur Urol. 2015;68(5):824–32; discussion 35–6.

Patterson BO, Holt PJE, Hinchliffe R, Loftus IM, Thompson MM. Predicting risk in elective abdominal aortic aneurysm repair: a systematic review of current evidence. Eur J Vasc Endovasc Surg. 2008;36(6):637–45.

Pavlovich CP, Levinson AW, Su LM, Mettee LZ, Feng Z, Bivalacqua TJ, Trock BJ. Nightly vs on-demand sildenafil for penile rehabilitation after minimally invasive nerve-sparing radical prostatectomy: results of a randomized double-blind trial with placebo. BJU Int. 203;112(6):844–51.

Pedersen M, Stafoggia M, Weinmayr G, Andersen ZJ, Galassi C, Sommar J, Forsberg B, et al. Is there an association between ambient air pollution and bladder cancer incidence? Analysis of 15 European cohorts. Eur Urol Focus. 2018;4(1):113–20.

Penson DF, McLerran D, Feng Z, Li L, Albertsen PC, Gilliland FD, Hamilton A, et al. 5-year urinary and sexual outcomes after radical prostatectomy: results from the prostate cancer outcomes study. J Urol. 2005;173(5):1701–5.

Perez MA, Meyerowitz BE, Lieskovsky G, Skinner DG, Reynolds B, Skinner EC. Quality of life and sexuality following radical prostatectomy in patients with prostate cancer who use or do not use erectile aids. Urology. 1997;50(5):740–6.

Persson B, Carringer M, Andren O, Andersson SO, Carlsson J, Ljungqvist O. Initial experiences with the enhanced recovery after surgery (eras) protocol in open radical cystectomy. Scandinavian J Urol. 2015;49(4):302–7.

Pesch B, Nasterlack M, Eberle F, Bonberg N, Taeger D, Leng G, Feil G, et al. The role of haematuria in bladder cancer screening among men with former occupational exposure to aromatic amines. BJU Int. 2011;108(4):546–52.

Philip J, Manikandan R, Venugopal S, Desouza J, Javle PM. Orthotopic neobladder versus ileal conduit urinary diversion after cystectomy—a quality-of-life based comparison. Ann R Coll Surg Engl. 2009;91(7):565–9.

Pieras Ayala E, Palou J, Rodriguez-Villamil L, Millan Rodriguez F, Salvador Bayarri J, Vicente Rodriguez J. Cytoscopic follow-up of initial G3t1 bladder tumors treated with Bcg. Arch Esp Urol. 2001;54(3):211–7.

Pignot G, Irani J, Bastide C, Ravery V. New concepts in management of Nmibc in 2010. Prog Urol. 2011;21(Suppl. 2):S34–7.

Ploumidis A, Gan M, De Naeyer G, Schatteman P, Volpe A, Mottrie A. Robot-assisted radical cystectomy for female patients. the O.L.V. Vattikuti robotic surgery institute technique. J Endourol. 2013;27:A307–8.

Ploumidis A, Volpe A, Ficarra V, Mottrie A. Robot-assisted radical cystectomy for female patients. The Olv Vattikuti robotic surgery institute technique. Eur Urol Suppl. 2014;13 (1):eV16.

Ploussard G, Daneshmand S, Efstathiou JA, Herr HW, James ND, Rodel CM, Shariat SF, et al. Critical analysis of bladder sparing with trimodal therapy in muscle-invasive bladder cancer: a systematic review. Eur Urol. 2014;66(1):120–37.

Ploussard G, Salomon L, Allory Y, Terry S, Vordos D, Hoznek A, Abbou CC, Vacherot F, de la Taille A. Pathological findings and prostate-specific antigen outcomes after laparoscopic radical prostatectomy for high-risk prostate cancer. BJU Int. 2010;106(1):86–90.

Ploussard G, Salomon L, Parier B, Abbou CC, de la Taille A. Extraperitoneal robot-assisted laparoscopic radical prostatectomy: a single-center experience beyond the learning curve. World J Urol. 2013;31(3):447–53.

Pluye P, Nha Hong Q. Combining the power of stories and the power of numbers: mixed methods research and mixed studies reviews. Annual Review of Public Health, 29–45. 4139 El Camino Way, P.O. Box 10139, Palo Alto CA 94306, United States: Annual Reviews Inc.; 2014.

Porpiglia F, Calza E, Poggio M, Fiori C, Cattaneo G, Morra I, Cossu M, et al. "Enhanced" recovery program in patients undergoing radical cystectomy: our experience. Eur Urol Suppl. 2015;14(2):e434.

Power NE, Izawa J. Comparison of guidelines on non-muscle invasive bladder cancer (Eau, Cua, Aua, Nccn, Nice). Bladder Cancer. 2016;2(1):27–36.

Prasad SM, Shalhav AL. Comparative effectiveness of minimally invasive versus open lymphadenectomy in urological cancers. Curr Opin Urol. 2013;23(1):57–64.

Preston MA, Lerner SP, Kibel AS. New trends in the surgical management of invasive bladder cancer. Hematol/Oncol Clin N Am. 2015;29(2):253–69.

Psutka SP, Boorjian SA, Moynagh MR, Schmit GD, Frank I, Carrasco A, Stewart SB, et al. Mortality after radical cystectomy: impact of obesity versus adiposity after adjusting for skeletal muscle wasting. J Urol. 2015;193(5):1507–13.

Pukkala E, Martinsen JI, Lynge E, Gunnarsdottir HK, Sparen P, Tryggvadottir L, Weiderpass E, Kjaerheim K. Occupation and cancer—follow-up of 15 million people in five nordic countries. Acta Oncol. 2009;48(5):646–790.

Puppo P, Introini C, Bertolotto F, Naselli A. Potency preserving cystectomy with intrafascial prostatectomy for high risk NMI bladder cancer. J Urol. 2008;179(5):1727–32; discussion 32.

Pushkar P, Taneja R, Sharma MK. Total intracorporeal robot-assisted laparoscopic radical cystectomy with ileal conduit (Bricker) urinary diversion. Indian J Urol. 2015;31:S102.

Quan H, Li B, Couris CM, Fushimi K, Graham P, Hider P, Januel JM, Sundararajan V. Practice of epidemiology: updating and validating the Charlson comorbidity index and score for risk adjustment in hospital discharge abstracts using data from 6 countries. Am J Epidemiol. 2011;173(6):676–82.

Quintens H, Guy L, Mazerolles C, Theodore C, Amsellem D, Roupret M, Wallerand H, et al. Treatment of infiltrating nonmetastatic bladder cancers in elderly patients. Prog Urol. 2009;19(Suppl. 3):S135–41.

Raina R, Agarwal A, Allamaneni SSR, Lakin MM, Zippe CD. Sildenafil citrate and vacuum constriction device combination enhances sexual satisfaction in erectile dysfunction after radical prostatectomy. Urology. 2005;65(2):360–64.

Raina R, Lakin MM, Agarwal A, Sharma R, Goyal KK, Montague DK, Klein E, Zippe CD. Long-term effect of sildenafil citrate on erectile dysfunction after radical prostatectomy: 3-year follow-up. Urology. 2003;62(1):110–5.

Raina R, Pahlajani G, Agarwal A, Zippe CD. The early use of transurethral alprostadil after radical prostatectomy potentially facilitates an earlier return of erectile function and successful sexual activity. BJU Int. 2007;100(6):1317–21.

Rajendran R, Cummings M. Erectile dysfunction: assessment and management in primary care. Prescriber. 2014;25(12):25–30.

Ratert N, Meyer HA, Jung M, Lioudmer P, Mollenkopf HJ, Wagner I, Miller K, et al. Mirna profiling identifies candidate mirnas for bladder cancer diagnosis and clinical outcome. J Mol Diagn. 2013;15(5):695–705.

Raz O, Arianayagam M, Varol C. Intracorporeal ileal conduit reconstruction following robotic radical cystectomy. Video highlight of technique. BJU Int. 2014;113:141.

Reason P. The Sage handbook of action research: participative inquiry and practice. Edited by H Bradbury, 5–10. California: Sage; 2008.

Reilly DF, McNeely MJ, Doerner D, Greenberg DL, Staiger TO, Geist MJ, Vedovatti PA, et al. Self-reported exercise tolerance and the risk of serious perioperative complications. Arch Intern Med. 1999;159(18):2185–92.

Rentsch CA, Birkhauser FD, Biot C, Gsponer JR, Bisiaux A, Wetterauer C, Lagranderie M, et al. Bacillus Calmette-Guerin strain differences have an impact on clinical outcome in bladder cancer immunotherapy. Eur Urol. 2014;66(4):677–88.

Rintala E, Jauhiainen K, Kaasinen E, Nurmi M, Alfthan O. Alternating mitomycin C and Bacillus Calmette-Guerin instillation prophylaxis for recurrent papillary (stages Ta to T1) NMI bladder cancer. Finnbladder group. J Urol. 1996;156(1):56–9; discussion 59–60.

Ritch CR, Cookson MS, Chang SS, Clark PE, Resnick MJ, Penson DF, Smith JA Jr, May AT, Anderson CB, You C, Lee H, Barocas DA. Impact of complications and hospital-free days on health related quality of life 1 year after radical cystectomy. J Urol. 2014;192(5):1360–4.

Rivers BM, August EM, Gwede CK, Hart A Jr, Donovan KA, Pow-Sang JM, Quinn GP. Psychosocial issues related to sexual functioning among african-american prostate cancer survivors and their spouses. Psycho-Oncol. 2011;20(1):106–10.

Rodriguez Faba O, Gaya JM, Lopez JM, Capell M, De Gracia-Nieto AE, Gomez Correa E, Breda A, Palou J. Current management of non-muscle-invasive bladder cancer. Minerva Med. 2013;104(3):273–86.

Rodriguez Morales-Bermudez AR. Fluorescence imaging technology for robotic assisted partial cystectomy and ureteral reconstruction minimizes lack of tactile feedback. Eur Urol Suppl. 2015;14(2):e980.

Roobol MJ, Bangma CH, el Bouazzaoui S, Franken-Raab CG, Zwarthoff EC. Feasibility study of screening for bladder cancer with urinary molecular markers (the Blu-P project). Urol Oncol. 2010;28(6):686–90.

Rose TL, Deal AM, Nielsen ME, Smith AB, Milowsky MI. Sex disparities in use of chemotherapy and survival in patients with advanced bladder cancer. Cancer. 2016;122(13):2012–20.

Rosen RC. Sexual function assessment in the male: physiological and self-report measures. Int J Impot Res. 1998;10(Suppl. 2):S59–63.

Rosen RC, Cappelleri JC, Smith MD, Lipsky J, Pen BM. Development and evaluation of an abridged, 5-item version of the international index of erectile function (Iief-5) as a diagnostic tool for erectile dysfunction. Int J Impot Res. 1999;11(6):319–26.

Rosen RC, Riley A, Wagner G, Osterloh IH, Kirkpatrick J, Mishra A. The international index of erectile function (Iief): a multidimensional scale for assessment of erectile dysfunction. Urology. 1997;49(6):822–30.

Roswall N, Freisling H, Bueno-de-Mesquita HB, Ros M, Christensen J, Overvad K, Boutron-Ruault MC, et al. Anthropometric measures and bladder cancer risk: a prospective study in the epic cohort. Int J Cancer. 2014;135(12):2918–29.

Rutherford D. Erectile dysfunction: assessment, treatment and prescribing issues. Nurs Times 2002;98(51):30–33.

Rybotycka Z, Dlugosz A. Diagnostic significance of protein Nmp22 in bladder cancer. Pol Merkur Lekarski. 2015;38(228):309–14.

Sabaa MA, El-Gamal OM, Abo-Elenen M, Khanam A. Combined modality treatment with bladder preservation for muscle invasive bladder cancer. Urol Oncol. 2010;28(1):14–20.

Sacristan R, Gonzalez C, Fernandez-Gomez JM, Fresno F, Escaf S, Sanchez-Carbayo M. Molecular classification of non-muscle-invasive bladder cancer (Pta low-grade, Pt1 low-grade, and Pt1 high-grade subgroups) using methylation of tumor-suppressor genes. J Mol Diagn. 2014;16(5):564–72.

Sadetzki S, Bensal D, Blumstein T, Novikov I, Modan B. Selected risk factors for transitional cell bladder cancer. Med Oncol. 2000;17(3):179–82.

Saldana J. The coding manual for qualitative researchers. California: Sage; 2009.

Sanda MG, Dunn RL, Michalski J, Sandler HM, Northouse L, Hembroff L, Lin X, et al. Quality of life and satisfaction with outcome among prostate-cancer survivors. N Engl J Med. 2008;358(12):1250–61.

Sandblom G, Ladjevardi S, Garmo H, Varenhorst E. The impact of prostate-specific antigen level at diagnosis on the relative survival of 28,531 men with localized carcinoma of the prostate. Cancer. 2008;112(4):813–9.

Satyanarayana R, Kallingal G, Parekh D. Current status of robotic and laparoscopic techniques in radical cystectomy and diversion procedures for bladder cancer: review. Minerva Urol Nefrol. 2014;66(1):1–14.

Savin-Baden M. Qualitative research: the essential guide to theory and practice. Edited by C Major. London: Routledge; 2013.

Schaafsma BE, Verbeek FP, Elzevier HW, Tummers QR, van der Vorst JR, Frangioni JV, van de Velde CJ, Pelger RC, Vahrmeijer AL. Optimization of sentinel lymph node mapping in bladder cancer using near-infrared fluorescence imaging. J Surg Oncol. 2014;110(7):845–50.

Scherbring M. Effect of caregiver perception of preparedness on burden in an oncology population. Oncol Nurs Forum. 2002;29(6):E70–6.

Schiavina R, Borghesi M, Dababneh H, Pultrone CV, Chessa F, Concetti S, Gentile G, et al. Survival, continence and potency (Scp) recovery after radical retropubic prostatectomy: a long-term combined evaluation of surgical outcomes. Eur J Surg Oncol. 2014;40(12):1716–23.

Schmahl D, Osswald H, Prochotta L. Quantitative studies in rats on the resistance of various organs to inoculated tumor cells. Z Krebsforsch. 1967;70(2):130–7.

Schover LR, Fouladi RT, Warneke CL, Neese L, Klein EA, Zippe C, Kupelian PA. The use of treatments for erectile dysfunction among survivors of prostate carcinoma. Cancer. 2002;95(11):2397–407.

Schover LR, Friedman JM, Weiler SJ. Multiaxial problem-oriented system for sexual dysfunctions. An alternative to Dsm-Iii. Arch Gen Psychiatry.1982;39(5):614–9.

Scosyrev E, Yao J, Messing E. Microscopic invasion of perivesical fat by urothelial carcinoma: implications for prognosis and pathology practice. Urology. 2010;76(4):908–13; discussion 14.

Sediman I. Technique isn't everything, but it is a lot. Interviewing as qualitative research. A guide for researchers in education and social science. New York: Teachers Press; 1998.

Seisen T, Sun M, Lipsitz SR, Abdollah F, Leow JJ, Menon M, Preston MA, et al. Comparative effectiveness of trimodal therapy versus radical cystectomy for localized muscle-invasive urothelial carcinoma of the bladder. Eur Urol. 2017;72(4):483–87.

Seung CK, Sung GK, Choi H, Young HK, Jeong GL, Je JK, Seok HK, Cheon J. The feasibility of robot-assisted laparoscopic radical cystectomy with pelvic lymphadenectomy: from the viewpoint of extended pelvic lymphadenectomy. Korean J Urol. 2009;50(9):870–78.

Shelley MD, Wilt TJ, Court J, Coles B, Kynaston H, Mason MD. Intravesical Bacillus Calmette-Guerin is superior to mitomycin c in reducing tumour recurrence in high-risk NMI bladder cancer: a meta-analysis of randomized trials. BJU Int. 2004;93(4):485–90.

Sherer BA, Levine LA. Current management of erectile dysfunction in prostate cancer survivors. Curr Opin Urol. 2014;24(4):401–6.

Shimpi RK. Renal funtional deterioration after urinary diversion a retrospective comparison between ileal conduit and ileal orthotopic neobladder. Eur Urol Suppl. 2014;13(5):153.

Shoemaker WC, Appel PL, Kram HB. Role of oxygen debt in the development of organ failure sepsis, and death in high-risk surgical patients. Chest. 1992;102(1):208–15.

Siddiqui KM, Izawa JI. Ileal conduit: standard urinary diversion for elderly patients undergoing radical cystectomy. World J Urol. 2015.

Silverman DT, Levin LI, Hoover RN. Occupational risks of bladder cancer among white women in the United States. Am J Epidemiol. 1990;132(3):453–61.

Singh P, Dogra PN, Saini A. Robot assisted laparoscopic radical cystectomy: a minimal invasive approach for bladder cancer. Indian J Urol. 2014;30:S55.

Sivarajan G, Prabhu V, Taksler GB, Laze J, Lepor H. Ten-year outcomes of sexual function after radical prostatectomy: results of a prospective longitudinal study. Eur Urol. 2014;65(1):58–65.

Smith JL, Verrill TA, Boura JA, Sakwa MP, Shannon FL, Franklin BA. Effect of cardiorespiratory fitness on short-term morbidity and mortality after coronary artery bypass grafting. Am J Cardiol. 2013;112(8):1104–9.

Smith J, Pruthi RS, McGrath J. Enhanced recovery programmes for patients undergoing radical cystectomy. Nat Rev Urol. 2014;11(8):437-44.

Smith ND, Castle EP, Gonzalgo ML, Svatek RS, Weizer AZ, Montgomery JS, Pruthi RS, et al. The Razor (randomized open vs robotic cystectomy) trial: study design and trial update. BJU Int. 2015;115(2):198–205.

Smith T, Stein KD, Mehta CC, Kaw C, Kepner JL, Buskirk T, Stafford J, Baker F. The rationale, design, and implementation of the American cancer society's studies of cancer survivors. Cancer. 2007;109(1):1–12.

Snow R, Sandall J, Humphrey C. Use of clinical targets in diabetes patient education: qualitative analysis of the expectations and impact of a structured self-management programme in type 1 diabetes. Diabet Med. 2014;31(6):733–38.

Snowden CP, Prentis JM, Anderson HL, Roberts DR, Randles D, Renton M, Manas DM. Submaximal cardiopulmonary exercise testing predicts complications and hospital length of stay in patients undergoing major elective surgery. Ann Surg. 2010;251(3):535–41.

Somani BK, Gimlin D, Fayers P, N'Dow J. Quality of life and body image for bladder cancer patients undergoing radical cystectomy and urinary diversion–a prospective cohort study with a systematic review of literature. Urology. 2009;74(5):1138–43.

Song L, Northouse LL, Braun TM, Zhang L, Cimprich B, Ronis DL, Mood DW. Assessing longitudinal quality of life in prostate cancer patients and their spouses: a multilevel modeling approach. Qual Life Res. 2011;20(3):371–81.

Stav K, Leibovici D, Goren E, Livshitz A, Siegel YI, Lindner A, Zisman A. Adverse effects of cystoscopy and its impact on patients' quality of life and sexual performance. Isr Med Assoc J. 2004;6)(8):474–8.

Studer UE, Danuser H, Hochreiter W, Springer JP, Turner WH, Zingg EJ. Summary of 10 Years' experience with an ileal low-pressure bladder substitute combined with an afferent tubular isoperistaltic segment. World J Urol. 1996;14(1):29–39.

Sun JW, Zhao LG, Yang Y, Ma X, Wang YY, Xiang YB. Obesity and risk of bladder cancer: a dose-response meta-analysis of 15 cohort studies. PLoS One. 2015;10(3):e0119313.

Tashakkori A. Handbook of mixed methods in social and behavioural research edited by Teddie C. Calcifornia: Sage; 2003.

Takaoka EI, Miyazaki J, Ishikawa H, Kawai K, Kimura T, Ishitsuka R, Kojima T, et al. Long-term single-institute experience with trimodal bladder-preserving therapy with proton beam therapy for muscle-invasive bladder cancer. Jpn J Clin Oncol. 2017;47(1):67–73.

Tashakkori A. Handbook of mixed methods in social and behavioural research. Edited by Teddie C. Calcifornia: Sage; 2003.

Taylor SJ. An introduction to qualitative research methods: the search for meanings. Edited by R Bogdan. Singapore: Wiley; 1984.

Teloken PE, Mulhall JP. Erectile function following prostate cancer treatment: factors predicting recovery. Sex Med Rev. 2013;1(2):91–103.

Teloken PE, Nelson CJ, Karellas M, Stasi J, Eastham J, Scardino PT, Mulhall JP. Defining the impact of vascular risk factors on erectile function recovery after radical prostatectomy. BJU Int. 2013;111(4):653–57.

Tendera M, Aboyans V, Bartelink ML, Baumgartner I, Clment D, Collet JP, Cremonesi A, et al. Esc guidelines on the diagnosis and treatment of peripheral artery diseases. Eur Hear J. 2011;32(22):2851–906.

Tewari A, Grover S, Sooriakumaran P, Srivastava A, Rao S, Gupta A, Gray R, Leung R, Paduch DA. Nerve sparing can preserve orgasmic function in most men after robotic-assisted laparoscopic radical prostatectomy. BJU Int. 2012;109(4):596–602.

Tewari AK, Ali A, Metgud S, Theckumparampil N, Srivastava A, Khani F, Robinson BD, et al. Functional outcomes following robotic prostatectomy using athermal, traction free risk-stratified grades of nerve sparing. World J Urol. 2013;31(3):471–80.

The British Pain Society. Pain and problem drug use: information for patients. 2007. http://www.britishpainsociety.org/pub_patient.htm.

Thuer D, Mottrie A, Buffi N, Koliakos N, De Naeyer G, Carpentier P, Schatteman P, Willemsen P, Fonteyne E. Total intracorporeal robot-assisted ileal conduit. Urologe - Ausgabe A. 2011;50:153.

Thyavihally Y, Patil A, Dharmadhikari N, Gulavani N, Rao H, Pednekar A. Urinary diversion after radical cystectomy-our initial experience comparing outcomes of extracorporeal and intracorporeal technique. Eur Urol Suppl. 2014;13(3):40.

Tobis S, Houman J, Mastrodonato K, Rashid H, Wu G. Robotic repair of post-cystectomy uret-eroileal anastomotic strictures: techniques for success. J Urol. 2013;1:e886.

Tobis S, Houman J, Mastrodonato K, Rashid H, Wu G. Robotic repair of post-cystectomy ure-teroileal anastomotic strictures: techniques for success. J Laparoendosc Adv Surg Tech. 2013;23(6):526–9.

Todenhofer T, Stenzl A, Schwentner C. Optimal use and outcomes of orthotopic neobladder reconstruction in men and women. Curr Opin Urol. 2013;23(5):479–86.

Townsend A. Support for men newly diagnosed with prostate cancer. Nurs Stand (R CollE Nurs (Great Britain). 1987;25(4):40–45.

Traeger L, Penedo FJ, Gonzalez JS, Dahn JR, Lechner SC, Schneiderman N, Antoni MH. Illness perceptions and emotional well-being in men treated for localized prostate cancer. J Psychosom Res. 2009;67(5):389–97.

Truong H, Nix J, Smith K, Mittal A, Agarwal P. Perioperative management of radical cystec-tomy patients: a questionnaire survey of the american urological association members. J Clin Oncol. 2013;1.

Tsang Y, Brown L, Parker S. The value of taking non-sentinel lymph nodes during the sentinal node procedure. Eur J Surg Oncol. 2011;37(11):988.

Tuppin P, Samson S, Fagot-Campagna A, Lukacs B, Alla F, Paccaud F, Thalabard JC, et al. Prostate cancer outcomes in france: treatments, adverse effects and two-year mortality. BMC Urol. 2014;14(1).

van Griensven H, Moore AP, Hall V. Mixed methods research - the best of both worlds?. Man Ther. 2014;19(5):367–71.

Vemana G, Nepple KG, Vetter J, Sandhu G, Strope SA. Defining the potential of neoadjuvant chemotherapy use as a quality indicator for bladder cancer care. J Urol. 2014;192(1):43–9.

Verma S, Rajesh A, Prasad SR, Gaitonde K, Lall CG, Mouraviev V, Aeron G, Bracken RB, Sandrasegaran K. Urinary bladder cancer: role of Mr imaging. Radiographics. 2012;32(2):371–87.

Verze P, Scuzzarella S, Martina GR, Giummelli P, Cantoni F, Mirone V. Long-term oncologi-cal and functional results of extraperitoneal laparoscopic radical prostatectomy: one surgical team's experience on 1,600 consecutive cases. World J Urol. 2013;31(3):529–34.

Villavicencio Mavrich H, Esquena S, Palou Redorta J, Gomez Ruciz JJ. Robotic radical pros-tatectomy: overview of our learning curve. Actas Urologicas Espanolas. 2007;31(6):587–92.

Volpe A, Ploumidis A, Gan M, De Naeyer G, Ficarra V, Mottrie A. Robot-assisted pelvic lymph node dissection during radical cystectomy. The Olv Vattikuti robotic surgery institute tech-nique. Eur Urol Suppl. 2014;13(1):eV72.

Ware Jr J, Kosinski M, Keller SD. A 12-item short-form health survey: construction of scales and preliminary tests of reliability and validity. Med Care. 1996;34(3):220–33.

Wei JT, Dunn RL, Litwin MS, Sandler HM, Sanda MG. Development and validation of the expanded prostate cancer index composite (Epic) for comprehensive assessment of health-re-lated quality of life in men with prostate cancer. Urology. 2000;56(6):899–905.

Weizer AZ, Palella GV, Montgomery JS. Managing muscle-invasive bladder cancer in the elderly. Expert Rev Anticancer Ther. 2010;10(6):903–15.

West M, Jack S, Grocott MPW. Perioperative cardiopulmonary exercise testing in the elderly. Best Pract Res: Clin Anaesthesiol. 2011;25(3):427–37.

Whelan P, Britton JP, Dowell AC. Three-year follow-up of bladder tumours found on screening. Br J Urol. 1993;72(6):893–6.

Whelan P, Ekbal S, Nehra A. Erectile dysfunction in robotic radical prostatectomy: outcomes and management. Indian J Urol. 2014;30(4):434–42.

Whyte WF. Participatory action research. participatory action research. Edited by Whyte WF. California: Sage; 1991.

Wilson RJT, Davies S, Yates D, Redman J, Stone M. Impaired functional capacity is associ-ated with all-cause mortality after major elective intra-abdominal surgery. Br J Anaesth. 2010;105(3):297–303.

Witjes JA, Meijden APvd, Collette L, Sylvester R, Debruyne FM, van Aubel A, Witjes WP. Long-term follow-up of an Eortc randomized prospective trial comparing intravesical Bacille Calmette-Guerin-Rivm and mitomycin C in NMI bladder cancer. Eortc Gu group and the Dutch south east cooperative urological group. European organisation for research and treatment of cancer genito-urinary tract cancer collaborative group. Urology. 1998;52(3):403–10.

Wittmann DA, Monties JE, He C, Mitchell S, Rodriguez-Galano N, Hola V, Perry S, Wood DP Jr. A Pilot study of the effect of a one-day retreat on sexuality on prostate cancer survivors' and partners' information awareness, help-seeking attitudes, sexual communication and sexual activity. J Sex Med. 2013;10:143.

Wittmann D, Carolan M, Given B, Skolarus TA, An L, Palapattu G, Montie JE. Exploring the role of the partner in couples' sexual recovery after surgery for prostate cancer. Support Care Cancer. 2014;22(9):2509–15.

Wyszynski A, Tanyos SA, Rees JR, Marsit CJ, Kelsey KT, Schned AR, Pendleton EM, et al. Body mass and smoking are modifiable risk factors for recurrent bladder cancer. Cancer. 2014;120(3):408–14.

Xu T, Zhu Z, Wang X, Xia L, Zhang X, Zhong S, Sun F, Zhu Y, Shen Z. Impact of body mass on recurrence and progression in chinese patients with Ta, T1 urothelial bladder cancer. Int Urol Nephrol. 2015a;47(7):1135–41.

Xu, W, Ahmadi H, Cai J, Miranda G, Shuckman A, Daneshmand S, Djaladat H. Post-operative pain management after radical cystectomy: comparing traditional and enhanced recovery after surgery protocol at Usc. J Urol. 2015b;1:e306.

Xu, W, Daneshmand S, Bazargani ST, Cai J, Miranda G, Schuckman AK, Djaladat H. Postoperative pain management after radical cystectomy: comparing traditional versus enhanced recovery protocol pathway. The J Urol. 2015c;194(5):1209–13.

Yamada Y, Kobayashi S, Isoshima S, Arima K, Sakuma H, Sugimura Y. The usefulness of diffusion-weighted magnetic resonance imaging in bladder cancer staging and functional analysis. J Cancer Res Ther. 2014;10(4):878–82.

Yang CK, Ou YC, Huang CF. preliminary experience of robotic assisted radical cystectomy with total intracorporeal urinary diversion in Vghtc, Taiwan. J Endourol. 2014;28:A70.

Young EL, Karthikesalingam A, Huddart S, Pearse RM, Hinchliffe RJ, Loftus IM, Thompson MM, Holt PJF. A systematic review of the role of cardiopulmonary exercise testing in vascular surgery. Eur J Vasc Endovasc Surg. 2012;44(1):64–71.

Yuh B, Butt Z, Fazili A, Piacente P, Tan W, Wilding G, Mohler J, Guru K. Short-term quality-of-life assessed after robot-assisted radical cystectomy: a prospective analysis. BJU Int. 2009;103(6):800–4.

Zaider T, Manne S, Nelson C, Mulhall J, Kissane D. Loss of masculine identity, marital affection, and sexual bother in men with localized prostate cancer. J Sex Med. 2012;9(10):2724–32.

Zee R, Schmidt KM, Polascik TJ, Steers W, Krupski TL. Prostate cancer partner perspective— unmet need. J Urol. 2014;1:e150.

Zhou G, Chen X, Zhang J, Zhu J, Zong G, Wang Z. Contrast-enhanced dynamic and diffusion-weighted mr imaging at 3.0t to assess aggressiveness of bladder cancer. Eur J Radiol. 2013;83(11):2013–8.

Zietman AL, Shipley WU, Kaufman DS. Organ-conserving approaches to muscle-invasive bladder cancer: future alternatives to radical cystectomy. Ann Med. 2000;32(1):34–42.

Index

Printed in the United States
By Bookmasters